Dentistry's Future

A Prescription for Success, Wealth and Joy

Dentistry's Future

A Prescription for
Success, Wealth and Joy

by John A. Wilde, D.D.S.

The Novel Pen
Hamilton, IL 62341

Although the author and publisher have made every effort to ensure the accuracy and completeness of information contained in this book, we assume no responsibility for errors, inaccuracies, omissions, or any inconsistency herein. Any slights of people, places, or organizations are unintentional.

First printing 1999

_____

ISBN 0-9648511-4-8

LCCN 98-92151

_____

ATTENTION CORPORATIONS, UNIVERSITIES, COLLEGES, AND PROFESSIONAL ORGANIZATIONS: Quantity discounts are available on bulk purchases of this book for educational purposes. Special books or book excerpts can also be created to fit specific needs. For information, please contact The Novel Pen, 210 Windy Hills, Hamilton, IL 62341, (217) 847-2816.

Dedication

To my family, Joann, John Jr., Heather, Megan and Rachel Wilde, the true blessings of my life, the source of my joy, the home of my peace.

And to my parents, Milton G. Wilde and Jeanne K. Wilde, who taught me to save and invest, and continue to reveal much of life's meaning.

To all of you I send my love.

P.S.

I offer special thanks to my extraordinary typist and skiing buddy, Ms. Rachel Wilde.

Contents

Introduction

My tortured reflections are interrupted by the sound of hurried footsteps ricocheting off the polished linoleum floor outside our room. I stretch aching muscles and shake my head vigorously—like a dog shedding water—attempting to clear some of the fog clouding a brain past exhaustion. I rub my tongue over the linguals of my coated teeth. Plaque, bad coffee and an upset stomach have coalesced to create the taste of rot, the stench of a tomb. I glance at my watch . . . 4 a.m. I do the groggy math— 45 hours since I last slept. God alone knows how long until I can rest. The least of my problems.

I gaze at the angel nestled in the bed below me and straighten the thin sheet that covers her frail body. My 5-year-old daughter, Megan, the third of my four children. Thick eye brows and long, curled lashes protect closed eyes and frame a cute, lightly freckled, button nose. Her face in the dim light is so innocent, still and pure. But instead of the pleasant scents of Megan's room—baby powder and candy—my nose is assaulted by the pungent odor of powerful disinfectants. The lovely nimbus of honey-blond, curly, thick, other-worldly hair is now dark, matted and clotted with her blood. A closer look—one I have no need or wish to make—reveals a face beyond repose.

The Injury

I'll never forget the day: Monday, May 11, 1987. Near twilight on this warm, spring evening my two babies—Megan and her 3-year-old sister, Rachel—were walking, hand-in-hand,

1

around the pond behind the country home in which our family had lived for 11 years. A 14-year-old neighbor boy was illegally racing his four-wheeler off his parent's property. He jumped an incline and didn't see my girls until he landed on them. Rachel was knocked aside, stunned and bruised, but not seriously hurt. The vehicle and rider landed squarely on Megan's head and chest.

Megan was rushed to the local hospital where x-rays were taken and 30-some stitches placed to reunite the nether edges of her torn scalp. There was concern about a badly bruised abdomen and leg, until the x-rays returned. The skull fracture was evident from across the room. Not much like the incipient Class 2 caries I'm paid to detect. Megan was immediately placed in an ambulance and hurriedly transported 40 miles to Quincy, Illinois, the nearest hospital with a neurologist on staff. During the ride she lapsed from grogginess into unconsciousness.

John's Story

Her daddy missed all this trauma. Unlikely as it seems, that very morning I had checked myself into the hospital toward which Megan sped through the dark of night. At 9 a.m. I stood, holding a steaming Styrofoam cup of decaf coffee for whatever meager warmth and comfort it could provide, in a strange place the hospital called its "sun room." Unable to endure eye contact, I stared at the worn carpet through misty eyes as I muttered to the 20 strangers seated around me, "Hi. My name is John . . . I'm an alcoholic."

This confession was but the most recent, if most painful, in a lengthy string of humiliations caused by my addiction to ethyl alcohol. I'd begun drinking a month before I turned 21. I worked my way through eight years of college, paying 100% of my expenses. I was married after my fifth year, and my bride, Joann (Jo) and I were blessed with a son, John Junior, during my seventh year at the University of Iowa. (Unfortunately, we were not blessed with medical insurance.)

Between full- or part-time jobs, dental school and family obligations, I had neither the finances nor the stamina to waste drinking or doing much of anything else. I completed eight years

2

of college (three of them married, one and one-half with a child), owing a grand total of $5,000 in education debt. This feat required perpetual 80- to 100- hour work weeks and a lot of doing without—sleep, food, fun—but I did what I felt to be necessary to avoid the quicksand of debt that engulfs so many of today's young professionals.

When I entered the army, in August of 1972, leisure time and sufficient money were available and I soon began to drink daily. A paltry 40-hour work week hardly caused me to break a sweat, and, when combined with a princely annual salary of $16,000, left me living in the lap of luxury! Fate placed my little family in military housing directly across the street from the base liquor store and officers' club. I made the most of this "opportunity," developing a circle of young dentist-physician friends and their "groupies," intent on partying hard to compensate for the good times we were forced to sacrifice upon the altar of professional education.

After my (technically, at least) honorable discharge, my wife, 3-year-old Johnny, and 1-year-old Heather moved to Keokuk, Iowa, in the summer of 1974. I began a practice from scratch. I worked six days a week, often 12-hour days, frequently working throughout lunch to provide emergency treatment. My drinking grew steadily heavier.

Despite my accelerating dependency on alcohol, my practice was a huge success! We'd spent a year searching for the ideal location, calling, writing, flying from my military base at Fort Lewis, Washington, back to Iowa twice, using almost all of my military leave time (paid vacation to civilians) to identify the ideal office location. In addition to performing the 40 hours a week of clinical dentistry requested by my Uncle Sam, I read management books, visited with any practicing dentist who would talk with me, spent hours studying and selecting equipment, designing an office plan and preparing a 60-page office policy manual. Our painstaking labors and four arduous weeks spent touring Iowa in search of the best possible practice location paid immediate dividends.

Keokuk desperately needed dentists. Most of the existing practitioners were near retirement and so busy they were not accepting new patients. During my first year in private practice we averaged over 100 new patients a month, many referred by other overly busy offices. From the Saturday we first unlocked the office doors I never had open time on my schedule, and the practice was immediately profitable. A more pressing and common problem was working in extra patients—often 10 or more a day. The four members of my little family huddled in a two-bedroom, upstairs apartment and existed on next to nothing, a talent we had refined during my school years. I paid off the office debt completely in March of 1975—seven months after we saw our first patient.

I worked seven days a week, five to six days providing patient care, with every evening and weekend devoted to studying my office and profession. After each long day, I drank to relieve my exhaustion and because "I work hard and deserve to relax and have some fun." I grew accustomed to beginning each day with a queasy stomach, headache and bad breath. As the years passed, the insides of my cheeks developed a numbness. This was joined by a tremor in my hands, an ill-defined but perpetual anxiety that included Sunday depression and insomnia among its blessings, and a growing predisposition to rage.

At age 35, my wife pregnant with Megan, I admitted my addiction to my parents and physician brother, Jim. I battled my foe alone for five years, using Antabuse to periodically stop drinking, drinking only beer, counting drinks, drinking only on certain days—behavior commonly referred to by alcoholics as "doing research"—all efforts undertaken to control my behavior sufficiently to allow me to continue to drink. At age 40, utterly defeated by Demon Rum, I stood before unknowns in that gloomy "sun room," staring hard at my worn tennis shoes, trying to keep my trembling hands from spilling coffee, as I confessed my utter powerlessness and shame. I believed this moment of tawdry ignominy to be as bad as things could possibly get. I had not a clue.

Maybe this is part of my disease, but I felt my condition to be much worse than that of those around me. Many of my "classmates," later friends, seemingly suffered more horrible situations than mine—lost health, families, homes, money, jobs, reputation and self-respect—but I had fallen from such heights.

An ancient Persian myth describes Satan as the most beautiful and faithful of angels, cast from God's presence into hell for refusing to serve humankind, determined to obey and attend only to the God he so deeply loved. The story is poignant due to the juxtaposition of eternal bliss transmuted to infinite banishment.

Or consider the fascination of the world with O.J. Simpson's trial. Many have been accused of murdering an ex-wife, but few fell from such power, fame and wealth . . . such a splendid state of grace. I was a boy from an impoverished background who struggled for education and success as a drowning person does for air, who appeared to achieve his every desire, only to face this disgrace and defeat. In my typical self-absorption, it seemed difficult to imagine a more tragic fate.

I stood on that gray May morn, clammy with nervous sweat, my heart thundering in terror and mortification, a millionaire at 40 with an enormously successful and still growing practice. I was not a "paper millionaire," who includes the value of his home, furniture, office, car, gold fillings in his calculation of net worth. My home, office, car and fillings were debt-free, and in 13 years of private practice I had accumulated over $1 million in stocks, bonds, money market funds, every penny earned by the sweat of my brow.

I owed no money, but my soul was in hock, as my addicted behavior provided many reasons for my family, staff and friends to hate me. No book or movie can portray the horror of living with the addicted, only offer a glimpse.

To keep drinking one must blame others for every problem, to justify one's behavior and allow the preferred form of abuse to continue. To accept responsibility for one's choices, as my trip to the unit finally forced me to do, means an end to blessed illusion and the beginning of sober reality. And I blamed—my wife, children, staff, patients and life—for causing the unbearable pressure and pain I chose to relieve with alcohol. Those closest to me suffered not only from the results of my erratic alcoholic behavior, but from the pain of my undeserved condemnation.

Most feel some compassion for the homeless drunk who has lost everything. The rich and successful addicted—as bloated with pride as booze—must be the hardest to forgive and love. Al Pacino, playing Satan in a recent movie, stated, "Vanity is my favorite sin." Members of 12-step programs, such as Alcoholics Anonymous, refer to this trait as grandiosity. The belief that the addict is the center of the universe. Speaking from the devil's perspective, no trait is more helpful to his cause than greedy self-absorption and the hubris it bequeaths. I was successful, wealthy, popular; how could my behavior be wrong? Even at the nadir of my drinking, I was as riddled with pride of my "accomplishments" as is a terminal cancer patient with tumors.

I had many "friends," all other alcoholics who would tolerate my drinking. I had no desire for sober relationships. It didn't take long, after leaving the hospital, to find my "friends" had no wish to be with sober people either. They especially did not desire to partake of the company of an old drinking buddy foolish enough to attempt going "on the water wagon."

One of the most painful aspects of dealing with addiction is, upon sobering up, realizing one has not a friend in the world, as my every acquaintance, every activity, revolved around booze. Conversely, one of the great blessings is the cognizance that, despite all the pain and damage one has inflicted, there exist family members who somehow are still able to love and support you. To these loved ones, who saved my life, I remain eternally and humbly grateful.

I suppose my accomplishments were admired by many. I had worked hard to earn the worldly trappings of success. A country home with a pond and in-the-ground swimming pool, vacations to paradises like Hawaii and St. John's, the new white and black Cadillac Eldorado I enjoyed. But I doubt anyone who knew the agony that finally drove me to this hospital, and the price of the utter humility with which healing must begin (the first step of the 12 step program of Alcoholics Anonymous is to "Admit I am powerless over alcohol"), would trade skins with me for any dollar amount.

Every alcoholic contemplates suicide, even the wealthy and successful. The pain of addiction is so great, it's understandable to wish the torment over; akin to a person on fire desiring death to end unbearable agony.

The Call

I'd lived through this first humiliating day of a scheduled three-week visit to the hospital's "behavior modification unit" (a more mellifluous title than drunk tank or sanitarium). I'd gotten acquainted with the 20 or so fellow unit members accompanying me on this arduous journey, met Pat, the unit's senior psychologist, assigned to my case, and survived group and individual therapy sessions. I was emotionally and physically exhausted as I crawled gratefully into my hospital bed, and had almost escaped to blessed sleep, when a nurse summoned me to her station to take a call. I still remember the sight of her amazingly long, glistening, blood-red fingernails as she handed me the worn, once-white telephone.

I was puzzled and frightened by a call at this place and at this hour. Has anyone ever received good news from a late-night call? And Jo and I had gone to great lengths to assure no one knew where I was, let alone why I was here. It was Jo on the phone. She was near hysteria. It took three tries before I could comprehend that she was in this hospital, two floors directly above me in pediatrics. That Megan had suffered an accident.

I raced up the back stairwell to find Jo crying, holding the hand of an unconscious and deathly pale Megan, lying in a hospital bed. A nasal cannula was in place, an I.V. bulged obscenely in the back of her tiny, red hand, her thin arm strapped to a restraining board. I held Jo and listened in incredulous horror as she sobbed the story of the accident into my chest.

The neurologist was foreign—Spanish his native tongue—and I had to listen carefully to understand. There was a skull

7

fracture and bruising of the brain. Megan was in a coma. There was no sign of excessive pressure on her brain, so the treatment of choice was to wait. The prognosis was completely unknown.

As my dazed mind began to clear, I asked Jo about the other kids. They were staying with our neighbors. I sent my reluctant and teary wife home to our little family, urging her to drive safely and promising to keep watch until she could get Johnny and Heather off to school, Rachel to a sitter and return in the morning.

The Watch

Thus began the vigil that forever changed my life. Each night I forced myself to remain constantly awake as Megan repeatedly vomited a clear, frothy liquid the medical staff feared she might aspirate. This could lead to strangulation or lung abscesses—either of which were potentially fatal. She also writhed in her dark, unnatural sleep, tangling and blocking her I.V. lines, triggering their jarring alarm system and setting me to frantic fumbling, attempting to restore the measured flow.

During the day I left Jo with Megan and performed my unit activities. I could have been excused from meetings and slept, but it was time for my weakness to end. After years of fighting a losing battle with booze on my own, I knew my treatment was essential. There has never been, nor will ever be, a more motivated and model patient than I, willing to do whatever was required to eliminate the now minor complication of my alcoholism.

I spent the endless nights praying, reading the Bible and big blue book of Alcoholics Anonymous, pleading with God to restore Megan, or take me instead, talking to my baby. I battled the seduction of sleep fiercely, horrified at the possible results of even a few minutes' lapse. I made promises Jesus couldn't keep, figuring I'd deal with the fallout later.

On the third day, Megan arose from her coma. She was too dizzy to even sit up and didn't recognize her parents or understand where she was, but she was awake!

This is no pulp-fiction thriller and I don't want to prolong the suspense. Megan quickly regained her faculties, and returned home in a week, sentenced to three months—an entire summer—of not being allowed to play while her fractured skull healed. She still has some minor memory problems, but is now an active, healthy, beautiful 17-year-old for whom I daily thank the Good Lord. (As she is a teen, I will admit to being more grateful on some days than others!)

The Lesson That Changed My Life

One privilege of writing is, like God and Albert Einstein, one is not constrained by the common linear notion of time. Allow me to revisit the second day after Megan's injury, during my private session with Pat, my insightful, dedicated therapist. The staff and other patients had been wonderful to me. Between Megan's coma and my personal problems, I can't imagine the mess I must have been! To begin our 50-minute session, Pat asked me, "How do you *feel* about Megan's injury?"

I explained her condition as the doctors had informed me.

Pat shook her head *no* firmly. Her heavy-lidded eyes bored into mine as she leaned forward in her worn, overstuffed chair, punctuating her query with stabs of her cigarette. "I didn't ask how Megan was. I asked, HOW DO **YOU FEEL?**"

Shifting uncomfortably in my chair, sensing danger, yet as paralyzed as a deer trapped in headlights, I muttered something about Megan's prognosis.

"John! You're not listening! Look here on the floor, by my feet. Visualize Megan lying there . . . Now, tell her *HOW YOU FEEL!*"

And on that stained, once green carpet, I saw her. Tears—my first—cascaded from my eyes and dripped to the floor as, in sob-racked words, I told Megan how terrified I was. How much I loved her. How I didn't think I could survive if she didn't recover.

It was quite some time before I could control my body sufficiently to talk coherently. I was frightened by the overwhelming, unmanageable power of my emotions, unlike any previous experience in my tightly controlled life. I listened intently as Pat, herself a recovering alcoholic and drug user, explained how addicts learn to block their feelings to allow them to continue their chosen form of abuse and how part of recovery was to become reattached to one's feelings and learn to use them in positive manners. In light of my recent experience, I had a strong hunch this was a portion of the journey I wasn't going to enjoy. Boy, was I right!

To survive the long years of college I'd developed an iron will and unwavering focus that allowed no time or energy for distracting, weakening emotions. Raised as part of a loving Christian family, I suffered great guilt over my drinking, but to enable myself to continue the behavior I craved, I refused to consider the pressure from my severely inflamed conscience. Under Pat's gentle tutelage—may God bless her soul—I grew to understand how and why I had separated my behavior from my feelings, and became aware of the ultimate price such deliberate distortion was extracting.

Accepting the pain and the guidance of my feelings—or reconnecting with my brain's right hemisphere, so long deliberately frozen from my awareness in my agony—was the key to unlocking untapped powers within me. Stimulated by my overwhelming emotional breakthrough with Pat, I slowly, painfully developed the strength and understanding to not only deal with problems objectively (left brain), but also intuitively (right brain). The resultant reunification of cerebral function restored my whole person.

Employing the resources of my emotional self enabled me to use my feelings to guide my behavior to more consistently follow my values. Absent such growth, I fear my drinking would have continued. Whole-brain integration was also the key to developing a level of wisdom that enabled me to envision solutions unattainable to my formerly left-brain, Mr. Spock, logic-based, rigid thinking; to tap previously unavailable creative resources to deal with whatever opportunity or crisis life presented.

A Touching Story, But Why Are You Telling Me This?

While Megan has recovered from her injury, I never have. I've become a different man—I hope a better one, certainly a happier one—since that experience. I want to share my journey to wholeness and delight in hopes of assisting others who sense their existence is less than completely fulfilling, who feel life can contain more.

There is great wisdom in the advice that, **to maximize a relationship, always tell the hardest truth first.** During a consultation appointment, this might mean discussing the unavoidable loss of some teeth, or the need to undergo endodontic or involved periodontal therapy, before explaining the patient's positive long-term prognosis. In a discussion with one's child it might take the form of, "I'm grounding you for two weeks . . . Now, let's review the situation." Once the barrier of the hardest truth is surmounted, the path to a positive relationship is revealed.

I'm following this sage advice now, as admitting my powerlessness to booze is my hardest truth. I'm willingly risking humiliation, judgement and rejection as I desire the development of a meaningful relationship between me and every reader of this book, based upon his or her knowing, understanding and thus trusting me to be completely honest and candid, and to always place the reader's best interests foremost. Without this visceral faith and understanding, the odds of meaningful change occurring in a reader's life are diminished. **And this book isn't meant to just inform or amuse . . . IT'S DESIGNED TO CHANGE LIVES!**

Even a few years ago I couldn't/wouldn't have revealed this story and admitted my greatest weakness and shame. I've always prided myself (Satan's favorite sin, remember?) on being candid and open in my writing. I feel, if I have the audacity to share my thoughts, I should support my assertions and theories with factual documentation. But while I never lied, I always shared half-truths—like the ones I presented to others when I

11

drank. Today, though my hands still sweat and tremble, I have attained the courage to stand again before a group of my peers and state, this time in writing, "Hi. My name is John, and I'm an alcoholic."

My dark secret robbed me of the most precious of gifts— the self-respect needed to achieve peace of mind. For many years I traded lasting joy for a few hours of mind-numbing relief; possibly the worst bargain since Jack exchanged the family's only cow for a handful of magic beans! The same bitter, soul-crushing loss was suffered by my friends in the unit, whether they were hospitalized for treatment of alcohol or other drug addiction, depression, eating disorders or anxiety problems.

I have not had a drink since Easter Sunday, 1987, some three weeks before I entered the unit. Sharing this message is a small portion of the daily battle I still fight to enjoy a positive sense of myself—the achievement of which gives meaning to all else. I pray my story might provide hope and guidance to others miserably mired, as was I, in self-destructive behavior of any form.

I've come to realize I was blessed by my alcoholism as, without it, I would have failed to learn many invaluable lessons. Some truths have helped my journey to wellness and joy. Other discoveries have enabled me to **create and refine a blueprint for dental achievement I believe portends our profession's future, as surely as Sam Walton's vision changed the face of retail stores in America with his revolutionary Wal-Mart super-store concept.**

A lesson contemporary society seems to have misplaced is that one must become worthy—earning the right by one's efforts and knowledge—before he or she may fully enjoy any accomplishment. To cite a too typical current example, when using debt to make a purchase, one attains something to which he or she has not, as yet, earned the right. Thus the joy inherent in the possession is tainted, diminished. (One might be enlightened by considering the false joy of alcohol or other drugs in a similar manner.)

By openly and honestly telling my personal and professional story, I hope to guide each person who shares this book to a level of success, wealth and joy his or her efforts indicate they desire and deserve; of which he or she has become worthy. I can offer no magic, only direction. Even with proper guidance, one must provide the energy and wisdom required to reach his or her goal. I agree with Bill Bright when he stated, "Inspiration without perspiration leads to frustration and stagnation." But, working hard to obtain a carefully selected, meaningful, and worthy goal is not something to avoid, but the very source that fills life with joy.

Selecting One's Goals

Among many lessons gleaned from my ordeal with alcoholism, Megan's injury and both our recoveries, I learned the danger inherent in not carefully choosing what one wishes for. Remember the classic short story entitled *"The Monkey's Paw"*? As a reward for an act of kindness, an elderly couple are granted three wishes from the talisman of a withered monkey's paw. They wished for money, to be told their only son was crushed to death at work and they would receive his insurance. Their second wish was to restore their son to life. When they heard the ghastly sound of his terribly mangled body approaching their door, they used their final wish to put him back in the grave.

I'd done little better than this fictional couple, as I'd wished for success, then wealth, and finally the grave. As a result of my writing I receive calls from dentists each week. During our discussion, I'm often horrified to sense—like my past self—my partner in conversation has confused, dimly defined goals, at best! The late, great Joseph Campbell, one of my heroes and source of inspiration, cautioned of the pain inherent to one who struggles valiantly to reach the top of his or her life's ladder, only to realize the ladder is resting against the wrong wall! I'd exerted every drop of energy I possessed to obtain my degree, business success and wealth—achievements beyond my wildest expectations! Yet my millionaire's view from the hospital "sun room" was certainly nothing other than the top of the wrong wall.

I had been working with my first associate for almost a year when I entered the unit. He is a fine and talented man, but not surprisingly, was planning to leave my office. A portion of the reason I chose to enter treatment at the time I did was to take advantage of the disappearing opportunity for my associate to keep the office open, thus employing my staff and caring for patients. I also wanted to avoid answering questions from those who suffered acute dental needs in my absence concerning where I'd been for three weeks. (Another compelling motivation was the awareness I was drinking myself to death!)

As soon as I completed my stay in the unit, I began to search for a new associate. One of the lessons I'd already learned was that I must cut back my long hours dedicated to patient care to allow myself and my family the long overdue attention we deserved. To continue to pay my staff and keep my commitment to patients would necessitate another dentist in the office. I've never practiced alone since finding that associate. (Two dentists, besides myself, are currently employed in my office. We'll deal with the pro and con of associates at length in the course of this book.)

It is virtually impossible to treat patients 36 hours a week, effectively manage a successful business, invest one's assets safely and wisely, spend quality time with your loved ones, and remain a fully functional human being. Yet, this is the impossible task many dentists have set for themselves, and yet we wonder why the addiction, divorce and suicide rates are so high within the profession!

In my struggle for sobriety, my lifelong quest for understanding of life's mystery intensified. I had drunk to relieve pain, but years spent battling on my own had shown that stopping drinking, **without eliminating the cause of my pain**, was not possible if I desired long-term sobriety. (In alcoholic parlance, a person no longer drinking, but still miserable, is referred to as a "dry-drunk." I had remained sober for as long as a year on my own, but was never free of the fear and anxiety that haunted me. Similar descriptions exist for those struggling with eating disorders, depression, etc., who control their behavior through sheer force of will, but still suffer from the root cause of their malady.)

My search of ancient wisdom, contemporary philosophy and psychology took on new importance, meaning and urgency. I realized the need to understand myself and the gift casually referred to as life not merely to be an interesting topic, but essential for my survival.

This shift in awareness led to my decision to invest energy in lengthy and regular segments of quiet time: reading, thinking, meditating, praying, eventually writing in a dedicated, deliberate effort to understand myself and the world I occupied. (This is my fourth dental book and I've had approximately 50 articles published in dental magazines and newsletters. I've had two short stories and a children's book of fiction published, plus a book on philosophy—*The Subject Is Joy*—co-written with my psychologist brother, Jerry Wilde, Ph.D. I've completed five drafts of a novel I believe will someday become good enough to be published. Writing is a hobby similar to gardening, in the sense that one never runs out of something to do!)

It seems spending quiet time alone is something avoided at all cost by the television, stereo, radio-playing, *let's have friends over* members of our culture. I believe many fear solitude, as within the quiet of one's mind, he or she may come face to face with the antediluvian dragon of self-doubt and fear. Better to whistle in shadowy unawareness, hoping one's deepest terror and insecurity might somehow pass us by.

But, it is within one's mind that the true hero's journey occurs. **Summoning the courage and energy to consistently, deeply and honestly reflect on life is the first critical step in a journey towards earning the self-understanding and wisdom necessary to enhance life's meaning and joy**. To experience life more abundantly.

To become all one is capable of being demands one be strong. It means deliberately facing the skeletons locked within one's mind, forgiving oneself and making friends with all the segments—those judged good and evil—of which he or she is composed. These "mental exercises" allow compassion, wisdom and love to grow. (It is also with the assistance of accurate self-knowledge and dedicated times of thoughtful reflection that powerfully innovative and accurate business decisions are reached that allow for the achievement of success, wealth and joy.)

Sharing What I've Learned

Intense self-study has changed my understanding, beliefs, values, existence. While this entire book is intended as a gift of what I've learned, allow me to summarize a few essential lessons and personalize them with examples of how they have worked in my life.

My most shocking, paradigm-shattering realization was that **the many professional and financial accomplishments I'd achieved while drinking proved meaningless, as I'd sacrificed joy for success.** Having 4,000 active patients and $1 million—achieving the American dream vividly described in books, movies and speeches, which had excited and motivated me for years—means little to one who is so tortured by life that eternal rest seems the only hope of peace. What a fool's bargain I'd struck!!! Once I accepted responsibility for my misery—that my pain accrued as the result of choices I'd made—my primary objective had to be reassessing the entire belief system that comprised the foundation of my existence.

While precise definitions will vary for each individual, I believe most dentists desire what I identified, after lengthy reflection, as my primary goals:

- **SUCCESS** (as with my highly profitable, 4,000-patient practice),

- **FINANCIAL FREEDOM** (which I define as having sufficient money to never have to work again, thus making labor a choice, not a necessity) and

- **HAPPINESS** (described by Aristotle thusly: "For man, a reasoning, purposeful creature, with a final endeavor in life, the supreme final end for the sake of which everything exists, is happiness.")

Few sacrifice as much as dentists to achieve their goals. Consider the exhausting and expensive years of education, the risk and effort required to establish oneself professionally, and the intense exertion demanded to provide continually excellent dental care.

Attaining any of the above three is noteworthy, but **the ultimate relationship of these entities is symbiotic**. The whole of the triune is worth many times the sum of the parts. I'd already proven this assertion, in a negative manner, by living a life that demonstrated *SUCCESS AND WEALTH WITHOUT JOY = MISERY!* Due to my personal experience, I'm not shocked or surprised to hear of someone who "has it all" taking their own life.

While happiness provides meaning to success and wealth, few professionals can find joy without simultaneously achieving professional and financial success. One doesn't go through the agony of years of education, building a business and working at a demanding, relentless job each day, to settle for "just getting by." Failure to feel adequately compensated for one's efforts leads to stress and resentment—the burnout to which so many dentists seemingly fall prey.

The Good News!

One doesn't have to sacrifice success and wealth to obtain joy! They are not mutually exclusive. Awareness, courage, wisdom, and right effort can allow attainment of an indomitable practice, achievement of complete financial independence, and joy within one's office and home. I can promise this is possible, as I've done it.

For the remainder of this book, I'll do my best to document how I've achieved these blessings, thus establishing a basic blueprint others may modify to suit personal tastes, then follow to assist in the attainment of their desires. Accomplishing all three goals has been great fun—a journey to the peak of my life's mountain! Besides enhancing personal joy, I believe examination of my passage will illustrate the optimal future practice mode that dentists who wish to survive in a form of practice we recognize, respect and love must adopt.

The Future Of Dentistry

I believe there are eight interconnected, symbiotic units needed to maximize success, wealth and joy within our dental universe. Each segment is important, and achievement in any of these venues bequeaths great rewards, making the varied stages of the journey more enjoyable. But, when all eight are simultaneously obtained, their power is geometric, the results astounding! Use the ideas within the book as you will, but attempting to achieve some of these goals, but not all, is akin to dismantling a Rolex watch for the parts!

No matter how exciting the following clinical concepts prove to be, never allow oneself to be distracted from the truth that self-understanding and courageous honesty provide the fuel that drives this powerful eight-cylinder engine and the gyroscope that sets an ideal course; that props one's ladder against the correct wall.

Many of the ideas we'll discuss venture outside the boundaries of conventional dental wisdom. Ask yourself, "Am I happy with the results following the status quo has gotten me? If not, am I willing to act to make changes?" It seems more acceptable among dentists to fail in a conventional manner than to succeed in a unique form.

Understanding the concepts we'll explore is essential, but remember Sophocles' admonition that, "Heaven ne'er helps the man who will not act." The harvest one reaps will be in proportion to the validity of one's insights and the might of one's labors.

To achieve more than normal results requires abnormal vision, dedication, action. Uniqueness and success threaten others. One may count on receiving criticism if he or she enjoys superior results. Take comfort in these words of Robert G. Allen. "Don't let the opinion of the average man scare you. Dream, and he thinks you're crazy. Succeed, and he thinks you're lucky. Acquire wealth, and he thinks you're greedy. Pay no attention, he simply doesn't understand."

18

Let's examine a brief overview of these "optimal eight," during which I will attempt to entice one's interest with a peek at some specifics of my personal achievements, thus motivating the weary reader to keep turning pages.

1. Clinical Excellence

Dentistry's Future is certainly not a technique book! And I'm certainly not a master dentist, motivated and able to describe the ultimate marginless bonded inlay or perfectly integrated implant. Yet performing to the very best of one's clinical ability (which is not to be confused with perfection; in that way lies madness!) is the foundational block upon which all other achievement rests.

Lucubration and hard work is demanded, but the key to obtaining a consistent level of maximum skill is a **decision in the heart and head of the dentist to stop doing less than his or her best.** Excellence is an act of will, available to all! The most expensive, intensive training, dedicated study, innumerable hours of continuing education are meaningless without this internal commitment to do and be one's best. Mix this decision of excellence with psychological health, honesty, a willingness to work and grow, and over time, one will develop to the optimal technical efficiency his or her talents allow.

Despite acknowledgement of my lack of any extraordinary clinical skill, I will avail myself of this bully pulpit to discuss a few suggestions of a behavioral type that can have an immense impact on practice success and personal satisfaction—such as the vital importance of, and techniques to assure attainment of, gentle, profound and predictable anesthesia, and how employing nitrous oxide can facilitate clinical and financial achievement.

2. People Skills

That the need for outstanding people skills in a successful office has become almost a cliche' does nothing to diminish the power and truth of this statement. The most extraordinary technical excellence is of little value unless the dentist and staff are behaviorally adept. Happy staff cannot be retained, patients will not accept treatment, personal relationships won't be optimized—your dog will run away from home—unless superb interpersonal skills are developed.

Awareness is the first giant step in attainment. Motivated by the knowledge of its importance, outstanding communications must become a major point of emphasis for the entire team. **Understanding that one may achieve everything he or she desires in life by helping others—and that SELF-ADVANCE-MENT IS SELF-DEFEATING—is essential.** To assure success, one need only find sufficient ways in which to serve. I-messages, active listening, and neuro-linguistic programming are among the communication techniques that can aid one in the refinement of these vital interpersonal skills.

3. Patient Recruitment and Retainment

No office can succeed without patients, but there exists a wide difference of opinion concerning how best to attract clients into one's practice. **A middle ground does exist between sitting in one's office willing the phone to ring, and studying marketing techniques from used-car and insurance salesmen!!!** I'll explain methods based on behavioral understanding and excellent communication skills that will develop quick and sustained patient flow. **Each strategy is professional, inexpensive and FUN.**

Examples include:

a) A chart audit system used daily by staff to express the dentist's concern and reactivate patients of record currently out of relationship with one's office,

b) A series of four direct-mail letters to quickly stimulate new patient flow, their efficacy supported by the documented success achieved in the author's practice,

c) A unique and revolutionary, value-based Yellow Pages ad,

d) Results obtainable from optimally employed Welcome Wagon (W.W.) membership (I wrote an article for Welcome Wagon's national newsletter documenting W.W. success in my office based on an outstanding welcome letter, a compelling-new patient offer and skillful follow-up),

e) Strategies to assure photos and articles about one's office appear in the local paper every month at no charge, and

f) Effective use of patient testimonials.

4. Business Systems

Was it ever acceptable for dentists to practice inefficiently and pass on the cost of their ineptness to the consumer? The question is moot, as the level of competition within the modern dental marketplace has eliminated this wasteful possibility.

Precise, easily understood and consistently monitored systems must be established and regularly consulted concerning every important facet of office function. It is the dentist's responsibility to provide the practice vision and design monitors to evaluate and accelerate passage toward the achievement of identified goals. **These systems must be in writing and mandatory for all staff to follow. (MEASURED BEHAVIOR IMPROVES!)** Each system must be constantly evaluated and adjusted to assure it continues to enhance profitability, efficiency and joy within the office.

To assist in monitoring systems, our office gleans and consolidates reams of computer data to generate five concise pages of internal monitors (which will be examined in detail in Chapter 4) to augment the seven pages of our accountant's monthly profit and loss statement. Our internal data is distributed and reviewed with every team member during our monthly ½-day staff meetings.

Many dentists are reluctant to share financial information, fearing that after surviving eight years of education, accepting the risk, dedication and sacrifice required to open an office and daily performing excellent care, the staff may suspect he or she makes a profit! I've got a news bulletin for you: Employees know dentists make more than they, as it is staff who count the money and deposit it in the bank each day. Doctors who refuse to be candid concerning money matters run the risk of allowing speculation to replace facts.

Developing a true team demands openness, honesty and a dollop of self-confidence and courage. Every member of my team is concerned with the office's financial health, as they understand their fiscal future is linked to the financial well-being of the practice. Sharing concise financial figures monthly, not just expressing my general concern, assures each team member is accurately aware of the documented specifics of office problems and motivated by this undeniable factual awareness to make needed adjustments. (Witnessing in writing that last month's collected dollars were 15% below the same month the previous year is of more value than the dentist stating, "We need to do something to improve production.")

Our data includes production of each provider (dentists and hygienist) on a year-to-date, monthly, and **hourly** basis, as well as hundreds of other items. I don't have to guess why the checking account balance is low this month, or what happened to make last month unusually profitable. Reasons behind pleasant and unpleasant results are obvious when our monitors are carefully reviewed. Such precise information allows our office to spot trends early and accurately work to enhance positives while rectifying negatives, thus maximizing potential.

5. *Expanded Hygiene*

Hygiene as a loss-leader service? Not in the aggressive marketplace of *Dentistry's Future*. I will discuss how expanded hygiene has been employed in my office, over the last 13 years, to allow our hygiene department to currently produce an average of $120 per hour, while **NETTING $62 per hour or in excess of $100,000 per year.**

By implementing expanded hygiene (two rooms and a full-time assistant dedicated to hygiene only), hygienists are better compensated and enjoy improved working conditions, office profit is maximized and, thanks to the availability of a chairside in hygiene, more time can be devoted to each patient.

Our current excellent hygienist has worked in three offices over the course of her nine-year career. During her three years in our office, she has driven 70 miles one-way, five days a week, to participate with our team—a living testimonial to the power and appeal of our office and systems.

6. *Multiple-Dentist Offices*

Successfully implementing the above five steps prepares the way for the major breakthrough of multiple dentists sharing office space, staff and supplies. This arrangement reduces overhead (our office overhead averages below 50%), increases production and profit, while enhancing patient convenience. New patient numbers increase because of expanded, more convenient office hours, and employing multiple dentists allows a wider variety of dental techniques to be performed in-house, thus increasing office production, while reducing the necessity of referrals to specialists which all patients hate.

However, if technical skills are deficient, communications poor, business systems imprecise, staff turnover common, hygiene a money-loser and patient flow and retention less than ideal, a multiple-dentist office is not a viable option.

All one's ducks must be concisely in order before this multi-provider step into dentistry's future can be undertaken successfully. One must manage an excellent office to achieve excellent results. Instability within any of these essential foundational units explains the many failures of associate relationships. **Adding a dentist to a disorganized office results in CHAOS.** It's like having a baby to "help" a failing marriage, dousing a spark with gasoline, or building a house upon sand.

I will detail remuneration possible within an efficient multiple-dentist setting extensively, but let's consider two brief examples:

During July and August of 1997, I saw patients for a total of three six-hour days and had a **total net income of $52,000 for that two-month period, a $2,889 NET PER HOUR AVERAGE.**

During 1996 I enjoyed **an average Net INCOME of $6,700 per day** I treated patients—approximately **10 TIMES THE**

NATIONAL AVERAGE. As unattainable as these figures seem, if someone is doing it, chances are it's possible.

7. How To Find, Hire and Establish Successful Associates

There are many systems extant to identify, hire and employ an associate. Most are designed by non-dentists who receive a fee for providing these services to dentists. Few of these arrangements prove fruitful, and this lack of success discourages many established dentists from employing associates, despite awareness of significant possible benefits.

The success of group practices increases dramatically when the founding dentist ACCEPTS PERSONAL RESPONSIBILITY to identify and employ the ideal associate for his or her unique office. We'll discuss all the important ingredients: recruitment, interviewing, hiring, contracts, working with staff, technique and languaging to assure patients will accept this newest team member. Associate dentists, practice owner, staff and patients must all win for group practices to be successful.

8. Investing/Financial Planning

The above steps effectively implemented, the question becomes, "What do I do with all this darn money?" It's a nice problem to face, but **if financial matters are handled incorrectly, even the most impressive practice success can be squandered.** I've visited with many dentist-owners of highly successful and profitable offices who, because of improper financial management, have a negative net worth.

Developing a philosophy of how to employ money, establishing the discipline to eliminate debt, then save first (before spending, not saving what's left!), learning techniques of successful investing (**in 1996 I enjoyed an income of $338,000 from investments alone**), and much more will be covered to illustrate how to get your cash working so you don't have to.

The American taxation system makes it difficult to earn one's way to wealth. But, while spent income is always taxed, savings can be positioned to grow tax-deferred, even tax-free.

Learning to create safe, maximum earning, tax-advantaged, wealth accumulation strategies is essential to the achievement of financial freedom.

Refocus

Following each of these eight chapters dealing with the creation of an optimal dental practice, a short segment I've entitled **Refocus** appears. These essays discuss various topics related to personal growth. Although deliberately brief, they consist of material unfamiliar to many dentists, and may prove challenging. Due to their vital, yet difficult nature, I've been deliberately redundant at times, approaching important topics from a variety of directions in hopes of enhancing understanding of this fundamental information.

Refocus sections are interspersed throughout the text to assure each reader continues to concentrate on the essential task of enhancing personal power, understanding, growth and joy. That way one doesn't become blinded by visions of clinical success and wealth, as I once did, and, as a result of such limited understanding and vision, risk forfeiting JOY.

Despite our perpetual grumbling, dentistry has richly blessed most of us. There is no question our profession faces significant challenges to which it must respond, but I agree with the opossum sage Pogo in his summary of the state of dentistry: "Gentlemen, we are surrounded by insurmountable opportunity."

We are members of a professional monopoly and among the top few wage earners in the most wealthy nation in our planet's history. Pursuing careers in dentistry has provided us with freedom in many forms. Yet, polls reveal the majority hate their chosen profession and outside powers threaten to wrest it from our control.

We live in times of impending crisis, but also during an era of immense opportunity. Such is always the case during times of rapid change. As we journey together, take time to reflect on your life and dreams openly, courageously. Dr. Hans Selye—the famous stress doctor—stated, "To have a great dream come true, you must first have a great dream." Dare to dream bravely, as I believe the information within this book can help direct one toward achievement of rewards consistent with one's efforts, and possibly, as it has for me, beyond one's greatest expectations.

A vital component of a successful life's journey must be the awareness that what one does, and what one fails to do, controls one's destiny. Abandon the Walter Mitty existence of daydream and fantasy. Act! Gladly accept the challenge—the agony and the ecstasy—that is life. Commit to playing this greatest of games with courage and passion.

Albert Camus said, "If there is a sin against life, it consists perhaps not so much in despairing of life as in hoping for another life and in eluding the implacable grandeur of this life." Seize the divine gift of the glorious day that no man or woman can earn, with a vigor worthy of one aware of its blessing. Proceed with me from this departure point on the trip you were placed on earth to make—the journey to the attainment of your dreams.

Let your battle cry on this crusade toward a fuller, more rewarding life be Logan Pearsall Smith's immortal words, "There are two things to win at in life; first, to get what you want, and, after that, to enjoy it. **Only the wisest of mankind achieves the second.**"

Employ these thoughts to challenge yourself to become one of the elect few, both happy and wise. How can you settle for less, when such wonder is within your grasp?

Chapter One

Clinical Excellence

Allow me to reemphasize the critical message that **nothing is more foundational to a dentist's success than his or her ability to consistently provide excellent dental care.** Maybe this seems too obvious to require mentioning? To me, the fact seems too essential not to stress by presenting it as the first segment of the optimal eight.

With so many books, magazines and newsletter articles devoted to the nuances of dental success—from sending patients birthday cards to skillful employment of aroma-therapy—it's possible for one to become so engulfed in subtlety as to ignore the **glaring certainty that no peripheral knowledge or skill can, or should, allow a dentist who performs poor treatment to survive, let alone thrive.**

This is a topic that demands attention, as every experienced clinician can attest a great deal of substandard care is being inflicted on trusting patients. **Never forget, the mouth is the entrance to the sacred temple of the body, and dentists are entrusted with the essential position of gatekeepers.** Thus there exists a moral as well as legal obligation to provide the best possible treatment one's skills allow.

The unquestionable need for technical expertise established, I'd like to expand the horizons concerning this pivotal topic by examining a pattern of thought I've never heard expressed by another soul. (That this hasn't been previously discussed may be the borderline over which fools rush in, while angels—and smart folks in general—fear to tread. If so, it appears I'm the perfect man for the job. I won't admit to being a fool—each reader will be afforded ample opportunity to make that call for himself or herself—and don't go asking my wife!—but I'm certainly no angel!)

The Lord God made us all, but, similar to His concept of the snowflake, no two humans are created exactly alike. I'm unsure concerning the fate of individual snowflakes. I hope this isn't construed as bias, but, despite their acknowledged uniqueness, all snowflakes look alike to me. I have studied humans' innate abilities extensively, because I find the topic of individual potential fascinating, enlightening, and amazingly rewarding; and as research for two psychology and philosophy books I've co-written with brother Jerry. I'd like to bring some salient points concerning the topic of individual variation in ability to the reader's attention.

Dentistry and Basketball

To more clearly illustrate my contentions concerning human potential, I'll use basketball—a sport to which I'm devoted—as an analogy. I apologize to non-basketball fans (who apparently don't realize what you're missing!), but the parallels between basketball and dentistry are so obvious, I believe I can make my point clear, even if one is uncertain if this is the game with the pointy ball, or the round one.

I love basketball and played until age 49, when bad knees, old age and a chronically deteriorating attitude forced me to retire. As a kid growing up in a Mississippi River town of 1,000 souls (Lansing, Iowa), I started spending hours shooting baskets as soon as I was tall enough, and strong enough, to throw the ball as high as the rim.

A VALUABLE ASIDE: (If you're uncertain what you truly love, reflect on where you spend your time. I recall teary conversations during long nights in smoky bars where I expressed love for my family, while said loved ones sat at home, uncertain

28

where I was, and worried. Where one devotes his or her time (in my case, a bar, despite my protestations to the contrary) accurately identifies the true temple at which he or she worships. Only a little honest reflection is required to determine one's authentic interests, and decide if these are consistent with one's values. **Indulging in behavior that is contrary to one's personal beliefs results in certain unhappiness.**)

I'd shovel snow off our gravel driveway all winter long and be outside for hours, or at least until my gloved hands lost feeling, often alone, working on my shot. (Winters are long, cold and snowy in the northeastern corner of Iowa where I grew up, and if one can handle a ball on snow-packed gravel while wearing gloves, he or she can handle a ball anywhere!)

I'm 5-feet 10-inches tall. (My weight is beyond your need to know, and slightly beyond my belt's capacity.) I'm not blessed with burning speed and can't jump a lick. To my dismay, I learned very early in life, as regards basketball at least, there exist finite limits beyond which no amount of study, practice, savvy and want-to could take me. I never was, never could be a star, but, despite my limitations, I loved the game, played a lot, and for forty years basketball blessed my life with great joy.

Even at age 49 I competed vigorously, with great intensity and knowledge of the sport, doing everything within my power to assure my team would win. But that's just me. I reluctantly quit when I could no longer defend younger players (who didn't seem to be carrying the two invisible buckets of sand I was forced to haul) and I knew my play was hurting my team.

Over the years I played with thousands of athletes. Many of them were, like myself, focused, hard-working; loved and understood the game, including being accurately aware as to the finite extent of their skills. Such limited, but hard-working athletes are often referred to as "role players." Not stars who excel at every facet of the sport, but people who can do some things well—play defense, rebound, pass the ball, hit the open shot—and thus positively contribute to their team.

I also played with a plethora of more skilled players, often younger athletes with great quickness, coordination and leaping ability that enabled them to make spectacular plays. Quite often these talented folks were lazy and selfish on the basketball court. They played hard at times, usually on offense, and were more concerned with looking good personally than winning. Despite their innate talent, they had no clear concept of the game itself. They were capable of astonishing individual plays, but due to their lack of overall understanding of the game, were seldom on the winning team.

There exist a few players who combine great skill with the dedication, knowledge and willingness to sacrifice as needed to win exhibited by role players. When this fortunate combination exists, in dentistry or basketball, you have something special, such as a Michael Jordan, or a Dr. Peter Dawson. The Good Lord just didn't make many like Mike or Pete—supremely gifted talents with great work ethics, willing to do whatever is necessary for the team to succeed—in any venue.

I was forced by fate (i.e. short, can't jump) to be a basketball role player. Here is the point our profession seems unwilling to discuss: **Not all dentists are created equal**. Some doctors are born with talents that no amount of effort or education by less skilled dentists can allow them to equal. As one who isn't happy about it, but will admit to being "less equal" in the skills required for clinically excellent dentistry (another hard truth!), allow me to open a frank discussion concerning this uncomfortable, if not totally taboo, topic.

I taught senior students at the University of Iowa College of Dentistry a few decades ago. I was stunned by the degree of variation in talent among members of this class. I had no sense of this gradation of ability among my classmates as a student (possibly in self-defense). People who averaged 70% on biochemistry examinations didn't seem appreciably less gifted than those who scored 90%, and I was too busy to observe other students' crown preps. (In my own defense, I got pretty good grades, especially considering I'd worked all night while the majority of my classmates slept and studied. As you'll soon see, my dental shortcomings aren't caused by my head, but my hands! . . . Not that my head hasn't caused trouble enough.) Teaching these almost-dentists, I was stunned that some could barely complete a simple restoration, while others exhibited a wide range of clinical competence.

A Short Trip to the Johnson O'Connor Foundation

Let's take a small detour to help clarify our discussion of excellence. At least a dozen years ago, I heard of a unique institution called the Johnson O'Connor Research Foundation Human Engineering Laboratory. They are an organization that has invested all their efforts for many decades to refine their ability to measure a person's innate skills (those talents with which one is born—not those learned or developed).

My oldest child, John Jr., was a high-school junior, not a dedicated student, and had no sense of career. (I perhaps should have left well enough alone, as he's now a lawyer!) I was being forced by my increasing distress to face the issue of why I was so unhappy, despite having reached, reset, and again achieved every goal I established. (These events occurred before I sought help with my alcoholism.) I decided to take the five-hour trip to Chicago (one of Johnson O'Connor's twelve locations) for Johnny and me to take the tests. The information gained has been **INVALUABLE!!** (So far three of my children have completed these examinations. Rachel, our baby, will take the test around her junior year of high school.)

I won't try to detail the twenty-plus segments of the test sporting such strange, archaic names as graphoria, ideaphoria and silograms. All of the segments are nonverbal, except the vocabulary test.

(An interesting aside: The Johnson O'Connor team has determined the level of one's vocabulary is directly related to income, no matter what skill level one displays on other test segments, or what one's career. Let me stress that the more developed one's vocabulary, the greater will be one's income, compared to others in the same profession. No other test segment has a positive correlation with income. If one wishes to make MORE MONEY, years of Johnson O'Connor studies show increasing one's vocabulary will help achieve this end, regardless of one's circumstances. And yes, I am a student of words and have a dictionary by my side every moment I'm writing.)

The tests explained a lot to me. Stating I scored in the bottom 5% on both portions of the manual dexterity test is self-explanatory. (I don't believe they go below 5% for any score. I assume it's a matter of delicacy!) These results clarified the difficulty I experienced in freshman lab carving wax teeth, and why an entire universe of clinical procedures exist that are **hard for me**. Carving wax was the first time I was faced with a task that, no matter how hard I worked, I couldn't do well.

(The dexterity test also explains my problems with chalk carving. Thank God I was accepted into dental school BEFORE I TOOK MY APTITUDE TESTS. How that happened is a longish story, not even of interest to me anymore, but I bet the dental college was less than thrilled when they finally got those entrance examination carving results.)

I'm not trying to abuse myself. The Johnson O'Connor test showed I had areas of great ability, but certainly not in ANYTHING that required using my fingers! I showed potential as a writer, editor, businessman, or teacher. These traits may explain my financial success, despite severe skill deficiencies (including, but not limited to, possessing hands of stone and no opposable thumbs!)

The Johnson O'Connor folks are quick to point out that lacking innate ability doesn't mean one can't master a subject—it will just prove more difficult, take longer to learn and probably never be as satisfying for one to perform as would the same task for someone blessed with more natural talent in that area.

They also indicated that people with major talents who don't find an outlet for these abilities are often troubled by a vague but implacable sense of un-ease. As I said, they explained a lot. (Like why I now spend a great deal of my day blissfully working away at the computer keyboard, losing all sense of time, while I could be cutting precise holes in dentition for a *FAR* superior remuneration. Writing is challenging, lonely, intense work that I love as it somehow fills a hole in me.)

You may reach the Johnson O'Connor Boston office by calling 617-536-1584. They will gladly forward information on all their office locations. The tests require a full day to take, a second morning to discuss, and cost about $500. (A significant fee, but less than the investment required for a single hour of college credit at many institutions of higher learning.) I couldn't recommend these services more highly for any dentist concerned about his or her career, or for EVERY CHILD. I've never spent better money on myself or my children.

The tests indicated Johnny's talents were ideally suited for a career in law. Our indifferent high-school student finished his college undergraduate work in 3½ years with honors—having achieved the top grade-point in his major—and is now practicing law in our home town.

Heather was directed to the world of business by Johnson O'Connor and completed her undergraduate work in THREE YEARS with a 3.90 GPA. (She'd been considering a career in pharmacy because she worked as a clerk in a local pharmacy as a teen and thought the pharmacist was a pretty cool guy. Why and how did you pick dentistry? I just sort of stumbled in.)

Heather's now a very successful investment broker, frequently ranked number one among her large training class in their monthly ratings, and has also moved back to Keokuk, where, at age 25, she was allowed to open and manage her own satellite branch office.

(Here's a thought. Maybe the ADA would be interested in compiling and publishing monthly rankings comparing the success levels of each member of a dental school class. How would such information, that Heather's firm, A.G. Edwards, is thoughtful enough to supply each of their brokers monthly, affect one's performance? One's sanity?)

I'm thrilled and humbled that my two eldest chose to return to our community to live! My behavior while drinking, and probably still today, affords them an excuse to flee to any coast or continent to avoid their difficult father. I'm grateful for their love and generosity, and the fact that life isn't fair. How many among us wish to get what they deserve?

All Dentists Aren't Created Equal

Back to dentistry and basketball. It may be self-serving, as one whose life experience and test scores indicate limited ability in both these venues (and many more, as well!), but I think it is important to one's mental health, happiness and personal sense of peace to accept the fact that undeniable differences in people's abilities exist.

I can't dunk a basketball and no exercise—short of trampoline work—will help. I am equally unable to do the excellent job of carving wax some of my peers seemed able to perform naturally, almost effortlessly. If I worked hard—maybe hired a personal wax-carving trainer—I'd get better. I'd probably always dislike carving wax teeth, and I'd never become great, but my skills would improve.

Do you see where this line of logic leads? Like the snowflakes, all humans are blessed with a diverse set of aptitudes. THIS ABSOLUTE TRUTH, **THAT SOME DENTISTS ARE INNATELY MORE GIFTED IN THE PROFESSION THAN OTHERS,** SEEMS TO BE UNIVERSALLY IGNORED WITHIN DENTISTRY. To pretend that all dentists are capable of being "in the top 10%" of the profession defies reality, as well as the inflexible laws of mathematics. Only 10% can be in the top 10%, which means, like kids at Thanksgiving dinner, the remaining 90% must sit at another, lower table.

One essential point must be made: While some enjoy more natural talent than others, **EVERY DENTIST IS CAPABLE OF PERFORMING AT AN ACCEPTABLE LEVEL OF CLINICAL SKILL.** No dentist lacks the skill to remove every bit of decay from every tooth. All can fabricate an acceptable crown, given honest, diligent effort and adequate time. But the same crown prep might take one dentist an hour, while another, who enjoys greater natural ability, can prepare a superior preparation in half the time. Such is life.

Let me summarize the discussion to date: Despite the guarantees of America's Declaration of Independence, and the impression created by virtually every dental lecturer I've ever heard, we are NOT all created equal. I believe many writers and lecturers are blessed with great dexterity and perhaps honestly believe all can perform to their level of skill. (I'm generously assuming naivete over disingenuousness.) To those of us with lesser ability, being held to their standards is like going through a two-hour basketball practice where all one does is attempt to dunk! Despite what the coach says, it makes no difference how hard one tries, how positive one's attitude—lacking the required jumping skills assures failure. This discouraging reality seems difficult for the naturally gifted to grasp.

Stating the fact of our humanness, our uniqueness, seems to violate some unwritten prohibition. It's a topic polite dentists don't discuss. While it may be true in some circumstances that ignorance is bliss, being unaware of this truth, and failing to comprehend how it affects one personally, seems less than optimal preparation for one's life journey toward success, wealth and joy.

I'm not suggesting any dentist give up, but rather arguing for a painstakingly thorough self-examination of technical skills by every member of the profession, just as I've beseeched each to carefully consider personal values. What is the dentist who discovers he or she is blessed with fewer innate gifts to do?

What Are Less Skilled Dentists to Do?

HONEST AWARENESS of one's strengths, one's weaknesses, is the first critical step toward significant achievement. Unflinching reality is the basis upon which optimal decisions must be reached, not the treacherous, if more comfortable, sand of self-deception.

Over the last decade-plus, almost every potential associate with whom I've talked has assured me his or her clinical skills are exceptional! I believe the majority of dentists would rank themselves well within the top half of their profession as regards clinical skills. This would make the top 50% a crowded neighborhood, indeed! **Denial ain't just a river in Egypt!**

If you love dentistry and are devoted to it, but in complete candor realize you lack talent in some aspect(s) (as was my fate in basketball), or find yourself stuck in the profession, aware this may not be the ideal place for you, but financial and family obligations make a career change unrealistic (as I was in dentistry), I wish to offer some precise advice. (To any of the Michael Jordans of our profession reading this . . . go do a flawless full-arch fourteen-unit prep in the next 30 minutes while the rest of us muddle on.)

The superstars dismissed—both of them—let's continue this discussion among the spear carriers, the role players without which there would not be a profession. To compensate for lack of basketball ability I had to abandon my dreams of superstardom and work hard, doing the little things that lead to success and happiness. I set great picks, then rolled to the hoop. I blocked out to rebound, compensating for my lack of jumping ability. I defended with all my energy, and learned to get the ball to the scoring stars at the right time, in the right place. I did all the little things, within the framework of my ability, that enhanced my game's success. I avoided more difficult feats, where odds of my success were diminished.

How does this translate into dentistry? Same concept. **Be honestly aware of what you can do, and more importantly, what you can't.** (If I took too many shots, my team lost. I have never attempted, nor will I ever attempt, a full mouth reconstruction. I don't have the skills—and I break out in hives when I receive mail from attorneys. If one will pardon another mixed metaphor—this of the fishing/dentistry variety—my doing full mouth reconstruction is a form of trolling for litigation. Yet I've heard many successful dentist-lecturers exhorting every member of their audience—even me—to go back to the office and "sell that full-case dentistry.")

Let me reiterate that none of what I've said can be construed as license to justify providing treatment that is less than one's best. One compensates for skills limits all face in some

facets of life with knowledge and effort. Read books, visit other offices, develop mentors and ask questions, go to meetings, study harder and work more painstakingly than those who are blessed. It's not fair! But then I should have been tall, muscular and good-looking!

A major blessing bestowed by a professional degree is freedom. (This book is written, in large part, to help assure dentists may choose to retain this great gift, currently in genuine peril.) Use this freedom to create an office environment ideally suited to one's strengths and weakness by:

1. Identifying and focusing on the areas in which one is best able to perform. (Sealants under a rubber dam for me.) In the complex world that is modern dentistry, it is impossible for any one dentist to provide optimal treatment in every facet of possible care. **It is easier to excel by maximizing one's gift than by strengthening one's deficiencies**—and a hell of a lot more fun!

2. Time procedures, not to work faster and make more money, but to create the *office pace ideal for the talent and temperament of each dentist*. (Chapter 12 of *Bringing Your Practice into Focus*—hereafter known as *Focus*—is completely devoted to timing procedures and creating a scheduling ruler.)

3. Deliberately develop a staff who can compensate for one's shortcomings. (The degree of my deficiencies explains my need for a large staff. No two or three people could possibly compensate for my lack of talent!) If one suffers from a lack of dexterity, he or she may hire chairsides blessed with more gifted fingers—having hobbies that require fine coordination, such as sewing, is a sure indicator of such gifts—then delegate every legally allowed clinical procedure.

If a dentist is quiet, he or she may compensate for this inherent tendency by hiring naturally gregarious staff, easily detected in an interview. One should strive for a balance of talent within a dental staff, just as a basketball team requires a mixture of ball handlers, rebounders, defenders and scorers to succeed.

4. Fearlessly identify areas one doesn't enjoy or isn't good at (they are usually the same thing) and either work to improve skills in these venues, or quit performing that care. (If one is unsure what these areas might be, ask staff. They will only tell you if one has established a relationship that can bear the truth, but they know!)

A blessing of multiple-dentist offices is the freedom to allow each dentist to specialize in the treatment at which he or she excels, thus avoiding the temptation to offer care where skills are less than ideal and which one hates to perform, or having to frustrate patients and lose revenue by referring them outside the office.

For example, the Johnson O'Connor tests revealed I lacked the innate ability to visualize in three dimensions, a skill essential for surgery. This deficiency at least partially explained my dislike for oral surgery. I used to shudder every time I saw a surgical procedure on the day-sheet. After considering the Johnson O'Connor information, as well as my emotions, I have not extracted a tooth in years. Patients and I are both blessed by this decision.

These are important general strategies, but, as I mentioned in the Introduction, the primary ingredient to excellence in any endeavor is the **decision, in the heart and mind of the individual, to accept nothing less than the best care of which one is capable.** To achieve excellence requires rigorous honesty, but not extraordinary talent. Forgive my redundancy, but it is critical for every reader to understand that **excellence is an act of will, available to all.**

I'm not talking about providing the best care when one feels great, has a cooperative patient, and an extra 30 minutes to devote to the procedure due to a cancellation. I am talking about CREATING AN OFFICE ENVIRONMENT THAT CONSTANTLY PLACES ONE IN A POSITION TO PERFORM AND BE ONE'S BEST. I'm also referring to the doctor accepting personal responsibility to correct every situation that detracts from this optimal atmosphere. (Such as running behind schedule.)

But, in this high-overhead, competitive dental world, who can afford the time to always offer ideal care? Every dentist who desires success must. No dentist can "afford" to provide substandard care. Your practice can't afford it, your stomach lining and arterial walls can't afford it, your bank account can't afford it. Lifetime success (and happiness) ultimately depends on forsaking the possible quick buck and working to create excellence in all one does.

If one qualified for dental school, graduated, and passed boards, with dedication, effort and time, one can achieve excellence, that I define—not as perfection—but as consistently doing the best of which one is capable.

The remainder of this chapter is a potpourri of clinical data. Since I've been pretty candid in indicating I have virtually NO DENTAL SKILLS, it should come as little surprise that the great majority of the following information has more of a behavioral slant.

I have been, and will continue to be, candid in sharing the numbers—documentable facts of my office performance—despite my awareness that I will offend some with seeming bragging. (Only the naive believe honesty is without price.) We've mentioned a few generic suggestions to aid the less than ideally skilled practitioner. How I specifically created an optimal environment in which even one who scored in the lowest 5% of dexterity has a chance to succeed and become wealthy through my efforts is a fair and valid question. The answer to that query encompasses this entire book and the three dental books I previously wrote, but allow me to present a few highlights:

1. As mentioned, finding and training ideal staff is critical. (Someone must be skilled if I'm not). Nothing is more essential to the attainment of success, wealth and joy than surrounding oneself with the right people. I thank the Lord

each day for the current staff that blesses my office and keeps me smiling. It hasn't always been thus.

Chapters 7, 8 and 9 of *Focus* detail sophisticated and precise staff recruitment, selection and team-building techniques. I'm hardly an unbiased source, but I'd strongly recommend researching at least these three chapters of *Focus*, as the creation of an optimal team is ESSENTIAL TO DENTAL SUCCESS.

2. Attention to detail—willingness to do the little things needed to win—such as:

a) The previously discussed timing procedures to create the ideal pace, so one is always running on schedule and never forced to battle time pressures that reduce quality and increase stress.

b) Having excellent equipment available in every room, as using magnification, fiber optic handpieces, caries detect, etc.

c) Education. I am and always have been an information junkie. It means giving up television most of the time (except for ball games), and trying many new concepts, the majority of which don't work, but, among the debris, discovering a precious few that help. (A process called learning.) In basketball, dentistry, and damn near everything else, one can compensate for physical deficiencies through mental development and increased effort.

d) Establishing an optimal patient environment to get these folks as relaxed and comfortable as possible. I'm aware that I need all the help I can get! A few examples: We make fresh bread in the office daily, primarily for the great smell! Entering an office, only to suffer a Formacreosol assault to the olfactory region, does little to calm patients' anxiety. We use warmed neck pillows for long procedures, have cable television connected to each of our five intraoral cameras, and also to our virtual reality glasses; nitrous oxide is available in every operatory, and we offer a host of other patient-friendly behaviors we'll touch on in the course of our discussions.

Let's now proceed to the more purely clinical aspects of excellence.

Gentle, Profound, Predictable Anesthesia

We begin our clinical considerations by focusing on a subject few dentists would dispute is critical to both practice growth and clinical excellence, yet one infrequently discussed. It's the art and science of *gentle, profound, and predictable anesthesia.*

I've written about this foundational topic before, including Chapter 13 of *Focus*, from which some of the following material is borrowed. I feel the information bears reexamination, as the most gifted and skilled dentist can't provide his or her best dental work on a squirming, screaming patient. **If one can't numb teeth well, one can't provide excellent care.** Soon this critical lack of skill won't matter, as, **if one has trouble obtaining profound anesthesia, or causes pain when he or she injects, no patients will be coming to see you anyway!**

But don't all doctors provide "gentle, profound, and predictable anesthesia"? Not according to some of the patients I see. One sweet lady in her 70's told me, after I'd completed giving anesthesia, "That's the first shot I've gotten in my life that didn't hurt." (Seventy years is a long time to wait . . . for anything.) Do you think there is a chance she alluded to this blessed event in conversation with anyone else? Is it *possible* the people to whom she mentioned it also prefer injections that don't hurt and will consider leaving their current dentist in search of this painless Mecca?

I believe most doctors assume "my shots don't hurt" (at least not much), but start to *observe* your patients. Do they tense, close their eyes (or occasionally kick their feet and scream)? All these behaviors could be subtle clues that things aren't as comfortable as one had hoped. Possibly I'm unique, but I can feel the tension in a patient, and *it doesn't feel good.* Their pulse becomes my pulse and their blood pressure, mine. And the dentist gets to experience this sensation 10 times a day! The patient at least only has to put up with it once.

This brings me to a second major point about anesthesia: "gentle, profound, and predictable anesthesia" can save or at least prolong a life . . . yours. Nothing in dentistry is as stressful to me as treating a patient who can "feel it" or even a patient who has psychic powers and suspects she may be about to "feel it."

I once traveled 200 miles to watch a noted endodontist ply his trade. During the course of his day, he incised and drained an abscess in the number 30 area for an elderly emergency patient. The procedure didn't take long, but this lady "felt it." When the abscess was opened and the screaming and kicking stopped, I found myself out in the hall with sweat on my lip and a bad headache. Thank God I was only watching!

To me, the most amazing part of this whole scenario was the behavior of patients in the reception room . . . they were still there! Such unhappy occurrences are not good for the profession of dentistry, or for the dentist, staff, and patient involved.

So, I hope you'll grant me these two points:

1. Treating patients without profound anesthesia, or hurting them during the injection, is stressful to everybody in the room. It's something dentists would like to avoid, if for no other reason than saving wear and tear on our bodies and souls.

2. The ability to provide gentle, profound, predictable anesthesia may be the biggest practice builder in existence. (Or lack of this skill may have the most negative impact on a practice possible.) My years of clinical experience have allowed me to become acquainted with a lot of people whose *former dentist hurt them*. Most of us don't want to be the next former dentist, so let's explore how to avoid this fate.

Allow me to begin with this disclaimer: As with about everything else, I'm no expert on local anesthetic. However, the critical act of numbing teeth is an area where the playing field is level. Any dentist, of any skill level, given sufficient motivation and concern, can learn to give painless and effective injections. **A major reason behind my unlikely success is I am a dentist who doesn't hurt.** It should also be stated that any dentist who does give painful shots is **guilty of not doing one's best to avoid hurting another human being.** The awareness that I was indifferent to causing others avoidable pain would not help me fall asleep at night!

Despite my lack of manual dexterity, I do possess a secret weapon. I have the good fortune to be terrified of needles (the sharp, pointy end of same, at least). This has given me an empathy that borders on the supernatural and explains my selfish reasons (namely personal psychic terror) for trying so diligently not to cause any discomfort when injections are given.

I was a terrified child who screamed his way through every injection (while my baby sisters smiled and didn't even blink . . . the traitors!) It's difficult for me to comprehend that this very dread is a trait that significantly explains the success I've enjoyed in dentistry! As my grandmother often inquired, "Will wonders never cease?"

That clarified, I believe we have two separate subjects to address:

1. Gentle anesthesia.

2. Profound and predictable anesthesia.

Gentle:

I've often wondered, do my patients love me, or is it my nitrous oxide? I suppose, if nitrous oxide sedation were outlawed, I'd still practice dentistry, but I try not to think about things like that. Nitrous plays such a central role in my war against dental pain that we'll devote the entire next segment of this chapter to a detailed discussion of N_2O—a blessing no office should choose to function without.

My next best "gentle" helper is a good topical anesthetic, placed on dried tissue for about 30 seconds before injecting. I've had doctors tell me topicals don't reduce discomfort. It's easy to find out. Just inject yourself with a few drops of local (you big chicken), applying topical on one side and not on the other. There's no reason one should take my word for it, and this experiment should eliminate all doubt as to topical's effectiveness.

I think most topicals work well, so I select them more on the basis of smell and taste. Even the sensation of numbness before the needle, and the knowledge that the dentist is concerned enough to provide this extra care, are important practice builders when brought to the patient's attention.

During the examination appointment I explain that we numb the gums before we numb the teeth, thus most patients will feel nothing during the injection. Placing a small dollop of topical on the tongue is a convincing demonstration, as the entire mouth feels numb in a few seconds. This simple act probably reduces our failure rate.

I always "wiggle" the tissue vigorously while placing the needle and injecting. As I understand it, this concept is part of the "gate" theory of pain. If nerves are relaying a movement or pressure sensation to the brain, they can't carry the "ouch" message.

The last point about "gentle" is the most critical: **GO SLOWLY!** One can gauge ideal injection speed by the patient's reactions. If one injects too quickly, he or she will feel the patient tense. I've watched lots of dentists give anesthetic and they invariably inject a lot faster than I. After the injection, they wait for the anesthetic to take effect (and the patient's back to unarch—"Don't treat them until their butt is back in the chair"—I guess).

I always carry on a conversation, as I'm patiently injecting, to help distract the patient. (If you know the patient's spouse is having an affair, mentioning the situation during the injection would be an almost perfect distraction!) At first, it's a little hard to find something to discuss at a tension-filled moment like this, but with experience and effort, this conversational diversion becomes second nature. (I have become master of the rhetorical question!) Focusing the patient's mind on **anything** other than the needle's pointy end helps.

Profound and Predictable:

Here I'm *really* not an expert, but I'd like to humbly share a few of the little things I do that will help achieve complete anesthesia for each of your patients.

1. Occasionally upper molars, especially second and third molars, won't get numb, even for routine operative, without palatal anesthesia. (I suspect this situation is the result of a lingual root projecting unusually far into the dense palatal bone.) When a couple of buccal infiltrations hasn't proven effective, palatal anesthetic usually numbs the tooth almost instantly.

   THE PAD, invented by Dr. William E. Mason, a periodontist, but seemingly nice guy, has helped me give much more comfortable palatal injections. After applying topical, the instrument is used to place firm pressure directly over the foramen. Because The Pad has a hole in the center, one can inject while keeping pressure constant. Patients report feeling more pressure than pain. One may order The Pad from Dr. Mason by calling 517-792-4431 or faxing 517-792-4387. All three dentists in our office feel The Pad is helpful.

2. To achieve anesthesia painlessly on the maxillary central incisors, I inject over the canine, wait a minute, then infiltrate over the central I'm going to treat. If one goes slowly, this *doesn't hurt* and the patient is usually amazed, as past injections in this sensitive area were so excruciatingly painful (from that "former" dentist).

   Once the buccal mucosa is anesthetized, one can achieve anterior palatal numbness painlessly! First, inject a few drops of anesthetic from the facial into the papilla on either side of the tooth one wishes to numb. The palatal tissue will blanch. If one is treating a primary tooth, this buccal infiltration is usually enough to achieve complete anesthesia. If not, after waiting a few seconds, one can inject directly into the blanched palatal area to augment the numbness already present. (The Pad, and the Patch we'll discuss shortly, are also helpful in assuring painless palatal injections.)

I clearly recall, as a dental student, numbing a maxillary central incisor as carefully as I could. The tears occasioned by the pain of that injection filled the EARS of my patient. There is no reason for anything like this to occur today with our tiny needles and excellent technique.

3. Mandibular blocks can present significant challenges. Here are the techniques I use in the sequence in which they are employed.

a) I've used the Gow-Gates block routinely for years. It's safer and more comfortable, in my opinion. It's also simple to learn.

b) Routine mandibular block. If the patient is "jumpy" I may give both the Gow-Gates and conventional block before I even begin a procedure.

c) Buccal and mental infiltration. If I were performing multiple crowns or molar endodontics on a new patient—or a nervous one—I use all three of the above listed techniques before beginning a procedure. I'm not recommending that for every patient. I know it's a lot of anesthesia and medically may not be the wisest, but I like my patients to be free of all discomfort. (No one ever says, "I think I was too well anesthetized." If they are not completely numb, one can count on them mentioning it.)

d) Mandibular lingual infiltration—this I rarely need—usually just for endodontics or removal of a lower molar. The mandibular lingual bone is much thinner than the buccal plate, so lingual infiltration is more effective. One needs to bend the needle at a 45-degree angle and employ significant pressure to inject into this thin, tough tissue.

e) When all these efforts haven't established complete anesthesia on a tooth scheduled for removal or endodontics, I use the Ligajet. I choose not to use this on teeth that are to remain vital, and I don't use it until the soft tissue is already numb. At least in my clumsy hands, the Ligajet seems to be more painful than the conventional syringe. It does, however, almost always establish instant anesthetic, even on the toughest of teeth . . . the sore lower molar. However, the Ligajet is least effective on mandibular molars, especially ones with very long roots.

I alternate between carbocaine and lidocaine, as this reduces toxicity and, I believe, increases effectiveness. **I use carbocaine first**, as the more neutral PH makes the injection more comfortable, then re-inject with longer-acting lidocaine, if required.

We are using **THE PATCH**, basically a strong topical anesthetic placed on an adhesive strip, more all the time. It works very well in hygiene, to allow thorough cleaning of a single sensitive area, and helps to numb the palate before an injection, or to provide adequate pain relief to place a rubber dam or seat a crown with a sub-gingival margin.

I have read about, but not used, the Stabident system. Interested dentists will have to explore this technique on their own. I will add that, were I the inventor, I would change the name. I'm a confessed needle-phobic, but I see no advantage to using the word "stab"!

So, there are a few "nuggets" from the creek bed of my experience. I believe taking the time to be sincerely concerned about patient comfort—and gentle, profound local anesthetic is certainly only one way among many where one can show one's commitment—is the "greatest practice builder" and one every dentist should think and talk about.

For some more recent graduates, an increase in skill or technique may be required, but for most experienced doctors, I believe achieving optimal patient comfort to be only a matter of carefully considering the benefits to them, their practice, and patients that more attention to painless local anesthesia can provide.

For many patients the single biggest concern of any dental appointment—more than fee, convenience, or pleasantness of the staff—is "Will it hurt?" It's very possible for any caring dentist to look any patient in the eye and say, "No, it will not."

Patients today, at least in Keokuk, seem to take our claim of painless dentistry seriously. That's great news to the offices that can fulfill these demands, but a death-blow to those that can't. Most patients simply won't tolerate being hurt, even a little.

Over the years many patients who have left our practice—usually as a result of higher fees—have returned after a single experience with a painful injection or a procedure performed despite failure to achieve complete anesthesia. Consistently numbing teeth thoroughly and painlessly gives one a tremendous competitive advantage with modern apprehensive and demanding patients.

Sure, it will take a little more time and effort on the dentist's part to keep this promise, but if you or a loved one were the patient, wouldn't it be worth it?

We'll continue our discussion of painless dentistry with the detailed examination of nitrous oxide I promised. N_2O is another topic near and dear to my heart, about which I've written several times including Chapter 17 of my third book, *How to Create the Dental Practice of Your Dreams*, henceforth *Dreams*.

Dreams was specifically written for those just beginning a dental office. I believe there will be very little overlap between readers of *Dreams* and *Dentistry's Future*. Also, it's rare to find information on the clinical use of nitrous oxide in print. For these reasons, and because I staunchly support the use of nitrous oxide as a wonderful adjunct to dental treatment, believing it to be of great value to patient and dentist alike, I'm including an updated version of comments I made in *Dreams* within *Dentistry's Future*.

Allow me to clearly state the following information is not intended to replace a course or detailed study of nitrous use, but is merely a discussion of my beliefs and personal techniques.

Laughing All the Way

Let us be candid. There are times (and for me their names are legion) when dentistry isn't much fun. It isn't fun for the patient, it isn't fun for the dentist or his or her staff—sometimes the birds outside my office are uptight.

There are a plethora of events and circumstances that conspire to rain unpleasantness on one's tooth parade, but I believe we can agree the two most common and severe storm-fronts to rock our dental world fall under the general headings of **anxiety** and **pain.**

Fortunately, modern dentists possess the capability to greatly subdue our profession's two ancient and implacable foes. Dr. Horace Wells unveiled this boon in 1844—shortly before I entered the profession—and it has been undergoing refinement ever since. I refer, of course, to nitrous oxide, N_2O . . . my old friend laughing gas.

I fancy myself a scientist, so the data that follows will be in the form of a classic pro-con discussion concerning the features, benefits and drawbacks of nitrous. But allow me to advise the reader that the overriding tenor of my comments will be a paean—a hymn of praise—to the wonders of this fine supplement to our difficult profession.

I retain hazy memories of my pre-nitrous days, these experiences occurring during dental school and two years of military service. But nitrous and I began private practice simultaneously in 1974 and we have been compatriots ever since.

Benefits of N_2O Use

As a behavioral adept—and all dentists who desire success must be—I realize it is most efficacious to begin our discussion by detailing the benefits of nitrous. Soon enough, as with all things, we will confront existing problems.

As we have discussed, I believe the single most essential ingredient to private practice success is the ability of the dentist to consistently provide quality care with **COMFORT. Nothing will retain patients whom one has hurt in his or her practice.**

For adult patients, I define comfort as demonstrating concern, gentleness and the ability to provide complete, consistent and painless anesthesia. Nitrous is an invaluable ally in the pursuit of these essential goals.

N_2O provides a sedative, or calming, and analgesic, or pain-reducing, effect. Thus nitrous both relaxes patients at the usually anxious moment of injection and elevates their pain threshold. Nitrous, when combined with the techniques we've just discussed, such as using a good topical, warmed anesthetic solution and a feather-gentle, slower-than-a-glacier injection technique, allows virtually every delivery of local anesthetic to be given painlessly. As a card-carrying member of needle-phobics of America, allow me to assure all that, to many of our species, the availability of painless injections is an **extremely** important issue—of surpassing more intimate concern than the national debt or nuclear disarmament.

Some of my adult patients prefer not to use nitrous. Others use it only during injections, then ask us to remove it altogether, or to reduce the level of sedation once anesthetic has been given. The majority find they are much more comfortable remaining within the relaxing influence of these soothing gases during their entire dental experience. We have no set procedure or rigid office policy concerning the use of laughing gas. I'm happy to comply with our patients' every wish concerning N_2O use, as our objective is to maximize their comfort during the course of care.

N_2O for Kids—a Miracle!

As helpful as nitrous is for adult anesthetic, **N_2O is close to a miracle for the treatment of primary teeth**. I haven't been forced to give local anesthetic to complete restorations on primary teeth for many years, even for deeper fillings. (Profound local anesthesia is required for extractions or vital pulpotomies performed on primary teeth.)

I vividly recall the first time I used only N_2O to restore primary teeth. On that fateful day, about 20 years ago, necessity was indeed the mother of invention. My patient was a tiny, barely two years old, with classic early baby bottle syndrome caries. I had started N$_2$O and already applied topical. As I sat with syringe in hand, I simply couldn't bring myself to inject the maxillary anterior region on this tiny child. The decay was fairly superficial, so I decided to attempt treatment without anesthetic. (I felt a referral of this 20-pound youngster with multiple caries to be imminent, anyway.) To my amazement, we restored four areas of decay without a whimper or wiggly from our Lilliputian patient. During that experience, my world irrevocably changed, and for the better.

The advantages of not requiring local for primary teeth are many and obvious. No one likes injections—not patients, not doctors—no matter how hard one attempts to make them comfortable. The fear of pain and of needles, the terror of a child whose face is "frozen stiff" (adults know the feeling will eventually leave, but a 3-year-old doesn't), the possibilities of lip biting, accidental inter-vessel injection and overdose, paraesthesia—are all concerns I can live very well without.

Using nitrous alone—without local anesthetic—primary teeth can be restored with complete comfort, and the relaxing sensation is especially pleasant for children. **Virtually every child I treat is enthusiastic and enjoys the dental experience!** Over the years, many youngsters have expressed disappointment that they had no more decay to be restored!!!! In stark contrast, I've worked on some wonderful adults, but I've never restored a single permanent tooth where I felt the patient had a marvelous time and regretted needing no additional treatment. (Of course, adults also get the bill.)

Years ago, the smell of the nasal hoods was objectionable to some kids and presented a barrier to getting them to use nitrous for the first time. Modern scented nasal hoods have eliminated that problem. I ask a child to sniff the bubble gum in our magic nose (my favorite flavor—of many available—for kids). After just a breath or two, he or she begins to relax. Modern nosepieces not only come in delicious scents, but are soft, comfortable, well-fitting and available in three sizes—so gas doesn't leak into patients' eyes and the air dental staff breathe.

The best nasal hoods I've discovered to date, the softest and most pleasant-smelling, come from the ACCUTRON company. You may reach these nitrous specialists by calling 800-531-2221.

At the beginning of treatment, the dentist must be certain the child patient is breathing through his or her nose. Some will tend to "sneak" air from the side of their mouth. I remind them to breathe through the bubble-gum nose, and sometimes gently lay a finger on their lips to be certain my patient is complying. The nitrous onset is so fast one can begin care within three minutes of the first breath—much quicker than is possible using local anesthetic.

Lest one think I have some unique hypnotic ability that allows me alone to restore primary teeth without anesthesia—seemingly a feat of legerdemain—let me hasten to add that the dentists who have toiled as associates in my office also routinely restore primary teeth without using local anesthetic.

Certainly, nitrous would be invaluable to my office if only for the above stated uses. But N_2O just keeps on giving! It eliminates the gag reflex in almost all patients, while retaining the protective cough reflex. Nitrous reduces salivary flow and tongue mobility, making my life decidedly more pleasant. The analgesic effect seems more pronounced on soft tissue, so prophys are much more comfortable. (Our office has nitrous plumbed to every operatory, including the two rooms dedicated to hygiene.)

Mobile primary teeth can be simply, safely and comfortably removed using just nitrous and topical anesthetic. Uncomfortable, yet not painful procedures, such as suture removal, dry socket treatment or crown seating, can be done more pleasantly, and without local, by using N_2O. Patients are grateful for the enhanced comfort of these procedures without having to endure hours with a numb lip—and making patients happy is what it's all about.

Contraindications of N_2O Use

But it is time to approach the dark side. The grim news: N_2O is not a panacea. Certain situations and patients exist where using N_2O is contraindicated. There is some debate concerning the safety of using nitrous during pregnancy. I choose to **never** offer it to pregnant patients. I also don't use nitrous on patients with a history of drug or alcohol abuse, fearing the sensation may trigger a renewal of their condition.

If a patient can't breathe through his or her nose, due to a cold or allergies, nitrous can't help us. (I reschedule kids unable to breathe through their noses rather than treat them with local. I'm thoroughly spoiled!) Claustrophobics can't stand to have their noses covered and some people find the N_2O sensation to be unpleasant. (Virtually no kids object to the "floaty" feeling.) N_2O is contraindicated for patients with chronic obstructive pulmonary diseases, such as emphysema, severe chronic bronchitis and tuberculosis. This entire list of patients for whom N_2O isn't a viable option accounts for less than 1% of the people I treat.

There are no known allergies to N_2O, and the gas is not irritating to the respiratory system. Because nitrous is not absorbed by the blood, but leaves the body quickly through the lungs, no organ system must break the drug down to allow the body to excrete it. Most patients feel no lingering effects of N_2O after the five minutes of 100% oxygen I give them as I complete the last portion of that day's treatment.

The most common side effect is nausea and vomiting. This occurs most frequently with children and is the result of too much gas, given for too long a time. Dentists need to learn to observe their patient for signs he or she is becoming too sedated, then reduce the gas level. This unpleasant side effect was once somewhat of a problem, but with experience, it has disappeared. I haven't had a patient vomit while on N_2O for many years. (Knock, knock!)

Clinical Techniques

As with every treatment topic, even after 25 years of use, I don't claim to be an expert on N_2O use. Not being one to shy away merely due to a lack of credentials, I do wish to relate specific techniques that have worked well in my office.

I begin all kids on five liters of oxygen and four liters of nitrous. (The two-day course on nitrous use I took in 1973 suggested starting patients at one liter of N_2O and slowly increasing the dosage. I never have a problem starting at the four-liter level, and see no reason to begin slowly.) On rare occasions, I need to increase the N_2O to five liters to get the desired effect, but I **choose to never exceed the 50% level for any patient**. If a child is too sleepy, reducing the nitrous to three liters invariably solves the problem.

I begin most adults on five liters of oxygen and two liters of nitrous. While N_2O acts as an analgesic on primary teeth, we benefit mostly from the sedative effect on adults. (One must achieve profound local anesthetic to treat all permanent teeth, no matter what the patient's age.) So lower doses are adequate for our purpose.

I find the level of nitrous needed to achieve the desired level of relaxation on adults varies from one to five liters, with 90% of patients feeling maximum comfort between two and three liters. Having started the N_2O at two liters, I ask patients to inform me immediately if they feel uncomfortably drowsy and I adjust the N_2O level down. If, after two minutes at two liters the patient feels no effect, I increase the nitrous level to three liters and continue on in one-liter increments until ideal relaxation is achieved. Once we have identified the personal comfort zone, I note the ideal N_2O dosage on the patient's chart and use that level at every subsequent visit.

I believe some medical conditions are aided by using nitrous. Room air has a 20.9 percent oxygen concentration. I never give less than 50% oxygen, so for any patient where enhanced oxygen flow is beneficial—such as angina and cardiac sufferers—N_2O is helpful. Nitrous acts as a muscle relaxant and reduces the stress of dental care for patients suffering from tender TMJs.

Dental Staff Concerns

There are concerns about the health of dental personnel repeatedly exposed to trace N_2O in the operatories. The studies available on this topic are somewhat confusing, and each dentist considering using N_2O would be wise to read them on his or her own. (The ADA library will forward a packet of articles dealing with nitrous use.) Many deal with hospital operating rooms where other gases are used in combination with nitrous. Some dental studies took place without scavengers being part of the systems evaluated. Let me stress that **scavengers—that greatly reduce the level of N_2O in operatories—should be a part of every nitrous system.** Rooms should be well ventilated, working with a rubber dam reduces N_2O leakage, and patients should be limited in their talking—all efforts that reduce trace gas levels within treatment areas.

The medical concerns for staff members exposed frequently to trace amounts of nitrous include reduced fertility, possibly greater chance of spontaneous abortion, and some potential tendency to increased liver and kidney problems. I have reread all available studies concerning dangers to staff from trace N_2O. When nitrous is used properly, as we've just described, I am not personally concerned about trace nitrous health risks.

Nitrous oxide recreational use and abuse is a problem limited almost entirely to doctors due to their ready access to the substance. Prolonged use at high levels will lead to neurological symptoms akin to those seen with multiple sclerosis. *Nitrous oxide is a drug and should never be used for social reasons.*

N_2O Cost

The cost of installing a system can also be a barrier to using N_2O. A portable unit can be obtained for around \$3,000, but I believe those who purchase such a system will find the inconvenience of dragging a single N_2O source from room to room will limit its use. If a plumbed or fixed system is installed, ACCUTRON (mentioned earlier as a source for nosepieces) will lease the flow meter, the main regulator of N_2O and major item of expense, for as little as \$10 per month, allowing an operatory to be totally equipped with nitrous for around \$700. Often dental meeting specials will allow a system to be purchased at a significant discount, sometimes as high as 50%.

N$_2$O Value

There are two advantages of nitrous that make it valuable to me, at almost any price. The first is the reduction in stress and distress for my patients its use provides. Relaxed patients greatly decrease the tension of providing care for my associate dentists, for me (a fragile creature) and staff. Certainly, the quality of my dental work is enhanced by working on comfortable, relaxed patients with reduced gag reflex, less salivary flow and tongue mobility—and remember—I need all the help I can get! N$_2$O even makes my jokes funny!

The second overwhelming advantage of N$_2$O lies within the realm of practice enhancement. I have no objections to those who assess a separate fee to administer N$_2$O, but I don't charge patients who choose to use nitrous. (For some apprehensive patients, I'd pay them to use N$_2$O!) It isn't full-page Yellow Pages ad, direct mail campaign, fancy office decor or even oh-so-tight margins that build a thriving dental practice. It is patients telling their friends that "My dentist doesn't hurt me." Creating this reputation within the community is of much greater value to me than any revenue forthcoming from a nitrous fee that could limit its use.

Not only is the ability to offer painless treatment the ultimate practice builder, but nothing gives me greater satisfaction than knowing I was able to provide optimal care in the most comfortable possible manner—especially to children. And the key to earning the right to provide care for every member of the family is often possessing the skill, technique and patience to successfully treat "Junior."

I have a dream. It is to live in a world where the words "I hate dentists!" are never spoken. Nitrous is one piece of the puzzle that moves my dream closer to reality.

The following is a controversial little essay I believe has merit for two reasons:

1. While our office places fewer amalgams each year, we still use the material frequently. I'm not ashamed of this fact (although, at a recent dental meeting, I dined at a table of eight

non-amalgam purists, and I would have enjoyed the exquisite meal more if the subject had not come up.) For whatever it's worth, I'd like what I believe to be the great almost-silent majority of dentists to know I share their use of amalgam.

2. More importantly, this is a short, but relevant example of how to use data from one's practice to assist in reaching **accurate business decisions**. Whether one is for or against amalgam, the simple technique demonstrated here will enable one to determine the profitability of every procedure his or her office performs.

Dentistry has to be one of the few industries where such basic knowledge of profitability is not standard. Can you imagine Wal-Mart not knowing the profit they make on a pair of sweat socks, to the fraction of a penny? Yet, rare is the dental office that devotes the few minutes required to determine if they are even making a profit on each of their procedures. Such unbusinesslike behavior has to end, or dentists deserve to call some lawyer working for a huge insurance company "Boss!"

Is the Crown Really King?

The following discussion timidly points out—from a management perspective—a few possible advantages of amalgam restorations. I'm well aware that many wish to read about the amalgam-less practice, where only gold and ceramic are judged to be of sufficient merit for their patients—offices where the receptionist drives a BMW and the day's receipts are picked up in an armored truck. I also realize, in the current mode of our profession, championing amalgam is considered in the same light as passing gas in a crowded elevator. Well, I've done that evil deed too, and survived, so I'll proceed bravely on with my topic.

It is not my intention to debate the pros and cons of amalgam safety. I will leave it to intellects greater than mine (no shortage of these!), and people with a lot more time on their hands, to dispute the safety of a material we've used for 150 years. I have a few amalgams in my mouth—some of you may too—but due to the state of my mental health, that may not be an argument in the material's favor.

My intent is to study the math—the potential profitability of placing amalgam restorations as compared to the Grail of quality dentistry: The Noble Crown. The figures and times I supply are actual data from my practice. Please substitute your numbers to create a personal analysis. **I promise, one way or the other, you'll learn something from the exercise.**

I schedule amalgams for four minutes per surface. (I allocate six minutes per surface for composite.) We allow 60 minutes to prep and 20 minutes to insert a single crown. (In Iowa assistants are no longer allowed to pack retraction cord, or fabricate or remove temporary crowns, thanks to a recent ruling of the wise solons in our state legislature.) These intervals were carefully and accurately determined by using a stopwatch to time multiple procedures. (Again, Chapter 12 of *Focus* deals with timing procedures and creating a scheduling ruler.)

Let's use, as our operative example, MO and MOD restorations, a total of five surfaces. We allow 10 minutes for anesthesia, so we would schedule 30 minutes for this appointment (10 minutes anesthesia, plus 4 minutes per surface for 5 surfaces). Our fee for an MO is $69, for an MOD $93. We would add $11 to each filling for amalgam bonding, so our total production would be ($69 + $93 + $11 + $11 =) $184. This works out to be $184/30 min. or **$6.13 per minute for the amalgam restorations**.

(We've been bonding amalgams for three years, and I'm pleased with the clinical results. Certainly, sensitivity is reduced, if not eliminated. I can't state categorically that bonded amalgam is the wave of the future, but I wouldn't place a non-bonded amalgam in a loved one's mouth. Perhaps, given time, bonding alone will change the fate of amalgams. If cusp support is enhanced, marginal leakage reduced and sensitivity markedly decreased, we are dealing with a vastly superior material. But, amalgam bonding materials are expensive, and *you have to charge for them*.)

Our single crown fee is $516, from which we must deduct a $90 lab charge. This leaves us with an after-lab net of $426. We schedule 80 total minutes to prep and insert, so our per-minute production will be $426/80 minutes or **$5.33 per minute**. This is a **15% reduction from our amalgam net**. Significant, if one's overhead approaches 70%.

I have no way of knowing your respective fees, or the times which you schedule for similar procedures. I can assure you, these figures are accurate for my practice. It should take only a moment to compare your calculations. As you do, reflect for a minute. Of the above named services, which has a higher rate of failure? Which is more difficult to perform, and thus more stressful for the clinician? Which is more likely to result in a non-vital pulp? In your own, or a loved one's mouth, would you prefer to have a conservative bonded MOD amalgam placed on tooth #4, or a crown? These are questions for which all must derive personal answers.

Certainly, a three-unit bridge is more productive than any operative dentistry. (I'm great at pontic preps!!) But consider the external pressures on our offices. The ridiculous and ubiquitous $1,000-per-year insurance limits. The alphabet soup of third parties, growing increasingly more disruptive to dentist-patient relationships. In my area, the farm families of six with no insurance, non-fluoridated water and a lot of restorative needs. As a profession, how are we to respond to these forces? By learning to more effectively "sell" crowns?

I'm an active investor in the stock market. One never goes broke buying stock in a company that is the most efficient, lowest-overhead producer in their industry. Our office has worked hard to become flexible and efficient and to be the **low-cost supplier** of dental care in our area. (Not low fee, or low profit, but low expense. Our overhead, not including doctor's compensation, averages below 50%.)

I'm not advocating replacing crowns with 10-surface amalgams attached to sky hooks. (Amalgam pontics are beyond my skill level, although I've witnessed overhangs roughly the size of a tooth.) I do believe, even in our composite and crown dental world, the lowly amalgam still has its place. I also believe, for those who labor to become organized, efficient and effective, this service can be performed profitably. Don't take my word for this. Be a **BUSINESSPERSON**—do the math. What do your numbers tell you?

Now that you've investigated the profitability of a single crown and amalgam, aren't you curious? How much does it COST YOU to perform a new-patient examination, or place a single one-surface restoration? What PROFIT do you enjoy from dentures or veneers? Do your fees, in any manner, correspond to the profit made from a procedure? Why not? What can you do about such craziness?

And while I'm asking, isn't it an interesting world in which we live?

REFOCUS ONE: THE ANSWER

Okay, you tell me. Does the "secret to success" in modern dentistry lie within the purview of the one-hour new-patient examination featuring Pankey clinical techniques plus freshly squeezed orange juice, gourmet coffee, freshly baked pastry and fruit to heighten the experience? Or is the solution to problems currently besetting our profession a volume-driven, 10-new-patients-a-day, low-overhead, low-fee, hard-scrabble dental existence?

I've been buffeted by these diverse crosscurrents of practice philosophy for the decades I've been earning my living putting my fingers in other people's mouths. Pressures placed upon the contemporary dentist—including steadily rising overhead, increasing government regulation, an abundance of dentists, and third-party interference—threaten our profession's existence, at least as we know and love it, and have intensified the demand to define the ideal practice form.

For me, the conundrum came to a head when I recently received two publications, both on the same day, both from outstanding dentists, each of whom I am proud to consider my friend. Both graciously shared the philosophy that had resulted in their respective, well-documented, glorious accomplishments. Both arguments were articulate and persuasive. **Yet their styles of practice were polar opposites.** Both could not be right!

One doctor's office featured a reception room composed of four private lounges for patients to enjoy, the walls of each displaying original art. Their patients were served refreshments on expensive china, while soft baroque music played in the background. The office has an **unlisted phone number,** and **no name on the door**, as patients are allowed into the practice by **invitation only**. Their financial success was outstanding!

The second practice featured multiple doctors, in multiple offices . . . multiples of multiples. They "worked" new-patient exams into an already bulgingly full schedule, sometimes as many as 10 a day. Overhead was vigorously restrained and efficiency honored. Practice locations were open 12 hours a day, six days a week. Each office had many operatories and featured large staffs. They marketed extensively and were proud to serve the entire alphabet universe (HMO, PPO, etc.) of third-party plans. Their financial success was outstanding!

Ingesting this exciting, enlightening, yet contradictory information in close juxtaposition was a shock to my system! As I sat, confused, bothered and bewildered, a possible solution came to me. I pass it along in the hopes of extracting other poor wet-gloved souls from the unpleasant tar-pits of similar confusion, and perhaps shedding light on their definition of the ideal form of dental practice.

There are NO ABSOLUTELY RIGHT BELIEFS—merely beliefs. For persuasions of any ilk to unleash the passion necessary to have a positive influence, they must be carefully considered and painstakingly clarified by their holder, and be consistent with his or her most closely held beliefs (an exercise that had obviously been accomplished by the two eminent author/clinicians). These beliefs evolve into the blueprints that become the physical plant and office systems. EVERY facet of an outstanding practice must resonate precisely with the core of values that makes each dentist a unique individual.

Beliefs "borrowed" from another, because one admires or covets his or her success, no matter how attractive-sounding, or how substantial the level of success promised by the presenter, won't produce the energy essential to create meaningful, long-term growth. One may achieve some transitory accomplishments from copying others, but these gains will soon drop by the wayside. **Sustainable growth occurs when the hard work of introspection results in clarified values that lead to authentic**

insight and vision within the heart and head of the practice leader. Anything less substantial is chimera, composed as much of spun sugar and air as is cotton candy.

How often have you been inspired by a lecture, book, article or conversation, and—brimming with enthusiasm— explained this exciting plan to your staff the next day . . . only to realize, in a few weeks, the changes one worked so hard to implement have been abandoned? And yet, some changes are sustained and improve one's practice. I'd like to suggest the ideas which result in meaningful growth are those compatible with one's personal values. The ideas dropped were attractive, but not in harmony with one's core beliefs.

The enemy of any system is inconsistency that leads to dissidence and confusion. If changes aren't based on the leader's authentic beliefs, but rather on who he or she wishes to be, lacking the pristine guiding beacon of internal truth, efforts toward achieving the desired end will fluctuate, depending on deliberate effort to be implemented.

The resulting inconsistency causes staff to doubt. When one doubts, one fails to act—at least with confidence and authority. Some occasional lapses—unnoticed and/or uncorrected by the office leader, as the behavior that sounded good doesn't reinforce an important portion of his or her values—lead to abandonment of the action. (Consider this example as it relates to an uncertain patient's likelihood of accepting and completing treatment.)

Attending a course, visiting with peers or a mentor, reading an excellent book or newsletter can provide valuable clues and stimulate one's thinking toward meaningful change. But, one achieves powerful beliefs by increasing self-knowledge through a deliberate program of personal and professional value clarification. This involves regular segments of significant time spent alone, pen, paper and perhaps a steaming cup of coffee handy, as one examines his or her beliefs and behaviors to determine, and to define in writing, what one most deeply affirms. From these clarified values comes the vision from which a dynamic practice is created, appearing first in the dentist's dreams, then in words, finally made manifest by action.

There is tremendous power—rivers of energy available—to employ on projects in which one believes. Think of the times in your life when you possessed great enthusiasm. It may have been during a school project, when courting the person of your dreams, as you engage in sports or hobbies you enjoy, or while performing particularly rewarding dental procedures. When one is involved in behaviors he or she loves, time goes quickly and one's energy level remains almost preternaturally high.

Now, reflect upon your emotional and physical state when compelled to perform tasks you did not value. For me, these include repetitive, noncreative tasks, fixing anything mechanical and removing teeth. Involved in these (and unfortunately, many other activities for which I possess neither talent nor interest), time seems frozen, energy plummets and attitude . . . you don't want to know. Such is the disheartening fate of those weary, forlorn souls, forced to act in a manner inconsistent with their values.

The answer to becoming happy, successful, productive—within one's practice or any other venue:

Determine what gives one joy and do those things.

Determine what robs one of energy and happiness, and work to eliminate these things from one's life.

The joy and power released by performing actions consistent with one's beliefs is infectious and will spread to staff, patients, even family. Everyone enjoys the companionship of happy people, obviously engaged in the performance of a task they love and will actively seek out such individuals.

The soul-numbing dread of being forced to act in a manner inconsistent with values is also contagious. Reflect on personal experiences when you have been forced to endure one who dislikes his or her job. Sharing time and space with such an unhappy soul is an experience most try to avoid at all costs.

The gauntlet has been tossed. The challenge to choose and achieve success, wealth and joy by charting a course as unique as one's values hangs in the air. This would be an appropriate moment to engage in an exercise in which (with no false modesty!) I excelled: namely, making up a long list of why such logical and exciting behavioral choices aren't possible for you.

Mumble all you want about low patient I.Q., lack of staff understanding and commitment, local economic conditions, the weather. When you cut to the chase, I believe you'll see many of the reasons deal with the "golden handcuffs" of dentistry. "I can't afford to take the risks necessary to establish the office of my dreams!" Many within this fiscally blessed profession feel compelled by financial considerations to prostitute themselves by practicing in a manner they don't value or enjoy in an effort to make more money. Yet, not a single event from one's history would suggest **money earned in misery is capable of purchasing joy**.

Another major reason to not choose a life of joy (as one's life is simply the result of the choices he or she makes) is a lack of self-confidence that leads to a crippling fear of failure. Low self-esteem results in one's following the advice of "experts," as miserable failure in a generally accepted manner is more palatable than daring to define what leads to bliss and trusting one's own thoughts, striking out on a unique path, thus risking the rejection of others for being "different," even if successful.

Realizing there is no such thing as failure—only actions and results—is very freeing. Sadly, the reality of individuals too frightened to even attempt success exists. They lack the clear values needed to provide enduring courage and effort, even—especially—in the face of disappointment, that is imperative to success. The chances of achieving mastery in any endeavor without a consistent master plan, pursued with vigor, are akin to the odds of standing with one's mouth open and having a roast duck fly in.

Is a miserable, stressed office, where people are asked to act in a manner in violation of their personal values, the epitome of success? If such working conditions create remarkable financial gain, is deciding to live in such a manner the choice a wise person would make? Would you choose to live with cancer because it paid rent? When office misery is traded for money, who benefits? The patients, the staff, the dentist or his or her family? Isn't the answer clearly NO ONE?

It is my contention that clarifying one's values, then consistently reinforcing these beliefs in everything one does—from surrounding oneself with staff who share similar beliefs and values, to the dental materials selected, to the magazines in the reception room—is the optimal manner by which one may achieve success, wealth and joy. But, how can one be certain his or her behavior is value-based?

One knows he or she has acted in a manner consistent with their values when they are happy. One knows he or she has violated their beliefs when they feel stress and discomfort. Unhappiness is a clue they have strayed from their true path and need to refocus their efforts. Such unpleasant emotions are long-term blessings, as they lead those who are aware to reflect and redirect behavior in a manner consistent with clarified personal values that will return them to happiness and peace.

Certain knowledge of the ideal behavior for any individual can be achieved only through painstaking reflection. This accurate self-knowledge forms the basis of wisdom. Acting with wisdom creates self-confidence and the energy of passion. Passionate energy enables one to achieve, no matter what obstacles must be overcome, in a manner that results in a lifetime of success and joy.

One doesn't create values. They exist in all of us, but must be identified through awareness and deliberate effort. One's personal path to meaningful success will vary by who one is. Allow me to illustrate this contention employing my life example.

I come from a blue-collar (and a soiled one at that) background. My dad worked in a factory all his career, often having a second job to sustain his family of seven. I'm not especially comfortable in a country club, caring for the dental needs of the local bank president or wearing a tie. I wasted a lot of time, endured a great deal of frustration, before I understood this is not good or bad, but merely a definition of who I am.

One can play-act to become who he or she feels they "should be," but the effort required to maintain perpetual disingenuousness is exhausting, and no level of exertion can fool oneself. Even mind-numbing doses of alcohol won't eliminate the distress, but only provide a temporary respite, akin to using perfume instead of taking a shower. **Honesty is extremely freeing; dishonesty confining, restricting, strangling.**

Another practitioner may have had a playpen reserved at "the club." The family's country club is an environment as comfortable as was the briar patch for Bre'r Rabbit. Can you see how the identical "good advice" given to such diverse souls might be excellent for one, a disaster for the other?

Shakespeare advised, to one's own self be true. The first step necessary to follow this wise counsel is discovering who you are. Once this essential question has been answered, it is possible to determine which paths have meaning for you. Set aside a minimum of one hour, once a week, and, at this regular time and in a regular place, allow nothing to distract you from the pursuit of your defining values. During this process, the flow of creative ideas that materialize will amaze you! The job will seem difficult at first, one's as yet undisciplined mind fights a tight focus, but as awareness and ideas grow, you'll soon realize you are mining a vein of pure gold! Dedication to this difficult task will allow clear insight into how every meaningful event and relationship in one's life should ideally be approached.

Such understanding allows one to avoid the painful, wasteful steps of following another's blueprint to success that has no relevance to one's values, no matter how enticing his or her journey seems. Not becoming lost in the melodrama of others is a major step toward achieving whatever possesses meaning in one's life.

The secret to dental success encompasses a practice tailored to the elite and one designed for the more common man. It exists within rural and urban settings, in 8,000- and 400-square-foot office facilities.

Carefully examine your beliefs. This is not a job one can hire a consultant for or assign to one's receptionist. Listen to the stories of others. They can advise, inspire and entertain. (And I hope this book is doing all three!) But, within your heart and mind, and only there, is the unique prescription for lasting success and joy in every facet of your existence.

One requires discernment and tenacity to seek the life of his or her dreams. Allow joy and pain to guide you on your way. If one summons the courage and determination to deliberately plot his or her path—admittedly no modest challenge—the forthcoming rewards will be beyond the imagination of most.

Chapter Two

People Skills

By whatever title one chooses to call it—people skills, chairside manner, communication ability, behavioral excellence—the art and/or science of optimizing interpersonal relationships has been a hot topic in the profession for decades. Reams have been written on the subject, including quite a bit by yours truly. And most dentists would agree that developing behavioral excellence is essential to the attainment of professional success and personal happiness. Despite this awareness, the ponderous majority have been able to improve people skills only when they remember to make a conscious effort—usually not often enough to meaningfully impact the results of an office or significantly elevate the dentist's joy.

The reason this intense attention has generated such a paucity of meaningful positive change is that the bulk of the discussion takes place on a superficial level, without awareness of the foundational truths that control critical behavioral skills. As is always the case, attempting changes that sound promising, without adequate understanding of the dynamic involved (and without complete understanding, no true commitment is possible), results in failed efforts and frustration.

We're going to delve into behavioral excellence at a substantive level, to provide more thorough understanding, and thus enable incorporation of these essential skills, which can make or break any service industry, into the value system of the dental team. Only through such deep-rooted changes can meaningful, consistent improvements be achieved.

Later in this chapter, I'll briefly review major points concerning people skills occurring in my past books, mainly from Chapters 7 through 10 of, *How Dentistry Can Be a Joyous Path to Financial Freedom*, henceforth *Freedom*. (I'm so glad this book has a short title!)

I want *Dentistry's Future* to be all-inclusive, yet don't think it wise, fair, or in the reader's best interest to include large segments of even the most pertinent of my past writings. (A compilation of five books and over 50 articles would combine to create a tome challenging to carry, let alone read!) When germane to the topic under discussion, I will continue to reference my past efforts, or add segments of updated and revised previously published information, for the reader's convenience. I believe some of my past comments concerning people skills will prove interesting and helpful toward our goal, especially when reanalyzed in the clarifying light of the new paradigm we are examining.

When this new, thought-provoking information has been ingested, I hope data and suggestions from many sources that, in the past, sounded inherently true, but which many found difficult, stiff, unnatural to follow, will be understood at a deeper level, and thus be more easily incorporated into routine dental team behavior.

Some of the REFOCUS segments are comprised of further, advanced or "graduate level" information probing ever deeper into the underlying principles of behavioral excellence. Fair warning: This discussion may reveal glimpses of new worlds of behavioral and self-understanding for one's consideration. That's exciting! It's also unusual, unsettling, confusing, perhaps threatening, and may require multiple readings to understand and implement this powerful, but "un-dentist-like" information.

Genetics Versus Culture

My second co-authored psychology book, currently unpublished, but under contract with an agent (he said hopefully), with a working title, *Of Balance and Bliss*, deals almost exclusively with the interaction between the forces of culture and genetics, and how this primal conflict significantly impacts the great majority of human interaction and behavior, but at a level usually beneath one's conscious awareness.

Of Balance and Bliss comprises over 300 pages, containing more information on the subject than most dentists might care to know, or I have space in this book to provide. Our dialogue will be restricted to examining the nature of people skills, why they are essential, what natural barriers exist to make them difficult to employ consistently, how interpersonal relationships can be maximized, and emphasizing why **behavioral excellence is critically important for dentists who wish to obtain success, wealth and happiness**. We'll also take a gander at the creation of a creature I've dubbed the "super-dentist." I hope even this severely truncated study of the effects of the omnipresent conflict between genetic drives and social restrictions will open new vistas of inquiry for the facile-minded.

The arch-enemy of people skills is genetic, consisting of DNA commands lodged in the deepest recesses of the human brain. (I'm not a neuro-anatomist, but I believe these instructions dwell in the limbic or ancient reptile portion of the human brain, below the level where verbal function is possible.) Here is the home of humans' most deep-seated, hard-wired genetic imperative: **Do whatever is required to survive and reproduce**. This primary directive is the guiding commandment of life and takes precedence over all other ideas and impulses. That we are seldom consciously aware of this command does nothing to diminish its authority and influence on our behavior.

To reproduce, one must survive—sort of a chicken-and-egg relationship. I'm grateful to be allowed to restrict my explanation to the survival end of this continuum. (I've already admitted to being unskilled at so many endeavors, I have no desire to go anywhere near procreation! I still retain a modicum of pride!) I'll leave the reproductive issue to many other willing entities, for example, *Penthouse, Playgirl* and their ilk, which have glossy color photographs available, for superior visual aids.

Essential to survival is the attainment of oxygen, fluids, food and shelter. (We'll stick to the basics, leaving Abraham Maslow's Hierarchy of Needs and the achievement of self-actualization for a later time.) It is **humankind's innate nature to accumulate anything that enhances survival opportunities**, as the more one has, the better one's chance of remaining extant. **Moreover, there is no naturally occurring brake on humankind's accumulation train—no genetically established point where one states, "I guess ten tons of chocolate, or $200 billion is enough."** The deepest regions of the human brain echo with the ceaseless cry: Get me MORE! And it is the power inherent within this demand that has allowed *Homo sapiens* to continue to exist, despite problems caused by this dictum within our modern world that we'll soon consider.

Human existence has been a constant battle for survival, at least until most recent times, in some more fortuitous portions of the earth. (Thank God I was born in a place and time of plenty. People perched on the spiny edge of existence seldom have time to read, let alone write a book. And I doubt they get much ice cream!) Throughout history, with the exception of a privileged few—kings and such—the concept of overindulgence didn't exist. The search for calorie-free substances that taste good, the struggle with obesity, are among our species' newer problems.

Natural selection—that old Darwin thing—mandated our taste for sweets, as this tendency led to consumption of fruits, which are great sources of nutrition. This food choice enjoyed genetic favor, as humans who ate fruits were generally stronger, healthier, and thus more prone to survive. (And it's hard to get fat eating apples!) Our genetic controls didn't anticipate the "empty calories" of cookies, doughnuts, candy and ice cream, or the sedentary nature of modern existence.

This natural tendency to accumulate all one possibly can to protect against the vicissitudes of life is labeled "the sin of greed" by society, which, as we'll soon see, must assure its members share possession if they are to peacefully coexist. But, despite culture's value judgement, wanting to possess the objects that enhance survival is not "evil," merely following the deep-seated imperatives of one's nature to maximize survival opportunities.

This explanation of genetically encoded drives is not meant to glorify greed, but is merely a statement of fact, at least as I perceive it. Modern humans have cerebral functions that allow abstraction and reason. We are capable of overriding these ancient drives, not only when pressured by the outside powers of society we'll soon examine, but when the personal perception of having enough is achieved.

This genetic-based, perpetual questing for more is the root of much of modern human unhappiness, as even billionaires feel joy and peace of mind lie in one more lavish possession, or obtaining another few million dollars. While these genetic commands were imperative for survival throughout most of human existence, today, in our plenty, we are blessed with choices beyond mere constant accumulation.

The concept of greed would be beyond the comprehension of our hunter-gatherer ancestors whose survival was at all times tenuous. These ancient ancestors lived in tribes of predominantly genetically related kin, before society, culture, community—humans living in large, heterogenous groups—burst on the scene. Non-genetically related *Homo sapiens* existing in close proximity required the creation, implementation and enforcement of rules of conduct to control humankind's natural behavior. Previously normal stuff, like killing, raping and robbing non-tribe members on sight (after all, despite our pretensions and protestations, humans are merely animals), caused rips in the delicate fabric that is society.

These myriad rules that allow humans to dwell in community take the forms of peer pressures, customs, manners, religion, laws, etc. Without such controls, chaos ensues and society can't exist.

Sigmund Freud, in the later writings of his amazing life, attributed the majority of modern humankind's mental anguish to individual will being in constant conflict with societal control. I believe his assertions contained more truth than poetry, as to live within large groups requires people to modify their innate behavior—an unnatural, stress-producing mandate. Referring to an individual as "cultured" or "civilized" is another way of stating he or she has lost touch with the animal they are, forcing their nature to comply with society's other-directed commands like a well-trained circus tiger.

The Development of People Skills

People skills, when reduced to their essence, are all various forms of exhibiting concern about others. But losing focus on oneself, or forfeiting possessions, decreases one's chances of survival. This violates our brain's most compelling command, and illustrates my earlier statement, that the mind is the chief enemy of behavioral excellence.

Our nature also explains why teaching children "nice people share" is such a difficult task. (All four of my kids learned the word "mine," and could say it with conviction and authority, at a very early age. It strikes me as sad that most people are so deeply conditioned by forces of culture as to view even natural behavior of children as "bad.") Except with one's genetic kin, sharing is an UNNATURAL ACT.

Please don't misconstrue these facts as a plea we all go "back to nature." I didn't create life in this fashion, but am merely reporting it. Allow me to repeat the Good News, so essential to happiness. As humankind evolved and the neocortex, cortex— all that gray, wrinkled stuff that sits atop the limbic brain—formed, we developed the ability to remember, reason and make choices. (Yeah, some of us a lot more than others.)

People skills are, in part, an enlightened realization that, as life is currently configured, one can obtain more of what he or she naturally desires by helping others. It's a **BRILLIANT** adaptation of the ability to fulfill individual needs within the purview of community.

The reason one disguises this other-focused behavior, designed to satisfy genetic demands, to make himself or herself appear as selfless and "good," is self-serving too. A behavioral advantage occurs to those who feel they are "right." That's why the cowboy in the white hat—a symbol of goodness—might take his lumps early in the movie, but eventually emerges victorious. Despite the preponderance of evidence to the contrary, humans desire and believe that good and right should triumph. Real power exists within beliefs. This personal advantage derived from helping others is the enticing reward—the **carrot**—within the behavioral milieu.

The Fear of Rejection

The **stick** driving people toward compliant social behavior is the fear of rejection by others. Let's take a moment and examine this power. In early civilizations, banishment from the tribe (a form of rejection) meant one would soon be fertilizing the forest, most likely compliments of the digestive system of some large, fanged, furry mammal. (If one was driven from the tribe, he or she would soon be DEAD, food for the many large man-eaters from which only those relatively feeble humans who lived in groups had protection. This explanation furnished for readers who suffer the form of dyslexia making it difficult for them to understand verbal imagery.)

This antediluvian, nonverbal awareness of the ultimate meaning of rejection is the root cause of why we fear speaking in public, asking someone for a date, or *presenting needed dental care*. In each of these situations, the deepest regions of one's brain understand one risks rejection—the emotional equivalent of death. (Under the circumstances, the sweating hands, pounding heart and fear diuresis occasioned by such confrontations make sense. In our brain stems, such situations are perceived as life-and-death encounters.)

The Teeter-Totter of Life Within Society

So nature's unceasing urge is for one to endlessly accumulate, thus maximizing survival and reproductive possibilities. (One hates the rich, simply because they have what we need. Nothing personal.) But, to live within society, these desires must be limited, controlled. (Genetic imperatives are eliminated only by death, regardless of how well trained and civilized one thinks he or she has become. A physical threat to your or your genetic offspring's (your DNA's) well-being, and one reverts to "jungle rules" with amazing speed and efficiency. Failure to do so may result in disqualification from the natural selection derby!)

Most individuals are smart enough to realize they must control their desires well enough to play within the boundaries created by these "new rules," or face modern society's varied forms of rejection, up to and including being sentenced to prison or death. This is the factual basis, the teeter-totter of genetic and social demands, upon which people skills must balance—even within a dental office. A bit more complex and unnaturally difficult than one is normally led to comprehend? **"Just be nice to people"—the level of advice provided by many dental experts—falls well short of being a complete or compelling suggestion in the face of contrary genetic demands.**

If one gives up power or possessions, he or she betrays genetic mandates. If one acquires excessively, he or she violates social codes. I believe this conundrum to be the root of the expression "damned if you do; damned if you don't." Successful and joyful modern living demands achieving an equilibrium between these primary forces of which few are even consciously aware.

Why are some people better able to play the people game? Part of this proclivity is genetic. Some are innately superior at detecting the subtle, nonverbal signs all humans emote with eyes, nostrils, lips, wrinkled brow, scent, posture, etc. Clues that, if detected, can help one identify another's emotional state earlier and more accurately than relying on words alone.

People skills can also be learned, both unintentionally as by a child, and deliberately as an adult. Weak individuals, or those who perceive themselves as relatively powerless, have to become more aware and sensitive to their environment, as stronger individuals and society's forces present a greater threat to them.

This diffident behavior, often adopted very early in life, is referred to as low self-confidence, or poor self-esteem. It consists of an acute awareness and fear of the opinions and emotions of others, as well as the powers of society, and is driven by fear of rejection. (An extreme example of such adoption occurs with abused children, whose ability to interpret subtle clues from the abuser may prove essential to remaining alive!)

The "sensitive" dentist will fear presenting treatment, as to offer is to risk rejection (psychic death). He or she will also have trouble facing up to unhappy patients, staff or family members, let alone archetypical authority figures such as parents, church leaders, or government officials. The mere sight of a police car may cause these law-abiding citizens acute apprehension.

Insensitive individuals—whether due to a genetic inability to read subtle behavioral signs, a powerful sense of self, low fear of rejection, or a combination of all—don't detect emotional states efficiently and, as a result, appear relatively fearless in their dealings with others. Because of their lack of awareness and concern for the state of others, they are often called callous, cold, heartless, uncaring, unfeeling, arrogant, jerks, and a whole lot of more colorful aphorisms. They might be described as "only caring about themselves," and, if lacking the minimum level of restraint demanded by society, can be imprisoned for a variety of "antisocial," or self-focused, behaviors.

(There seems no safe place to present the following information. I'll at least attempt to hide it behind a set of parentheses. Please consider this statement as illustrative of the genetic-culture interface friction we've been examining.

Part of being "civilized" today is not noticing men and women are different. Those who detect such variations risk being referred to by the pejorative of "pigs." Well—oink, oink—I do notice some differences. The females I know tend towards longer hair and generally smell better. There also exist some anatomical differences for which I've always been extremely appreciative—if not as much lately as I once was. But some innate behavioral tendencies also exist that are germane to our discussion.

Man's historic role in society is one of protector-warrior-hunter; women's of nurturer-planner. I mean to imply no advantage to any gender, as both roles are essential, and some males are nurturers, some females warriors. Yet even in our increasingly unisex society, the great majority of warriors are males, the preponderance of nurturers, female. This is neither good nor bad, right or wrong, but simply a description of our species' function, separated by gender.

It is advantageous for a warrior-hunter of either gender to act quickly, decisively when confronted with danger. Too long a consideration of a lion's motives results in the warrior's DNA, and that of his family and friends, becoming plant fertilizer.

However, in the role of nurturer-planner, a contemplative, ruminative, careful mind-set, unhurried and extremely sensitive to the feelings and desires of others within the group, proves most efficacious.

It bothers me to be apprehensive about stating behavioral facts as patent as observing females generally have larger breasts than males. I'm too timid to suggest general assumptions concerning male and female health-care providers based solely on these historic precedents of genetically determined behavior roles, but enlightened readers may feel free to attempt to draw personal conclusions.)

Super-dentist

Let's utilize this abstract theory to examine pragmatically the creation of a being I refer to as the "super-dentist." Two basic but diverse paths exist toward the origination of this formidable creature.

In the first scenario, this superior provider of care has excellent perception of people's emotions, possibly from a genetic predilection and/or a learned awareness of the emotional state of others acquired at an early age. (Acquired sensitivity derives from a lack of self-confidence, or diminished faith in the safety of the world. Natural selection has shown fear to be a viable survival mechanism, just as it has courage.) **This sensitive dentist will be perceived as "caring," because being aware and responding with concern to the feelings and needs of others is what defines caring in our culture.**

So far we have only a dentist with an awareness of others' feelings and an intense fear of rejection. Sadly, this is often the end point; a dentist willing to go to any lengths to please others—and this trait is an asset in any service business—but afraid to risk confrontation, and possible rejection, by suggesting needed care. This poor creature is the antithesis of a super-dentist, too fear-paralyzed to act, fortunate to merely survive in the modern, competitive dental jungle.

But suppose some motivation (debt, divorce, fear of failing, increased knowledge and understanding as might be gained from reading a book or newsletter) persuaded this sensitive soul to dare confronting the primeval fear of rejection and forthrightly recommend needed treatment to his or her patients. Under these circumstances, still rightly perceived by others to be caring and honest—thus trustworthy—his or her ability to gain patient acceptance of suggested care will be outstanding!

The dark side: here we have a person who confronts a deep fear almost daily. With repetition, he or she will become more skilled and less distressed by this behavior, but such encounters never become completely comfortable for these insecure-by-nature souls. Forced courage creates anxiety that may result in efforts to find solace, leading to such problems as alcohol or drug addiction, depression or other emotional problems, eating disorders developing. Sensitive dentists defying their nature and consistently daring to offer care can also enjoy incredible financial success, as they are intuitively trusted by patients. The end result can be a rich, fearful, addicted dentist. (This description sounds eerily familiar!)

Let's study the other theoretical track to super-dentist status—a path in which I have no personal experience, but one I believe I've witnessed while listening to and reading about many famous and successful dentists. We begin with an individual not well endowed with genetic or learned sensitivity to others. Due to this habitual pattern of self-awareness, his or her focus remains fixed on meeting personal needs, yet staying within limits of behavior allowed by society (or one's license, if not one's liberty, is forfeit!). So far we have only the self-centered jerk, referenced above. A person most will sense as inherently untrustworthy, the polar-opposite of a super-dentist.

Let's assume some motivation leads him or her to develop sensitivity to others, mastering the requisite skills, and adopting people-pleasing behavior. It will be easier for him or her to present needed care, as fear of rejection is minimal. They need only to become proficient in the behavioral skills required to enable them to relate ideally to others, thus achieving super-dentist status. This second track to great achievement is free of the psychic horror incurred when constantly forced to confront one's fears. One might refer to these individuals as "great salesmen."

Is such deliberately assimilated behavior manipulative, evil or dishonest? No, only adaptive—a method of learning to thrive in the existing environment that seems as natural to me as turtles learning to survive in the desert.

Assuming honesty and best efforts given, super-dentists of either ilk are optimally equipped to persuade people to accept needed care that is in the patient's best interests, and are richly rewarded in direct relation to their skills and contributions.

What Is a Dentist to Do?

This information should give one a lot on which to reflect. The first step toward becoming a super-dentist—should that be one of your goals—is to identify yourself as basically sensitive or insensitive to nonverbal signals of another's emotional state. One's level of anxiety in confrontational situations is a clue, as the innately sensitive will be more stressed. Also, someone close to you—family member, or trusted staff—after understanding the information we've discussed, can be a valuable source of feedback in determining one's status.

There is no black or white, as all fall somewhere on the continuum between these sensitivity extremes. Once one's primary orientation is identified, one must seek motivation to confront (if sensitive), begin to learn people skills (if insensitive) or some combination of both behaviors—whichever course is most appropriate, given individual circumstances.

Again, it is imperative to understand that such learning is not disingenuous. Rather, it is honestly facing the facts of existence, and in the social structure within which one must abide, adjusting one's behavior to maximize survival opportunities. Such changes involve utilizing awareness to achieve personal growth. The other alternative is remaining stupid!

If innate drives are fulfilled within the strictures of culture—by the rules—both genetic and cultural mandates are satisfied. And please understand this critical point: **Both social and genetic needs must be fulfilled for success, wealth and joy to exist**.

This new paradigm doesn't invalidate all other behavioral information. It does create a bedrock of factual data from which one may judge the accuracy and potential efficacy of other ideas. Can you comprehend how confusion and consternation can result when one hears genetic-based data (It is the job of each individual to work hard and achieve to the maximum of one's ability!) and it sounds valid, then one hears societal messages (Humankind is all one, it is only right and fair that we share everything with each other.) that are just as compelling—but the two contradict impossibly? No wonder so much uncertainty and painful confusion exists.

Partly to illustrate these points, I'd like to review some updated and revised information I've previously published—as stated earlier, mostly from Chapters 7 through 10 of *Freedom*—now considering this information from the perspective of our enhanced understanding.

The Teacher

The word *doctor* comes from the Latin verb, *docere*, meaning to teach. Thus, the historical precedent of every doctor/dentist is a teacher, yet few contemporary patients or dentists consider dental-care providers to be educators. Dentists are perceived as men and women of deed and action, not erudition. We make our living by cutting teeth, not mincing words. With the nature of our training, and the technique and materials available today, it appears to make little sense to waste time teaching!

I'd like to advance a vision I believe to be more powerful than seeing ourselves as gifted fixers of teeth: When modern technical abilities are united with the behavioral excellence we are diligently examining, **dentists may achieve the power to change lives**.

We have discussed clinical excellence and I will assume technical competence for every reader. Developing this life-enhancing ability demands the implementation of solid people skills, based on self-discovered wisdom, that allows education to occur on a level that can effect changes in behavior.

Carl Rogers stated, "**The only learning that significantly influences BEHAVIOR is SELF-DISCOVERY**." Ingestion of data is of little value unless it enhances self-awareness. This is a foundational truth, both for patient and dentist.

I can't speak for others, but I judge my influence on patients by changes in their actions . . . not words. I look to behavior—like maintaining consistently good oral hygiene, keeping appointments, referring others, paying bills in a timely fashion—as benchmarks of patients' authentic values. I have little confidence in a client who thanks me effusively, then engages in none of the above.

On a personal level, the premise is unchanged. Reading a book on nutrition has not impacted my values unless my diet (behavior) changes—no matter what I wish to believe. A dental book has little worth unless its study results in changes within my daily office comportment. **One may judge substantial value shifts by the resulting changes in behavior**. Changed behavior means changed lives. Anything less substantial is self-delusion, mere vacuous dialogue.

Self-discovery—the quintessential ingredient in change—occurs when a behaviorally adept dental team member makes a conscious effort to aid a patient in detecting his or her preferred dental health future. By skillfully assisting a patient in clarifying his or her oral health values one employs the power to change lives, by doing all that is possible to motivate the patient to accept a goal of maintaining teeth in a state of comfort, health and beauty for a lifetime. (Few experienced dentists would argue the contention that optimal oral health significantly enhances quality of life. And recent research linking oral and cardiac health wasn't needed for veteran dentists to reach this conclusion.)

We've all witnessed our finest restorative work fail (come on, 'fess up!) in the unhealthy, unclean mouth of a patient who hasn't kept recare appointments. No matter if she is the wealthiest person in town, the dollar amount of her dental investment is of no concern, and her dentists have been allowed to provide the optimal care their skills allow, breakdown will occur if **behavior demonstrates the patient doesn't value her oral health**.

All dentists have also witnessed people making authentic financial sacrifices to obtain care they can't easily afford, then performing every act we request to maintain optimum dentition, because excellent oral health is consistent with who they see themselves to be. (Both scenarios illustrate how values are reflected in behavior.)

Helping Clarify Values

Dentists must respect patients' beliefs and refrain from judging (provide **freedom**) while allowing the patient **time** to gather information and engage in the reflection required to clarify the dental future he or she desires. As educators, the dentist and his or her team's task is to artfully guide patients along the path to discovering dental health goals consistent with deeply held personal values.

(Universal Truth: One doesn't create values, they exist within us all. But often beliefs are unclear or confused, and careful questioning and quiet thoughts are needed to precisely identify them. The power within clear values results because they consistently guide and energize one's behavior.)

The **Socratic Method** is a technique of promoting self-discovery by guiding another with precisely formulated questions. (Where I received my dental education a variation of this ancient method, technically known as "making the student feel stupid—in front of others if at all possible," was employed. Say what one will about this system, but moments stuck in one's memory. Thirty years later I can still recall dental school instructors whom I despise!)

Let's consider a scenario where a dental team uses carefully crafted questions (Socratic Method) to assist a patient in consideration of his or her preferred lifetime oral health level. (dental health value clarification).

This is a technique of great power that can be used to crystallize beliefs and empower action in any venue of life—not just within the dental office. Once you've grasped this skill, don't hesitate to use it with staff, family—even the ultimate acid test . . . teenagers—to help elucidate their true beliefs.

The Behaviorally Oriented New-Patient Examination

Let's consider the dentist as educator from the perspective of the first, often critical, new-patient examination appointment. (Especially crucial if, due to lack of behavioral skill, the exam frequently turns out the last time one sees patients!)

Again, my new-patient examination technique—shamelessly stolen from the best—is thoroughly covered in *Freedom*, and I don't intend to repeat that information here. I would like to reinforce our study of people skills by briefly highlighting points illustrative of the behavioral techniques we're discussing using a pragmatic example—the new-patient experience—where excellence is vital to practice success.

I meet each adult new patient in my private office: a comfortable, quiet, non-threatening environment. The patient's medical history, including just-taken blood pressure reading, is completed and waiting on my desk. The results of a patient evaluation, conducted in interview fashion by my chairside, also await. (The patient isn't handed a form on a clipboard to be filled out, but asked a series of thought-provoking queries by a skilled assistant who is able to answer patient questions, thus planting seeds for the critical task of helping clarify his or her unique oral health goals, while building rapport.)

Two of the eight posers on our questionnaire are:

1. On a scale of 1-10, how important is it to keep your natural teeth for a lifetime?

2. What personal plans do you have to achieve this objective?

Asking questions forces one to focus on the other person. This is great behavioral technique, and, I believe, the source of the famous saying, "If you must speak during a new-patient interview, ask a question." (I think I first heard this statement many years ago from one of my dental heroes—Dr. Omer Reed.)

After reviewing the medical history, I sit back in my chair, focus my complete attention on the patient, look him or her directly in the eye, and, using their first name, ask, "How may I help you?" I try to make no statement, other than in the form of a question, until we reach the operatory and begin the clinical examination. I want to use these few invaluable quiet moments to get to know and understand the patient—not how many kids she has, or her hobbies—but what she desires, and in what she believes.

The above two questions are "Socratic," as they encourage the patient:

1. to consider how important oral health is to them, (and I've seen every number, from 10 to zero, given as a response), and to begin reflection on past behavior, examining how it has led to the present state of oral health he or she enjoys . . . or suffers.

We seem to live in a world of self-proclaimed victims—people who can endure anything, as long as it's NOT THEIR

FAULT. The first step in changing any behavior is assuming responsibility for one's actions and realizing how personal choices led to the current situation.

(Assumption of personal responsibility is a universal truth, vital for the enlightened dentist who wishes control of his or her life to internalize. Things do happen over which one has no control, but these events are rare, and even under such circumstances, one retains the choice as to how he or she responds to the occurrence. Basically, life is what happens as a result of the choices one makes.

Patients' teeth—your teeth—are in their current condition largely due to past behavioral choices. To change this condition requires NEW CHOICES. The dentist's life is also a result of the choices he or she has made. To change one's life condition requires ___ _____. I know this is a weary old saw, but it's still true—doing the same things and expecting different results is insane!)

2. The questions start the patient's thoughts focusing on his or her desired lifetime oral health future (clarifying values), beyond the acute need to have a sharp tooth smoothed, or a sensitive area evaluated. The realization their decisions and actions will determine the quality of their oral health is encouraged.

3. Such self-reflection is the first step in the critical process of the dentist and patient **co-developing a treatment plan that is clear, concise and consistent with the values of ALL PARTIES INVOLVED**. This common plan is the basis—the life's blood—of a developing dentist-patient affinity.

Think of interactions with your family, staff, friends. In any facet of life, nothing is more significant to a relationship than shared values. Identifying beliefs the dental team and patient share is the basis of a long-term, mutually pleasant affiliation. (This "value gap" explains why raising teenagers, who are struggling to forge a unique identity within those same beloved children whose values once perfectly mirrored yours, can prove such a daunting and potentially painful challenge!)

The Benefits of the Dentist-Educator

One can argue that being an educator consumes more time than a 10-minute examination where one dictates needed care and hopes the patient schedules to receive recommended treatment. But moments invested in education and value exploration are akin to working with a rubber dam, as the few minutes required to place the dam (or begin a relationship) are regained many times over during the course of treatment. It's much easier, more fun, and rewarding to work with patients with whom one shares common values and treatment goals. And your dentistry will be better!!

This brief glimpse of patient interaction during the early stages of the new-patient experience is consistent with behavioral excellence, and illustrates the sensitivity to others that is essential in achieving the high-trust, low-fear relationship with fellow human beings all desire. Of course, it is but one small example of how people skills are employed to enhance practice success and personal joy for all parties involved.

However, let me issue this stark warning: This technique offers no panacea—no guarantee—of professional triumph and personal happiness. Behavioral skills aren't a method of hypnotizing others into bending to one's will, or changing their existing beliefs. Sometimes one will find the patients' values, when clarified to themselves and the dental team, to be inconsistent with the dentist's personal beliefs. In such a case, I'd suggest immediately referring the patient elsewhere.

By carefully working to achieve mutual understanding (or the realization this patient and dentist have none) early in the relationship, lots of problems—failed appointments, unpaid bills, unhappiness with treatment results—are avoided. (It seems to me that endodontically treated teeth, no matter how they appear on x-rays, are never completely comfortable for patients who demanded an extraction, but who were coerced into saving a tooth without first clarifying their values. Also, many seeming money problems are really value mis-communications where currency just happens to be the issue over which the debate occurs.)

Referral of a patient with dissimilar values isn't a loss, as treating a patient with widely differing beliefs will result in frustration for all involved. While treating such people may seem to bequeath short-term benefits—as a busier office and increased production—such gains are a chimera and will not lead to the attainment of personal goals. **Attempting to be all things to all people means one must stand for NOTHING!**

During the early years of my practice I spent significant time, emotion and energy debating endodontics versus extractions, or discussing why bother to fill "only baby teeth." These were unpleasant, often confrontational conversations that threatened the office goal of timeliness, not to mention tranquility. As my values became clearer, the community—slowly but surely, as if by osmosis—became aware of them. Today, I seldom see new patients whose basic beliefs aren't compatible with those of our office.

But it requires courage, consistency and time to achieve this identity. Its basis must be the concise understanding of values in the heart and head of the dentist, arrived at after the careful awareness building we are discussing, and shared with his or her team. If values aren't clear to the doctor and team—and it's best they be in written form as an OFFICE PURPOSE—there will occur weak moments when one gives in to the demands of others and violates his or her beliefs. Such variations from one's values cause confusion and attenuate the team focus. (The essential task of creating an office purpose is described in *Focus*.)

As a personal example of professional values, I believe in retaining every restorable tooth, but our office performs a wide variety of dental care, including amalgam restorations, and even an occasional stainless steel crown. I don't limit my practice to bonded inlays, implants and full mouth reconstruction. If I did, in Keokuk, Iowa—at least with my skills and personal values— I'd only have patients to see about two days a year . . . but at least my average daily production would look great!

This personal explanation is in no way intended to suggest my beliefs are the correct ones, as there are no right or wrong values. I state these facts merely to illustrate my values, thus presenting a more comprehensive picture of my identity and beliefs, that strengthens the relationship between writer and reader. (Good behavioral technique, huh?)

In the language of the first section of this chapter, the key to behavioral excellence, as illustrated with the new-patient interview, is to develop sufficient understanding and skill to avoid the genetic mandate of focusing on the dentist's needs (such as money and ego gratification). One is guilty of that offense if one spends new-patient exams talking about himself or herself, rather than asking questions. It seems intuitively correct to impress the patient with what a fine, talented, caring person the dentist is, but the behavioral adept realizes **such behavior is counterproductive.**

Behavioral brilliance is understanding that by focusing on others' needs, one can receive anything he or she desires. It is the road less traveled, but the very scarcity of competition makes one who has incorporated these essential truths more likely to achieve success, wealth and joy.

Let's examine an advanced technique that contains the power to enhance people skills and allow quick, sure development of trusting relationships—the key to teaching on a level that effects behavioral change and treatment acceptance.

The Magic of Mirroring

The skill of Neuro Linguistic Programming (henceforth NLP) was developed within the realm of psychology. When sophisticated communication techniques are combined with the depth of understanding of human behavior we've been examining, a dramatic short cut to forming relationships can occur, allowing one to consistently make friends with strangers in about two minutes, almost as if by magic.

This alchemy is made possible by understanding the concept of MIRRORING. Along with our five intraoral cameras, we use a hand mirror to aid in co-diagnoses during clinical exams.

Our little mirror is a valuable educational tool, but the mirroring I'd like to discuss is a behavioral, not a physical, reality.

Think about the last time you were with a group of people and came away especially pleasantly impressed by one individual. It may be impossible to precisely identify why anyone prefers one person over another, but upon reflection, one will usually discover you perceived the person you felt the affinity with . . . to be a lot like yourself!

Opposites may attract and some people love to argue, but after some cogitation I believe you will agree—as discussed in the preceding new-patient examination segment of this chapter—all enjoy the company of people who have values, interests and beliefs similar to their own.

If you will concede this point, how can any information help one to "make friends with new patients in two minutes?" The secret to almost instant rapport is to develop one's awareness of the behavioral hints (that are picked up subconsciously) which inform us this person is indeed "like us." These clues, detected by the more primitive portion of one's brain, are much more powerful than the mere spoken word. Anyone can agree with a statement, if for no better reason than to be pleasant. The "clues" to which I refer are nonverbal and encompass a wide range of behaviors, from very obvious to extremely intricate.

From the moment I enter my office to begin a new-patient interview, I observe the patient closely and soon begin to mirror her behavior and mannerisms. The first things I note may be posture, or the rhythm and speed of her speech. If the patient talks slowly, so . . . do . . . I. If the speech is quick and concise, so is mine. If she is seated erectly, I am likewise. I don't mind a comfortable slump, if that is what the patient prefers. In short, I copy every facet of her behavior as closely as possible. (I won't indulge in poor grammar or vulgarity, but I'll be happy to throw in a little slang if such will prove beneficial to forming a positive relationship.)

I have discussed only the most superficial of mirroring behaviors. NLP can be very complex, and one can become as adept in this discipline as he or she feels the need to be. For example:

NLP informs us that people relate to the world by using primarily either their sense of vision (visual), hearing (auditory), or touch (kinesthetic). Each of these three basic relational types will give multiple clues as to their individual orientation. Some are obvious. When a point is made, visual people say, "I see." Auditories might acknowledge, "I hear you." Kinesthetics may remark, "I feel you're right."

Some clues are subtle. As one makes an effort to recall information, the position of the eye's focus varies with each relational type. Visuals shift their eyes up to recall, Auditories look straight ahead, while Kinesthetics access memory by looking downward. One can detect the relational type he or she is dealing with by asking a simple question—such as the date she last saw a dentist—and watching her eyes as she searches her memory.

Rate of speech differs greatly by types and also offers a significant clue regarding relational type. Visuals speak quickly. Auditory people speak more slowly. Kinesthetics' speech is so protracted it's akin to watching glaciers race.

I am visual. I speak rapidly. Listening to a very slow (to me at least) -speaking Kinesthetic about drives me nuts! If I interrupt in an attempt to speed the conversation to the level of my comfort, I have offended my slower-speaking friend. The reason one feels at home with some people more easily than with others is often because the person with whom you're comfortable accesses information by the same primary mode as you.

Once one has identified how the person with whom he or she is conversing processes data, the knowledge can be employed—not to change the meaning of the message one wishes to give—but to couch the communication in optimal terms for that particular patient to assimilate. For example, the aware dentist will match the patient's rate of speech, and offer feedback such as "I see" to visual patients.

This is a complex subject, but let's cut right to the chase. Mirroring is simply the act of copying the behaviors of the person with whom one is developing a relationship as closely as possible. One's efforts will be rewarded by an almost mystical ability to quickly make people feel comfortable, be it patients, friends or even family. Comfort will facilitate the formation of trust that is essential for education, and possible behavioral changes, to occur.

There is a hidden payoff that results from attempts to mirror another's behavior. As one makes this effort, he or she begins to observe people more closely. One begins to detect subtle clues and listen at a deeper level than before, thus developing the critical (but genetically unnatural) other-focus of sensitivity essential to compatibility. As a result of these efforts, one becomes more comfortable with others, and starts to see them as the unique and wonderful creations they are. This growing awareness diminishes the fear of rejection and facilitates closer relationships.

For those who wish to delve more deeply into NLP, for our brief discussion has barely touched upon the subject, allow me to recommend two introductory-level books:

Frogs Into Princes, by Richard Bandler and John Grinder—Real People Press, and

Trance-Formation, by the same authors and publisher.

The Bond of Trust

Let's consider another facet of behavioral excellence that allows one to employ people skills to optimize case acceptance, realizing that without case acceptance, dentists are unable to help patients.

There's been a lot of manure spread on the topic of how best to gain patient enthusiasm for suggested care, yet it seems but little growth has occurred, despite liberal application of nitrogen. (Forgive the earthy analogy—I'm from Iowa—the Tall Corn State?)

I've heard about magic slides (a variation of the magic beans of Jack and the Beanstalk fame), dressing for success (I listened to one respected lecturer advise 200 dentists against putting anything in their pants, like keys or wallet, as that would ruin the line of their slacks!!), and so many other "tricks of case acceptance" it gives me a headache to think about them!

There is some validity to many of the techniques in which I've been coached. (There is a saying in writing circles that, whatever the general guidelines, whatever works . . . works. The same is true within dental offices.) But most of these behaviors are merely hacking at the leaves of assuring patient compliance. I want this information to strike deeply, to the root—the base cause—of human conduct. I contend a **primary ingredient to high case acceptance is the evident trust, caring and mutual respect between dentist and all members of his or her team.**

The corollary—the spear in the heart of case acceptance— is the patient's perception of a poor relationship between ANY MEMBERS OF THE DENTAL TEAM.

Such affiliations are the living embodiment of the high-trust, low-fear environment in which all desire to live, but that perspicacious readers now understand to be abnormal, as natural selection favors innate wariness. (Survival odds are enhanced for those who run from noise in the jungle, rather than peeking through the grass to investigate what's making that awful growling sound.)

Forgive yet another aside, but I've been troubled for over a year by the succinct advice of a well-known lecturer I eagerly looked forward to hearing. His key to success was that every dentist with whom he worked made a commitment to present at least one $20,000 case per month!

I know I'm from Iowa, and fees are lower here, but not only have I never suggested anywhere near that amount of care, I still can't figure out what one can do for—or to?—a patient to justify $20,000 worth of treatment. Are there people—perhaps giants—existing in other sections of this great land with 64 teeth?

But beyond the problem of my personal lack of imagination in getting to $20,000 ($10,000 worth of fluoride treatments?), I believe this advice to be based entirely on fulfillment of the dentist's needs. Such a tactic is inherently appealing, as it is consistent with one's genetic mandate to acquire, but what of the trust of staff, patients, nation? If such self-serving behavior is commonplace within the profession, *Reader's Digest* had us centered in the cross-hairs of their scope, and we deserve the shot we took.

I'm not as concerned with the moral implications of over-treatment—unsavory as those are—as I am with the fact that such obvious self-serving behavior does not prove effective over time. Consider this situation, but let's return more directly to the topic of trust.

The difficulty with trust is one can't buy it for any price, like the magic slides; or simply remember to do it, like smiling, shaking hands, wearing slacks free of wrinkles (sporting creases with which one could slice bread!), keeping one's hair neat and shoes shiny all day; or delegate obtaining it to a staff member. **Trust must be earned by consistently exhibiting trustworthy behavior**. (Isn't there always a catch?)

Virtually all dental treatment, with the possible exception of acute pain relief and post-trauma care, is optional and accepted primarily based on trust. Doesn't it amaze you when asymptomatic periodontal patients accept unpleasant, time-consuming, expensive care based almost entirely on their belief in what the dentist and/or hygienist they might have just met told them? Or when patients agree to spend thousands of dollars to enhance their smile with anterior veneers, based on the slender vine of a few photos and faith in the care provider?

The first step in developing a high-trust office is the effort so central to success—the clarification of the dentist's values. Forgive my redundancy, but only one who has labored to discover his or her personal guiding principles can consistently make and follow through with value-oriented decisions.

The next step is to develop and implement a values-based hiring and training program to allow identification and employment of people with basic beliefs similar to those of the dental team. While one can force another to behave in a manner inconsistent with his or her beliefs short-term, the strain is constant, and adopting such unnatural behavior beyond long-term tolerance. The inherent conflict of people with varied beliefs required to work in close proximity destroys happiness and diminishes mutual trust.

Recall that a core of basic beliefs exists within each of us, even if one has never gone through the difficult process of value clarification. One can choose to modify values by the long, slow process we've been discussing, but NOBODY undertakes the lengthy, arduous task of self-examination because another—even a boss—asks them to. (It required a calamity of almost Biblical proportions to propel me down that pain-filled path.) Despite what promises might be made in an interview, the newness soon wears off, and existing personal values will control behavior of the seemingly perfect new team member in the long run. It's much better for all involved if skills are honed to allow identification of team members who already share office beliefs.

We won't discuss construction of a values-based want-ad, staff recruitment, selection, training, or staff meetings that exemplify the art of team building. These essential topics comprise Chapters 7 through 9 of *Focus*. I suggest even one familiar with the book reread these sections in light of the newer level of behavioral awareness and skills he or she is developing. There is no topic more important, or more deserving of one's attention, than employing staff with beliefs consistent with one's own. Working, marrying, or raising children with differing values makes the possibility of achieving success, wealth and especially joy unlikely.

After the doctor has clarified his or her values, and hired and trained a compatible team, the next step in the development of confidence is the doctor's constantly proving, by his or her behavior, to be **worthy of the team's trust.** One's lofty education, practice achievements, substantial net worth, neat car, well-creased slacks and status as a health care provider mean nothing. Staff evaluate you in the same manner as do your children—not by what you say, but by what you do.

(Recall the old rhyme—"Children more attention pay to what you do than what you say." Or the wisdom, shared by Ralph Waldo Emerson, I believe, that what you do speaks so loudly, I can't hear what you say. You'll seldom be exposed to any statements teeming with more truth.)

This means being fair . . . always. Not playing favorites, or making decisions based on the whim of the moment—rather than long-term beliefs—even when one is tired, stressed, hungry or in an acute financial crisis. It means being painfully honest and accepting complete responsibility, a portion of which is always doing one's best clinically. (Recall the decision one makes in committing to performing nothing but the best of which one is capable, as discussed in the clinical segment?)

One can't be perfect, but one can always choose to be honest. In the (too frequent!) times when treatment I provide doesn't go as planned, I never blame another (well . . . hardly ever), but look the patient in the eye and say "I'm sorry, but this hasn't turned out to my satisfaction. I can accept nothing less than my best, and I'll do whatever is required to get this right. **I'm not perfect, but I am honest.**"

It's hard for anyone to contend with this statement (especially the "not perfect" part), and staff frequently hearing me say this reinforces my commitment to always do the best of which I'm capable. (I'd be happier if everything went right the first time, but as you all know, most failures really are the lab's fault!)

What does team trust look like? As with pornography, trust is hard to describe and define, but one knows it when one sees it. (More critically, so do patients!) Perhaps the best indication of mutual trust is the ability of staff to joke and kid with each other. (The dentist teasing staff without back-and-forth exchange is bullying—considerably south of trust.)

Faith is also manifested by sincere compliments given both by dentist and staff. Unsolicited praise occurs naturally among people who respect and admire each other.

Trust is also illustrated by what's missing within the office—conflict, tension, blaming—especially when things go wrong. People who trust and like each other work as a team to reach common goals. They don't judge each other, as they understand that **fixing the blame doesn't fix the problem, and they desire results!**

Do you enjoy the company of hypocrites and liars? When problems occur, is it excuses you desire? How do you react to another when you know they are lying—even if only to save embarrassment? Are these disingenuous folks the type with whom you wish to continue a relationship?

Why would you assume your staff and patients don't feel the same way? Most people sense dishonesty, even if they can't prove it, just as you do. They also deeply resent being lied to—treated like a fool—as do you.

(This chapter ends with a short, but vital essay concerning the power of apology and honesty. Please consider that information carefully as regards staff trust and patient acceptance.)

Couched in the special language of this chapter, one must develop the wisdom and courage to forfeit short-term gain—as the time saved by seating an inferior crown—to create the long-term value of trust. To the unenlightened, such decisions seem to be in defiance of the genetic mandate to accumulate all one can. The wise realize the best way to achieve every goal he or she desire is by embracing trustworthiness. One can debate "right" and "wrong" of moral behavior—and I hope you do—but here is my message: **Honesty is the best guarantee of success.** It requires a long-term focus, clear values and an accurate perception of human behavior to firmly grasp this truth.

Let's turn our attention to people skills in another common venue by answering the query: How does a behavioral adept best employ the opportunities inherent within anger?

Are You Mad at Me?

Every human who has walked the face of Planet Earth has experienced the emotion of ANGER. This is a hormonal reflex, its existence favored by natural selection as it enhances one's odds in the face of danger by triggering the famous "fight or flight" reaction, critical in humankind's early days when deadly predators perpetually surrounded them.

Today, thank God, one is seldom faced with authentic life threats. (I've been in three life-or-death situations—the most recent last fall when the boat in which my father, son John and I were duck hunting overturned in 12 feet of water, tossing us into the swift current of a very chilly Mississippi River. All of us were wearing chest-waders, which filled with water to create a significant weight. On the boat ride home, after all of us were pulled to safety, I shook "like a dog crapping bones," to borrow one of my father's colorful aphorisms, my system saturated with adrenaline. Thus, I can personally assure you the fight or flight reflex still exists when needed. Apparently, unlike many of my other organ systems, it isn't vulnerable to disuse atrophy.)

A more prominent contemporary problem is having a situation trigger anger where one's autonomically controlled hormonal response occurs, but one has no opportunity to vent the chemicals and emotions that accumulate. (I had plenty of activity on which to burn energy during my recent short stay in the Mississippi.)

A common misconception is that one can control the existence of emotions. It's not true. One can govern his or her reaction, and choose to be honest or dishonest about feelings, but as I learned in "the unit," feelings exist, whether one approves or desires them . . . or not.

One of the hardest, unhealthiest, unavoidable portions of the dental profession is to have one's body dealing with acute stress (maybe the lab really did make an error on a six-unit bridge, and the patient is leaving for an extended stay in Spain next week—as happened to me!) and having to plaster a smile on one's sweating mug, will one's pulse rate down, swallow acidic bile and cheerfully move on to treat the next patient as if nothing untoward has happened.

As we've discussed, these emotions don't disappear because you choose to deny or ignore them—they just lie in wait until your resistance is low—then seek you out as unerringly as did Charles Dickens's Christmas ghosts.

We'll touch but lightly on the biology of which all dentists are aware—that anger damages one physically, emotionally, behaviorally and mentally. From diminished immune response to cancer, from depression to despair, from alcoholism to suicide, one pays a dear price for unexamined emotions.

The Buddha told us, "We are not punished **for** our anger—we are punished **by** our anger." As the above listing of physical problems associated with anger certifies, this is an undeniable biological truth, but this book's—admittedly wavering—focus is on people skills, so let's eschew other internal ramifications of rage and examine how one ideally confronts anger in another. (The following advice assumes the "other" to be unarmed!)

Here is the technique that has worked almost perfectly for me when forced to confront an angry individual:

1. **Touch.** This is usually a handshake, but can be a finger laid on a shoulder or arm. It's tough to initiate contact when one knows a person is upset—perhaps our protective reflex counsels to keep distance between ourselves and the potentially dangerous—but it's more difficult to remain angry with a person after touching.

2. **Look the angry person directly in the eyes.** Again, tough. The tops of one's shoes seem much more interesting in such uncomfortable situations. I'd guess this step is imperative, as similar to not running from an angry dog; one must not reveal his or her fear, especially to someone already angry, or one's danger is increased.

3. Asking—hopefully in a calm, steady voice—"**Are you mad at me?**" This candid query is disarming, shocking, and almost always results in a stammering denial of anger. (It's up to the angry person to deal with his or her emotions honestly on their own time. I simply desire—for selfish reasons entirely—for the uncomfortable anger to disappear. I'm a dentist, not a psychologist or the patient's mother.)

I follow up the denial with a broad, hopefully contagious smile (and silent whoa!) and state, "Good, because if I ever do or say anything to upset you, I'd be grateful if you would inform me of it at once and give me a chance to set things right."

The result of this behavioral excellence is **MAGIC**. An angry person is INSTANTLY TRANSFORMED into a docile one. The patient is forced, by my actions, to confront his or her attitude, and, almost always, discovers being angry is not socially acceptable in this physically non-threatening situation. (Displaying behavioral skills such as these goes a long way toward building admiration and faith among staff, as well as reducing the acidity of gastric contents, and relieving dangerous pressure coalescing on assorted sphincters.)

BEHAVIORAL MASTERY is the ability to instantly change the emotional state of others. (I speak of behavioral accomplishments—not drawing a weapon—which also works, technically.)

If you need to use this technique often, you'd better examine your office and team conduct. In a well-managed, behaviorally aware office, one shouldn't be forced to deal with an angry person more than a few times in his or her career. (At least this is true in rural Iowa.)

But some folks go through life angry, and occasionally one will inadvertently stumble into your path. (Such unpleasant occurrences are still an improvement over our ancestor's occasional up-close-and-personal moments with a saber-toothed tiger!) Here is a skill that can transform that unfortunate situation and make one appear a magician to all who witness such legerdemain—including the angry person.

Facing anger is difficult due to the fear of rejection we've discussed. Recall that being cast out by the tribe is the psychic equivalent of death, and one understands why confronting this dark emotion can be terrifying. (I was raised rather roughly in a little river town. I've had my nose broken five times, and can assure you the physical danger of anger can also be a concern.)

Behavioral excellence displayed in the face of anger and possible violence depends on one's ability to draw upon acquired wisdom to avoid the normal or genetic instinct to defend or attack. One must reach beyond primitive reflexes to engage the advanced portions of one's brain to define a new and better manner of behavior, consistent with the current rules of culture.

(Have you ever heard of a dentist who punched his or her way to success?)

I hope you are developing an increasing sense of the importance of behavioral skills and how vital they are to achieving our three-part goal of success, wealth and joy. Let's study one last example of how understanding people can result in choosing behavior that seems to place one at a disadvantage, but which, over time, results in accelerating one toward his or her life's goals.

The Power of Apology

As hoary veterans of the dental wars (please don't get excited—the word means gray-haired, old; the one you're thinking of is pronounced the same, but starts with a "W"), you're all familiar with the following scenarios. It may be a patient who appears to have a denture delivered, and you discover the lab work has not yet arrived. It might be a chipped bonding, veneer or crown you recently completed. Perhaps a new MOD amalgam on tooth number four has fractured through the midline.

Your loyal staff has informed you of the problem. You must face the patient, possibly an unhappy one, in a matter of seconds. As you complete care on your current patient, your pulse accelerates as your mind wrestles with the "best possible approach" to the predicament. How can you most efficaciously deal with this lack of perfection? You could blame the lab, a staff member, site material failure, or chastise the patient for doing something you *strictly forbade them to do,* that resulted in the demise of your carefully crafted dental perfection. All tried and true remedies from our profession's history.

Or, you could accept full responsibility, apologize to the patient for his or her inconvenience, and do whatever is needed to set things right without an additional charge. (Behaving in such a manner is worthwhile just to witness the shocked reaction of someone observing a person stepping up and doing what is right. I'd suggest trying this at least once, if for no other motive than to enjoy observing the result!)

A VITAL ASIDE: I believe a sincere apology to be more essential than not charging a fee, as it is more authentically personal, thus of greater emotional import. As with any meaningful communication, one's message should be delivered after using the patient's name, establishing direct eye contact, and some form of touch. Allow me to reiterate that using a person's name, looking them in the eye, and touching—and one must perform all three—will geometrically increase the effectiveness of every communication. Don't believe for a minute that re-treating at no charge takes the place of understanding, courage and the skill of a proper apology.

"But if I admit it's my fault, don't I risk being sued?"

I'm not an attorney, so the following comments represent only my feelings. I will confess to fixing teeth since shortly after the end of the most recent Ice Age and (the rhythmic tapping you hear is me knocking on wood) having never been sued. Legally, those qualifications count for naught, but it is my hope that readers will be kind enough to consider my thoughts anyway.

My lack of legal status established (I consider the ponderous list of skills I don't possess to be merely the narrowing of my focus), it is my belief that those who admit to error and/or accept responsibility are seen by others—not as idiots, weaklings, cowards and failures—but as people of courage, character and strength. It is possible such an act of candor may make it more difficult to win a malpractice suit, but I contend this forthright approach will allow one to avoid most legal problems.

Reflect on personal experience. When something you've purchased or a service you paid for fails, how do you react to excuses? When the dental unit that has just been repaired continues to drip water on everything, everywhere—including the upper-midline of your wrinkle-free, perfectly creased slacks (thereby placing your zipper in jeopardy of rusting)—is it an explanation you long for? What you want is a knight in shining armor to appear and masterfully resolve your dilemma.

We live in a world short of perfection. (Although damn near every dentist I know is working feverishly to correct God's seeming oversight.) Mistakes happen to us all. (But a lot more often to me since I turned 50!) When predicaments occur, the primary issue isn't who's at fault, but who will step forward, be responsible, and proactively put things right.

In every dental catastrophe, one is presented with an occasion to show patients and staff what kind of person he or she is. There is wisdom available in understanding why the Chinese use the same word for crisis and opportunity. Anyone can do well under ideal circumstances. **Mastery consists of achieving excellence in the face of adversity.** Within every crisis is the chance to display behavior that will enhance trust and strengthen relationships.

Mark Twain advised us to tell the truth, as it's easier to remember what we've said. As I age, and my memory (and the rest of my body) sags, I agree ever more with Mr. Twain's sage sentiments. I also wish to advance the theory that one lies from a self-perceived position of fear and weakness. One tells the truth from a posture of moral strength. Often, one's veracity reflects the level of one's self-confidence and courage. In plain words, **to lie is the act of a coward.**

Even if you prevaricate with adequate conviction and skill to fool a patient, you won't trick your staff (one's dishonesty thus decreasing trust and respect) and you won't deceive yourself. (See you at 4 A.M.!!) You'll not fool many patients either. In the behavioral clues of downcast eyes, trembling voice and sweating skin, others can accurately perceive deception, even if they can't prove it.

How would you react if you strongly suspected your doctor wasn't telling you the truth? Would your perception of him or her be altered? In which manner—honesty or dishonesty—do you wish to be seen by your patients, staff and family? How would you prefer to be dealt with by others? The Golden Rule, to treat others as we wish to be treated, is not only an ideal formula for the next existence, but is a guaranteed prescription for a calm stomach, a good night's sleep, and a life filled with success and joy.

In the situations we've described, and countless others, we make choices. I urge you to claim the path of fortitude and honesty, not only because it's "the right thing to do," but because it is the surest path to success and realization of one's dreams.

Often, doing the correct thing seems frightening, daunting. I believe you'll find the opposite to be the case. Once accomplished, the internal relief forthcoming from an act of courageous integrity is palpable. People's reaction to an apology and good-natured acceptance of responsibility will astound you! Your strength of character will be noted and appreciated—it is indeed a rarity in our it's-not-my-fault victim's world—and for it you will realize the blessings you deserve.

REFOCUS TWO: THE EQUILIBRIUM OF JOY

Do you ever suffer the frustrating thought that no matter what you do, it's impossible to make everyone—including yourself—happy? Take today for example. A pleasant young mother of three was scheduled at the end of a long Monday for emergency treatment of a sore tooth. She had not been a patient in your office before. Her medical history was involved and complex, her dental symptoms vague. You eventually diagnosed a leaking MODL amalgam on 14 and reluctantly decided it would be best, in this case, to place a permanent restoration.

During the course of the examination the patient tearfully admitted her husband is laid off. She has no insurance, no money and several other obviously decayed and sensitive teeth. You refuse to even think about the crowns—minimum of four—she requires. You feel you have little choice but to reschedule her and at least restore all her decay as a charity case. This is what your staff expects, what your church and friends assume you'd do, and is consistent with the type of person you'd like to think you are.

And yet you can't help but consider the time required—you should have been home an hour ago already—the earnings you'll forfeit as you're providing free care, not to mention the out-of-pocket expense. And past philanthropic treatment you've provided hasn't always proven rewarding. You've even had charity patients fail appointments! All these thoughts leave you with a definite sense of frustration you hope doesn't indicate that, at heart, you're a bad person.

If you weren't so lost in thought you might have noted and been concerned by the frown on your faithful, uncomplaining chairside's face. Let's listen in on her internal dialogue:

I know it's my duty to help care for this person in pain, but it is almost an hour past our normal closing time. It clearly violates our office policy—we just discussed this at our last staff meeting—to place a permanent restoration in an emergency situation. I'm dead-tired, still need to stop at the store, fix supper, and the kids will want help with homework. I promised myself I'd begin the week enrolling in that new aerobics program. I've gained a few pounds, and I feel so lethargic any more. Looks like I won't be able to start exercising tonight either. I get so tired of helping others, and never having time for me. I hope these feelings don't mean I'm a bad person?

The patient is thinking: I really like this dentist—he's so gentle—and the office is real nice. I have a feeling he'll offer to help with some of my other bad teeth, and with Jock laid off, I don't know how else I could get the work done. I'm relieved and grateful . . . yet I feel so guilty! I wasn't brought up to have others take care of me. What will people think when they discover I'm receiving charity? What if my neighbors found out!? I hope accepting the dental work I need doesn't make me a bad person?

All the protagonists of our little melodrama seem doomed to less than complete contentment. The dentist and assistant have made the choice to do what they perceive to be "the right thing," yet feel disappointed that their personal desires must be sacrificed. The patient is getting her personal needs met—for dental care in this example—but is concerned about how she will be perceived by others within her community. Everyone has some of their needs fulfilled, but at the seeming expense of other desires. Instead of happiness, all three suffer a sense of loss, disappointment and anxiety.

Our examination of this common scenario illustrates how each of us spends our lifetime torn between two powerful and divergent forces, of which few are even aware. The counter-stresses of these perpetual drives create a swirling undercurrent that frequently leaves one perplexed, frustrated, unhappy. Allow me to illustrate the effects of these dynamics in action.

Imagine humankind suspended by the wrists between two powerful horses. The steed to the right is ridden by a naked youth and represents instinct—**the power of one's nature**—the hard-wired genetic imperatives that tell one to do everything possible to enhance and ensure one's survival and the passing of one's unique genetic legacy to his or her offspring.

The massive animal to the left is ridden by a mature, clothed person and represents the **forces of culture** that have existed since humans began to live in community. These directives create and enforce the restraints of instincts that must be present for people to coexist in close proximity. They command all to share, cooperate, be nice, in stark contrast to one's innate genetic commands to seek personal gain and well-being. These social powers are codified in the form of superstition, custom, religion, social mores and law. Humans can't live together in society without such controls.

Can you grasp the ultimate fate of all humans living in community? If one follows his or her instincts, to acquire all possible power in its every form, and thus enhance one's odds of survival and successful reproduction, culture punishes—with penalties as subtle as nagging guilt and peer disapproval—or as substantial as criminal charges and jail sentences.

If one obeys the dictates of culture—to share, obey the rules, allow others to go first—one feels resentful and cheated of the individual needs one's nature and every cell of one's body are demanding he or she achieve. Why must I always be giving to others? What of my inherent needs?

Increased pressure from either "horse" must be countered by similar pressure from the opposing "steed" to restore a balance that prevents disorder. But tender humankind is dangled, painfully torqued between these ancient forces. Personal liberty run wild ultimately leads to chaos—war in the streets and the complete breakdown of society. To illustrate the damage of societal pressure unchecked, consider Hitler's Germany or Stalin's Russia, where personal liberty was forfeit to the out-of-control power of the state.

This age-old conundrum is illustrated by the familiar cartoon portrayal of a moral dilemma. In the center of the scene stands a poor, confused, impacted person (with perhaps a mirror and explorer clasped in one hand?). On one shoulder sits the devil. His advice: Care for one's personal needs and leave others to fend for themselves. "Get all you can, as it's a cruel world you must face alone!" (The caricature of a devil is unfortunate, as there is nothing innately evil about wanting one's requirements met. As we've seen, the drive to achieve personal needs is instinctive—part of one's nature.)

On the other shoulder, the forces of culture, represented by an angel, counsel one to be kind, loving, follow the rules. "It's your duty to be a good citizen, and that means considering the needs of others first." (The image of an angel is also inaccurate, as Hitler and Stalin have illustrated the potential disaster of excessive cultural control. The point of the demonstration is not good versus evil, but to establish the essential need of balance.)

What's a person to do? There exists no simple, pleasant, easily reached middle ground. No matter what one decides—to obey the dictates of culture, or satisfy individual needs—there is a nagging sense that he or she has been deficient in the choice.

Our opening paragraphs revealed one small example of the dental office as a microcosm of the world, its inhabitants tormented in a variety of ways by the two powerful, contrary and ubiquitous forces of natural instinct and cultural demands. Each team member has personal needs, and the insistence they be fulfilled is as strident in one's career as in every other facet of life. At the same time, the requirements of patients, society and the culture milieu within one's office create restraints that interfere with one's fulfillment of these personal imperatives.

(Remember, not only do external forces support societal demands, but the need to be accepted within a group is primordial, as banishment from ancient tribes was, in effect, a sentence of death. In prison, solitary confinement is the ultimate of punishments. Infants not touched, talked to and acknowledged can die from "failure to thrive syndrome." Thus we see the old song spoke ancient truth . . . people do need people.)

So in life, and within our offices, people are asked to live on a teeter-totter. If one puts too much weight to the side of office demands, personal requirements go unfulfilled and one suffers the dark poisons of resentment. "Why must it always be me sacrificing for others?"

If one satisfies individual needs and defies the commands of culture, one feels guilt and risks the displeasure, and even abandonment, of the group. "The dentist is selfish and greedy, concerned only with getting more for herself. She isn't the kind of person I choose to work for." (Or provide my care, from a patient's perspective.) Or, "My chairside thinks only about his needs. I'm afraid he isn't a team player and doesn't fit in our office."

These ancient forces aren't likely to disappear. It seems the only possible solution to this problem is to achieve and maintain a comfortable **balance** between these two undeniable and unavoidable forces, but such a valuable achievement isn't easy. Let's consider plans by which a stable counterbalance may be achieved, thus enriching one's life.

The first step to establishing this pleasant and critical equilibrium is achieving full **awareness** of these divergent requirements of the individual and community and of the continual stress they create. (Simply considering this problem puts one well ahead of the great majority!) One must never lose sight of the reality that these are powerful, omnipresent forces whose constant conflict daily influences our lives in numerous ways.

Conscious realization allows one to carefully, deliberately chart an ideal middle path, not totally fulfilling genetic desires—thus risking expulsion by society—yet not ignoring the needs and demands of our beings, a behavior that eventually leads to mounting frustration and rage. (Yes, there is danger in being "too good," not that an old lone wolf like me feels at risk in this regard.)

The second step is to develop strategies wherein **the needs of the individual can be met within the boundaries of community, rather than in conflict with them.** Pardon my redundancy, but it is essential to understand that if BOTH personal and cultural desires aren't to some degree assuaged, the individual suffers. How can one achieve peer and societal acceptance, **without relinquishing the ability to meet personal needs?** No single answer exists, but allow me to advance some ideas.

If one desires to be accepted within his or her dental community, one should recall the brilliant and innovative Australian dentist Dr. Paddi Lund's contention that **politeness is the oil in which cultures smoothly function.** (We'll discuss my friend Paddi's ingenious concepts in detail later in the book.) This basic truth is most imperative for a leader—for example, the head of a dental office—to assimilate.

Be unfailing in one's praise. Catch others doing something right, and reward them with loud and frequent approval. SAY PLEASE AND THANK YOU! Overspend on positive reinforcement, not in a manipulative, disingenuous way, but from one's heart, with full awareness of your and your fellow worker's needs to enjoy community support. **Avoid talking in a negative manner behind a team member's back (behavior our office refers to as SUBGROUPING). This is a cancer that will destroy any group—especially a small, intimate and intense society, like a dental office.** One sacrifices none of his or her genetic demands by generously offering praise and thanks to others.

But acceptance is only half the victory. (The chair one sits upon is accepted—yet who envies the seat—at least mine—its duty, let alone its view?) To joyfully attain the PERSONAL RECOGNITION THAT CREATES IDENTITY, one must find creative ways to satisfy genetic demands that establish his or her uniqueness, and are sanctioned within the office culture.

The ideal path to meeting personal needs within community varies by one's skills, interests and level of awareness of how essential this step is to the attainment of success, wealth and personal happiness. To achieve our tripartite objective, one must create **a niche of value** where uniqueness can be highlighted while **enriching** the culture in which he or she exists.

Perhaps one's identity is established through the exceptional level of skill with which treatment is provided. Care can be delivered in an honest and compassionate manner that will gain society's approval. The rewards that redound from such valuable service will help satiate one's personal needs.

But balance is critical. If the care provider sacrifices too greatly in relation to the reward received, resentment results. (Consider the troubled mind-set of a dentist who labors diligently, but is unable to achieve financial success.) If the reward is too great for the service rendered, one will face resistance from society. (An office considered overpriced in relation to the service provided will be shunned by patients—a common, painful form of societal punishment for any business that, unchecked, results in bankruptcy.)

A staff member's uniqueness might be demonstrated by initiating and developing a chart audit system to help fill every provider's schedule. A wise employer will offer praise and a raise as a reward for this valuable achievement—thus providing fulfillment of personal needs and hopefully creating a loyal and motivated team member—and the entire office community will gratefully reap the project's benefits.

The specific details aren't important, as each can find personally appropriate and satisfying ways to establish identity, once one understands the imperative nature of the need to fulfill individual needs within the context of cultural acceptance.

A warning: No one can control the attitude and behavior of others. As you act on this wisdom, be cognizant that your personal awareness and performance are the only courts over which you have dominion. One has no ability to control the actions of those lacking this critical knowledge, but this enlightenment will allow one to observe the painful frustration and failure of others who fail to perceive and achieve this essential equilibrium.

One will be able to understand much of others' unhappiness that, before one became aware of this information, couldn't be fathomed. If one cares for another suffering from this essential imbalance, he or she could share this knowledge. (Or this entire book!)

These universal principles apply to everyone, in every situation—not just coworkers and patients—thus this wisdom can assist one in establishing the delicate balance needed to achieve joy in every facet of life. Maintaining equilibrium between personal needs and cultural demands is the secret to a happy marriage and family, to mutually satisfying friendships. Knowledge and thoughtful effort will allow one to meet his or her individual needs within the nurturing support, safety and approval of ANY caring community—family, office, club, city—to which he or she aspires to belong. This awareness and resultant behavioral adjustments represent a significant milestone upon the pathway that leads to life more abundant.

Consider the painful price you've paid the many times you've failed to maintain equilibrium between personal needs and societal demands. (In my case, alcohol addiction.) Make the struggle needed to comprehend this basic truth (I know it's not easy! What of true value ever is?) and every facet of one's future will be made more luminous by the effort.

Chapter Three

Patient Recruitment and Retainment

I hope *Dentistry's Future* shouts the message that the key to success in dentistry and life lies in **understanding and fulfilling human needs through insightful awareness and diligent effort**. Despite the bulk of this chapter dealing with activities designed to recruit new clients, never lose track of the ultimate reason patients come to, then stay with a dental practice: They believe this dentist can be trusted to provide the best possible care consistent with their best interests.

BECOME THAT TRUSTED PERSON!!

There is nothing wrong with making efforts to identify one-self to others as the dentist they seek (marketing), but any accomplishment less than achieving a thorough understanding of human nature and always trying to do one's best for another will eventually lead to professional disaster, no matter the hordes of patients attracted to one's practice by the most skilled and sophisticated marketing. I believe this is as it should be—both just and fair.

This general caveat in place, let's consider my personal philosophy and the techniques by which we assist patients in discovering our office is the perfect place for them to receive dental care.

I'll be honest. For the majority of my career, I haven't displayed much interest or expertise concerning the overt or external marketing of my practice. True, I've always marketed by working hard to please each patient and giving more than expected, I hope in a behaviorally adept manner (even if primarily motivated by fear of rejection). But as I've added associates and reduced my hours in the office, I've marketed a little more each year. As I do with every endeavor, once committed to deliberate patient recruitment, I became a student, attending courses and reading books on the subject.

It is ideal for an office to be so inundated with patients seeking care they have no reason to market, but such a fortuitous situation is seldom the case in today's ultra-competitive world. In painful candor, I believe our office's need to market developed as a manner in which we compensated for a reduced level of personalized services that led to diminished patient loyalty and thus lessened new-patient referrals—both results of a blurred office focus—a dilution in our level of commitment to our commonly agreed-upon purpose.

Part of this loss of clarity has to do with office size. In my practice's early years, when we had three staff and worked eight to five, Monday through Friday, and I was always present, it was easier to ensure every policy was precisely enforced. Today, with 10 staff (including dentists) and hours from 7 a.m. to 7 p.m. Monday through Friday, plus Saturday mornings—and the resultant rotation of team members needed to work these expanded hours—confusion as to who is to do what, and thus errors of every stripe, are more common.

For example, when one receptionist scheduled all patients—instead of seven staff using five computer terminals to schedule today—the chance of mistakes being made with appointments was markedly less. Also, if a misunderstanding concerning scheduling did occur, it was clear with whom to discuss the situation to assure our policy was completely understood and correctly implemented in the future. Partly due to the modern "wonder" of computers (I'm always wondering what happened since we've computerized!), today we're never quite certain how a patient mysteriously appears in the office, appointment card in hand, but their name not on our schedule.

However, the major cause of lost focus is weakened or failed leadership. I'm not present enough to **consistently define and enforce office policy and vision** (the duty of every leader), and my absence shows. Three dentists—no matter how bright, motivated, talented, cute—means three senses of direction and levels of dedication.

Today our office journey is akin to taking a car trip with a trio of rotating drivers, each with different maps and varied ideas as to the ideal final destination. It's not a lack of skill or effort on the part of the drivers (dentists) that creates the problems, but rather a lack of shared clarity as to exactly where we are headed and how best to get there.

(Chapters 6 and 7 of *Dentistry's Future* deal with multiple-dentist offices, of which I am a big supporter. At that time we'll discuss in detail what I consider to be the greatest threat to group practice—the loss of consistency and blurring of leadership—that must be continually addressed and boldly confronted if a multiple-dentist office is to achieve success.)

Another reason I never marketed as a solo dentist was because I was always too busy to handle the farrago of patients who wandered in, almost from the day I first opened the office doors. The precise historic details are a bit obscure (I didn't get much sleep in those days, and had not developed the office monitors we'll discuss in Chapter 4), but for four years our office did not accept new patients, as we were booked three or more months in advance. As I've mentioned, the pressure of constantly working patients into the schedule, starting early and always finishing late, about killed me, and was the major motivation for seeking an associate dentist to HELP!

The gurus of the industry might suggest I was scheduled months in advance because of office inefficiencies that "clogged my schedule." I would counter that I suffered from the effort to provide the best dental care I possibly could to over 5,000 very active patients—a staggering, impossible load!

Before adding an associate I did everything in my power to accommodate patient demand and maximize productivity. I had five fully equipped operatories, a staff of seven, implemented expanded hygiene (that will be the topic of Chapter 5), studied books and magazines, timed every clinical procedure (see Chapter 12 of *Focus* for specifics concerning the vital task of constructing a scheduling ruler), took courses and hired consultants to streamline every office system.

As we'll discuss later, BEFORE bringing in an associate, everything possible must be done to maximize office efficiency. Adding another care provider to a disorganized office is akin to having an affair to help a weak marriage—a recipe for almost certain disaster. Failure to refine all office systems before adding another dentist is a major reason associate relationships have such a dismal record of failure.

I was producing $40,000 per month as a solo dentist around 1982—when that was a significant amount of money. (Assuming 4% inflation during this 16-year interval, this would equate to approximately $75,000 per month in today's weakened dollars.) My office overhead had gradually drifted toward 70% as patient overload left little time for organization and inefficiency increased. When we added an associate, overhead dropped to around 50%, where it has generally remained. (The increased net/decreased overhead of a multi-dentist practice will be analyzed carefully at the appropriate time, as this booster rocket to net income is a major factor in my willingness to accept the problems inherent within a group practice.)

Once again, I've shared my personal experience to explain the context from which I present marketing data, thus helping this information to be more thoroughly and honestly interpreted. The history lesson completed for now, let's return our focus to patient recruitment.

I've written articles on marketing for *Dental Economics*, as well as for several dental newsletters. Chapter 12 of *Freedom* is entirely devoted to my early practice promotion efforts. Due to my short marketing history at the time of that writing, Chapter 12 is not lengthy. (Twenty pages, to be precise.) Though I freely admit to being no marketing maven, I want to include what information I can share to assist readers who feel inclined to market to do so in a professional, effective and fun manner. (All things—even marketing—are a portion of a joyous life's journey.) I'd also like to illustrate how clear values are critical to successful marketing, and how lacking clarity will doom any marketing effort.

Obviously, attracting patients in abundance is a critical portion of practice success. Marketing is one possible method whereby one may achieve this goal, especially helpful during the early years of a practice, or when adding an associate dentist—times when a robust flow of new patients is acutely needed.

Everyone Markets

Marketing encompasses every interaction any member of an office team has with another person. One "markets" when they smile and nod to someone on the street, as well as when they launch a $10,000 television advertising venture. Staff members market when visiting with a neighbor they happen to meet in the grocery store. Marketing includes views—good and bad—shared about one's office over the fence (where Iowa neighbors often converse in pleasant weather) or over the phone. In its broadest context, marketing is the way one presents himself or herself—clothes, speech, walk, behavior, etc.—in the efforts to gain acceptance, and avoid rejection, by other tribal members.

So, dentist or non-dentist, no one can avoid marketing. (In the final analysis, irrespective of occupation or motivation, all one has to sell is himself or herself.) One can choose to market with awareness and purpose, in a manner consistent with thoughtfully defined personal values, or stumble along, without clear direction, hoping everything somehow works out for the best. (Take a moment and consider which approach you have been employing, and how's it working to date? It might help to further define the premise to consider tongue-piercing as a form of marketing message—although glossal perforation is one signal the meaning of which I fear I'm too old to grasp.)

Allow me to share my personal definition of dental marketing—one unlike any I've seen in print:

Professional marketing includes any manner of displaying one's beliefs and values to the public to position one's business by defining to others WHAT ONE BELIEVES IN and thus attracting consumers with similar interests and beliefs.

Please consider this statement carefully. As we proceed, evaluate each topic considered as it relates to this standard. I think one will discover this definition describes and encompasses every effective marketing activity. Problems arise when one's values aren't clear, and thus the marketing message—in its varied forms—is changeable, muddled, sporadic and confusing.

I'll take no chance that this critical premise can be misunderstood. It should come as no surprise to those who have been paying attention so far, that the most critical segment of an effective marketing plan is the pristine definition of beliefs and values by the dental office leader—YOU, DOCTOR.

While form will vary substantially, here are the primary ingredients of every successful marketing concept:

1. Values are precisely articulated, then coalesced into written form by a unified dental team. This is the critical first step— the clarified statement of why an office exists—that creates the foundation upon which all success rests.

2. Clear values, combined with energy and some creative thought (aided, perhaps, by some external stimulation, as from an excellent dental book!), lead to developing an advertising scheme that defines one's mission to the public. This expression of office beliefs and benefits attracts patients, especially people with values similar to those of the practice.

3. IT IS CRITICAL THAT THE MESSAGE OF EVERY FORM OF ADVERTISING—from the hello and smile to a neighbor in the store, to the reception-room reading materials, to the expensive television campaign—be **consistent with these carefully defined values**.

4. To be effective, a marketing message must also be **consistently REPEATED**—not just activated when "things are slow" in the office.

Inconsistent marketing efforts were the norm in our office for years. Campaigns were mounted when increased new-patient flow was required, then abandoned due to enhanced office busyness, only to be laboriously resurrected years later when we again needed more patients. We kept reinventing and re-implementing similar marketing strategies, and these concepts require time, money and energy to employ and achieve results.

We ended this ineptness by designating one staff member as public relations leader and having her create a monthly calendar of PR events that we follow throughout the year, reviewing and discussing each month's plans, and assigning specific PR tasks to team members during our regular staff meetings.

(Please refer to a sample of our PR calendar, located at the end of this chapter.)

Developing an Effective Game Plan

I hope non-basketball fans will indulge me once again if I fall back on my old passion to illustrate a point. A great coach (leader) will assess his or her team (dental staff) and define what it is they do best, and in what areas they are deficient. Perhaps the coach discovers his or her team is quick, composed of good athletes, but small. This analysis carefully completed—because upon its accuracy the team will succeed or fail—a scheme is developed to optimize their unique blend of talents.

A quick, small athletic team might be best suited to play a full-court, pressing defense the entire game, thus employing their strengths to harass larger, more powerful teams into mistakes and turnovers that lead to easy baskets.

The same coach working with a big team may wish to slowly walk the ball up the floor, then work the ball inside, near the basket, to take advantage of their size and "pound the boards" for rebounds.

Whatever the scheme developed, every member of the organization must understand and enthusiastically support their portion of the plan. The strategy must be consistently practiced and constantly employed for the team to achieve the greatest possible success of which it is capable. Any deviation from this ideal course must be immediately identified and corrected.

If one has (I hope and pray) begun to clarify one's values, what is your dental scheme? (Marketing is merely a single facet of one's office values and identity.) Does the dentist wear a silk tie, the office play soothing baroque music and feature *Barron's* and *The Wall Street Journal* as reading materials in the reception area?

Or does the dress code consist of designer jeans, the music rock and roll and the reception room feature *People* magazine? **BOTH STYLES, AND ALL IN BETWEEN, CAN BE EFFECTIVE, IF CAREFULLY DESIGNED TO MAXIMIZE TEAM STRENGTHS AND CONSISTENTLY PORTRAYED.** But when a big team tries to fast-break, or a *Wall Street Journal* office goes to jeans, identity has been lost, and trouble soon ensues. Mixed messages confuse, and it is impossible to market effectively when one has not precisely defined what they are selling.

When office beliefs are clear to all team members, consistency in marketing and every other facet of office appearance and behavior will not present a problem. If unclear, office policy will change with every meeting attended, every book read.

Characteristics of the Wilde Marketing Program

Let's consider the universal or generic characteristics of what I consider to be an effective dental marketing strategy, before discussing my specific techniques and programs.

1. **Professional**—To me this means a marketing strategy in which:

    a) I am proud to have my name attached. (I believe each of the examples that follow will support and illustrate this contention—although a precise definition of professionalism will vary, profoundly influenced by individual values and taste.)

b) The focus of every message is on service to the public through dental health education.

c) Each message must enhance the strength of the entire dental profession. If one falls prey to an overt self-focus (allowing genetically mandated needs to cloud one's long-term vision), for example, by trumpeting self-proclaimed personal superiority over other dental health-care providers, such self-interest becomes apparent and results in decreased trust.

2. **Inexpensive**—I'm cheap. I also am concerned with enhancing my profit through marketing, not just "positioning my office," or making a name for myself in the community. I dislike using marketing programs where I can't measure results and where the money invested is not quickly returned multiple times. I consider marketing an investment, and as such, one should be able to measure results and expect to demonstrate a profit.

3. **FUN**—Every activity employed to promote the practice must be enjoyable for both patients and staff. Our team hasn't the discipline to continue working with concepts we don't enjoy. I doubt forced effort will yield desirable results anyway. Engaging in any activity that isn't genuine or consistent with one's beliefs usually results in the effort being abandoned and staff and patients becoming confused as to one's true beliefs. (Engaging in such unauthentic and ineffective efforts results from a failure to clarify values.)

4. **Not Perceived as Advertising**—This might just be personal bias—I'm over 50 and opinionated—but that which is obviously an ad reeks of self-service. I find such distinct self-promotional efforts, no matter how cleverly disguised, embarrassing to observe, and doubt they are effective. I believe an office positioned in such a manner is seen as greedy, desperate, or both.

A $1,920,000 Bargain

Our office monitors every important activity, as our team knows **measured behavior improves**. (If one wants to lose pounds, he or she needs the reinforcement of being weighed to monitor and evaluate progress—to cite a simplistic example of this powerful concept.) Consultants, with fees often in the $30,000 range, basically inform one:

1. What practice areas are important to monitor to maximize success.

2. How to measure said topics.

3. Consultants then harass their clients, demanding written feedback to document progress toward set goals, to be certain their suggestions are being acted upon.

What is the ultimate value of this $30,000? With a 10% return, money doubles every 7.2 years. If a 25-year-old dentist (my age upon graduation from dental college) put the $30,000 invested in consulting services into a retirement fund (where money compounds tax-deferred at our assumed 10% return) and never added another penny, how much revenue will this nest egg generate during his or her career?

> Age 25 ... $30,000
> 32 ... $60,000
> 39 ... $120,000
> 46 ... $240,000
> 53 ... $480,000
> 60 ... $960,000
> 67 ... **$1,920,000**

If one reads, comprehends and follows my advice, and invests the $30,000 consultant fee elsewhere, one might be embarrassed by the magnificent return on such an inexpensive book. If you'd feel better, send me the spare change—$920,000— I won't accept a penny more! That will still leave you with a million-dollar profit!!!

I hired consultants during my early years, and they can help one find answers. But if one hopes to employ another—at any fee, for any reason—to replace personal learning and growth, or to provide strength so he or she can avoid the need to confront staff concerning their commitment and obligations—they are deluding themselves. That's akin to hiring someone to exercise for you, thinking his or her efforts will get you in shape.

A personal trainer who shows one ideal exercise techniques and insists one follow up on the plan can prove helpful—but in the long run, to develop strength or achieve any other goal, the burden always has fallen, always will fall, four-square upon the shoulders of the individual who wishes to achieve.

The cardinal rule of most consultants is the client must follow the consultant's generic plan exactly. In other words, the dentist is asked to check his or her brains at the door. If one can accept this cookie-cutter concept—one plan being ideal for every office—you are potential consultant material. I wish it were so simple—that there existed a single philosophy of practice that would guarantee every dentist's prosperity. **If there was a concept that delivered universal success, don't you think every dentist would already be using it?** The unique path to a perfect marketing plan—to a perfect career and life FOR YOU—follows the tough but sure path of clarifying personal values and developing activities consistent with one's unique beliefs.

Forgive the sermon, but recall that a leader's task is to create a vision, then explain and reinforce that image. As office leader, you must follow my example of buttressing critical points of your beliefs at each opportunity and with every possible variety of example. Let's now consider specific marketing plans my office employs that I believe will clarify any of the above general points upon which one might be uncertain.

Defining the Office's Unique Selling Position

The first and most essential step in the development of one's marketing plan (I'm assuming value clarification has been completed—or you're wasting your time here!) is defining what is UNIQUE about one's office. This description is referred to as the office's **Unique Selling Position** (henceforth USP).

Please take no short cuts during this essential process, as the fate of every marketing venture hinges on the successful development of this step. I'd suggest devoting at least an entire staff meeting to the topic. Our office invested months in this vital venture.

Request each team member prepare a written list of positive features that are routine in your office. Assign a staff person to compile these ideas into one master list. Use a large pad of paper (big enough for the entire staff to read during the team meeting) on which to record these advantages in advance.

During the staff meeting, discuss and enlarge on each office benefit (piggy-backing on others' ideas). Have one staff member combine similar ideas and eliminate those considered inaccurate or not unique (using local anesthetic is not worthy of mention, but being able to consistently give painless injections certainly is), to arrive at a definitive list of the positive features of your office.

THE BENEFITS BEQUEATHED FROM THESE FEATURES ARE WHAT ONE MARKETS.

Our USP follows. It was helpful to our thought process to divide our office features into categories of:

Cost—Comfort—Convenience—Value.

Our USP should not be your USP, as our procedures and values differ from yours. Study our efforts with an eye on identifying the USP of your office. PLEASE NOTICE how every marketing effort we'll examine in the remainder of this chapter flows directly from the results of this office value clarification process.

Unique Selling Position
Cost

1. Providing written estimates for each patient before any major treatment eliminates unpleasant financial uncertainty and surprises.

2. Cash and senior citizen discounts available.

3. Financing available.

4. We firmly understand that dental health is cheap, dental disease is expensive, and

5. Quality dental care is a better value than inexpensive care over time.

Comfort

1. Pleasant, friendly, gentle, people-oriented staff who treat each patient like family.

2. FREE nitrous oxide (laughing gas) and gel to numb the gums, provided in an office famous for gentle, comfortable, predictable anesthetic.

3. Health and refreshment bar with free juice, soft drinks, tea, coffee, fruit, muffins.

4. Virtual reality glasses connected to cable TV allow dental care appointments to pass quickly and pleasantly as one watches a favorite program or VCR tape.

5. Proper use of N_2O means no shots are required to treat baby teeth.

6. Free SAGA games, toys, stickers, coloring books, coupons for French fries and milk-shakes, and stuffed animal give-aways every month all mean kids are delighted to visit our office!

7. Enjoy using our warm, moist towels to cleanse and refresh yourself after treatment.

8. Heated orthopedic neck pillows add to our patients' comfort.

Convenience

1. Multiple dentists allow our office to be open longer hours and every emergency patient to be seen the day they call for help.

2. Insurance is submitted for patients at no charge.

3. We have an 800 number and five phone lines, so patients don't pay for calls, and don't get busy signals when they need us.

4. We provide every type of dental care, including oral surgery, root canals, gum treatment, orthodontics, TMJ—so patients aren't forced to receive care at an unfamiliar specialist's office.

Value

1. Dr. Wilde gives a written warranty supporting all major work. This demonstrates our commitment to quality and removes the risk of dental care for the patient.

2. Our office is in total compliance with, or exceeds, all OSHA standards of sterilization and safety.

3. We use only the finest materials and best clinical techniques.

4. Staff dentists offer a combined 40-plus years of dental experience.

5. Dr. Wilde is an internationally known dental authority who has had three dental books and over 50 magazine articles published. He speaks on dental topics and is also a former University of Iowa College of Dentistry faculty member.

6. Our office is concerned about the satisfaction and well-being of every patient, treating them as we would our own family.

Can you envision how our USP becomes the basis for all office promotions? Can you detect reflected bits of our values within these features? The creation of our USP led to a totally new concept pertaining to our Yellow Pages ad. We retained the office logo and phone number, but decided to risk life without such catchy, motivational marketing phrases as "new patients welcome!"

As you study this copy, notice how our USP is employed to highlight the **BENEFITS** one receives from seeking care in our office. At least in our geographic area, no other office Yellow Pages ad is composed as a personal letter detailing the advantages our office provides for every patient we treat.

YELLOW PAGES
"Get a Taste of Truly Gentle Dentistry"

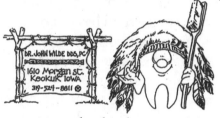

Please come visit our bright, cheery, modern office where up-to-date technology is combined with the personal touch of caring dentists and staff. Discover modern dentistry can be uplifting, lighthearted, even fun, for adults and children.

Relax in our family-atmosphere reception area. Enjoy complimentary snacks and beverages from our health and refreshment bar while your kids experience our special children's area, complete with giant Saga machine. (But don't expect to wait long—we are an **on-time office.**)

Soothing **laughing gas** means more comfort for you, **no shots for your kids**, and it's provided **FREE**. Watch cable television through our **virtual reality glasses**—something you must experience to believe—as time flies by while you receive care.

Three dentists mean **Prompt Emergency Care**, and **Evening and Saturday appointments.** You'll never be abandoned in time of need because no dentist is available that day—let alone for two weeks!

We feature **Painless, One-Appointment Root Canals,** plus the most modern in cosmetic care including bonding, veneers and easy, comfortable, affordable tooth lightening. **Today everyone may have the beautiful smile of his or her dreams!** Our infection control exceeds all requirements.

Every effort is made to **Achieve the Care You Need, Within the Framework of Your Budget**. We complete insurance forms for you, feature senior and cash discounts, have financing available and offer payment plans.

Please call 319-524-8811 or **Dial Toll Free** 1-800-742-WILD to make appointments for yourself and those you love today.

Master Card   Visa

Dr. Lowell K. Long   Dr. John A. Wilde   Dr. Joseph P. White

The Warsaw Letters

I decided to employ our USP in a really unique manner for our office. We had never sent any type of direct mail messages, but I felt our USP created a solid basis upon which to build, and an unusual opportunity existed.

The town of Warsaw, Illinois—population approximately 2,300—located five miles south of Keokuk, had been without a dentist for over a year. We decided the timing was ideal to target some of Warsaw's residents for a direct mail marketing campaign.

I considered opening a Warsaw satellite office, as a second office location is the one mistake I've yet to make in dentistry, and with a third dentist just coming aboard, we had the doctor time available for such foolishness. Direct mail—bring them to us—might not be as effective as opening an office in Warsaw, but it's one hell of a lot cheaper and less fraught with financial peril.

The ADA sells lists of dentists' names, addresses and phone numbers to multiple companies who are delighted to peddle versions of this compilation to anyone. Call the ADA (1-800-621-8099) and they will provide the names and numbers of these list companies. (Be sure to contact several companies and get precise, written bids, as to my surprise, the cost of purchasing identical ADA-provided lists varied by up to 100%!)

I use dentist lists for my book marketing, but the same companies, with the assistance of modern computers, will sell lists of any and every possible description and parameter. For our direct mail project we asked for the names and addresses of all in the

Warsaw zip codes with annual incomes in excess of $30,000. This request resulted in a list of 568 households.

We could have requested only left-handed people, currently involved in their third marriage, who own tropical fish—but I assume the list would have been shorter! Had I the opportunity to select my target population over again, I would include everyone over age 55. I think we missed a lot of senior citizens, due to the annual income limitation, and I consider these seasoned folks to be wonderful patients. The description of one's list criteria should be carefully and accurately defined to reflect office values and preferred type of patient—young families, seniors, wealthy, middle class, etc.—upon which one's office focuses.

We wanted to send a carefully crafted series of four letters, so we ordered four sets of pre-stick labels. The total cost of labels was $493 plus shipping. (One can also order a computer disc and print labels yourself, which is cheaper, provides better control and is a permanent record. I was unaware of this option at the time I placed my order.)

We mailed roughly 2,272 letters. (Four times 568 = 2,272.) I estimate our out-of-pocket expense (printing, stationery and postage) to be about $.50 per letter, so our total cash outlay was $493 for the list and $1,136 printing and mailing for a sum of $1,629. Of course, staff time to prepare the mailing and the cost of the free examination and bitewing x-rays offered must also be considered.

During the three months of mailings (we mailed the series of four letters at three-week intervals) and the month following we scheduled 16 new patients who received $17,558 worth of care—almost 11 times our out-of-pocket cost. With our 50% overhead, our net was approximately $8,700 . . . a **544% return on investment in about six months time!** And I thought the stock market was doing well!

In the months and years to come I hope these happy families will refer their friends and neighbors. I also anticipate that when others who received the letters require dental care they will remember our messages and call for appointments. (A dentist named Wilde isn't too hard to recollect!)

The focus of the following letters is on benefits to the patient and education. Please note we were careful to advise patients who were pleased with their existing dentist to stay in their happy dental homes. To the best of my knowledge, none of the patients we saw currently had a dentist.

Each letter contained educational handouts (a brief description of each follows the letter with which it was sent) and a full page of **patient testimonials.** Of course, we used different testimonials with each letter.

The letters took a long time to craft. Please feel free to copy or modify them as you see fit, if such an undertaking seems appropriate and worthwhile to you.

PLEASE DON'T SKIMP ON YOUR EFFORTS TO OB-TAIN TESTIMONIALS! I had a staff member (the head of our PR efforts) call and request patients write these powerful messages. (A dentist with less fear of rejection could ask for himself or herself.) We chose our testimonial targets with care, selecting patients with whom we related well, but everyone asked agreed to write something—some much better suited to our purpose than others. We sent an office mug filled with sugarless candy and a sincere note of thanks to each patient kind enough to pen a testimonial. If nothing else, these generous messages warmed my heart—even if we had to ask for them.

First Warsaw Letter
"A VALUE OF UP TO $500.00 FOR YOUR ENTIRE FAMILY—FREE!"

Dear Neighbor,

I'd like to take a moment in this too-busy world to introduce our office and talk to you friend to friend. And like any good neighbor, I'd like to offer you some sound advice about achieving excellent oral health. It's a topic I've studied for over 30 years. (If you're confused by my youthful good looks, I confess I entered dental school when I was 8.)

This advice concerns the number one reason people's "teeth" become plastic things soaking in a cup beside the bed at night. That villain is periodontal or gum disease. **Almost certainly you or someone you love has active gum disease right now!**

The early signs are seldom painful, and consist mainly of bleeding gums (ALWAYS a sign of active bacterial infection), bad breath (hard on both business and personal life), and finally loose and sore teeth with painful, pus-filled gum abscesses that quickly lead to tooth loss.

For those suffering from gum disease, **time is critical**, as the **infection is destroying your jawbone**. Often early, simple treatment can prevent or cure gum disease, but the problem must be caught in time.

As if you didn't have enough to worry about, recent medical studies have **linked periodontal and heart disease**. Need further motivation? The eminent physician, **Dr. Charles Mayo, stated that a healthy mouth can add 10 to 15 years to a person's life**. (The bad news is it's always added at the end. I'd prefer to have the extra years at about age 25!!)

How about some good news to follow all that dentist babble? **Today Almost Everyone Can Keep Their Natural Teeth in Health and Comfort for a Lifetime!** But, you need a dentist's help.

If you have a dentist, go see him or her. If you don't have a happy dental home, I'd like to offer our services to you. As a good neighbor, I'm going to make this proposal in a manner that takes away all your risk by offering your family a *FREE DENTAL HEALTH EXAM*. I'm not talking just a quick look around your mouth, but bitewing x-rays, gum check, blood pressure, **oral cancer exam** (a quick, easy, painless procedure that could save your life!), and cosmetic evaluation (we can do amazing things for your smile today). This can represent an **enormous savings of up to $500.00 per family**.

This is a *No Risk, No Cost, No Obligation* way to meet the friendly dental family at John A. Wilde, D.D.S., P.C. Please call TOLL FREE 1-800-742-WILD and let us welcome you to our happy dental family of 4,723 patients (and growing!)

Sincerely,

Staff of John A. Wilde, D.D.S., P.C.

P.S. We are a busy dental office, so there is a **limit to how many "let's get acquainted," free exams we can perform**. Please call immediately to avoid being placed on a waiting list!

Included with this mailing was a page of patient testimonials, a one-page article reprinted from *Consumer Reports* discussing periodontal disease and possible treatments, and a dental magazine article discussing the possible link between periodontal and heart disease. The figure for our patient population—4,723—was the number our computer registered as patients of record the day the letter was written.

Second Warsaw Letter

"THE SECRETS OF A BEAUTIFUL SMILE"

Dear Neighbor,

Hi. It's John Wilde again—the dentist who wrote a few weeks ago about periodontal disease and your dental health. We've heard from plenty of your neighbors—we've been burning some "midnight oil"—(working after 5 p.m. for a dentist) doing their "get acquainted" exams. It's been great fun, but we missed you, and we're concerned. The best reason for not calling is you already have a dentist you love, and that's great! We wouldn't want to change a positive relationship for anything in the world. But if some other reason has kept you from making an appointment, please listen to me once again.

The enclosed postcard is pretty dramatic. Look in the bathroom mirror and see which of these two images your mouth most closely resembles. Our office did a "scientific study" and discovered most folks don't prefer black teeth.

Let me get straight to the point: **Modern dentistry allows virtually everyone to have the smile of which they've always dreamed! Bonding** can make teeth look whiter, straighter, repair chips or close spaces and **is done without shots or cutting of teeth.** Porcelain veneers straighten teeth without braces and are three times as strong as natural teeth. We offer **comfortable, simple, affordable tooth lightening** to return your teeth to the color they were when you were sixteen. (Sorry, nothing I can do for the rest of your body. Sooner or later, gravity seems to win!)

Cosmetic dentistry can improve your career, increase your self-confidence and self-esteem, making you a happier, easier to meet person. Modern materials have given us the opportunity to dramatically improve patients' lives. Even dentists have to get excited about that!

Excellent modern dental care isn't cheap, but our office will do everything possible to allow you to **receive the care you desire within the limits of your budget.** We offer cash and senior discounts and accept credit cards. **Written estimates are given before any major treatment is performed,** and financing is available.

How you look, how you smile, affects every part of your life. There is no need to tolerate a smile that is less than ideal. Call **toll-free for a FREE EXAMINATION (at an enormous savings of up to $500.00 per family)** at 1-800-742-WILD.

Sincerely,

Staff of John A. Wilde, D.D.S., P.C.

P.S. We are so excited about seeing you that we are offering a **FREE DENTAL HEALTH KIT** to every patient. The kit includes an excellent toothbrush, toothpaste, floss and several other goodies. (We enjoy spoiling our guests!)

Along with a new page of testimonials, we included a post-card from High Impact Images showing a before and after photo of a quadrant, first with amalgam, then composite restorations. Phone 719-488-0808 to receive a copy of High Impact Images' brochure displaying their incredible dental photography.

Third Warsaw Letter

"DON'T FOOLISHLY RISK THE LIVES OF YOU AND YOUR LOVED ONES!"

Dear Neighbor,

John Wilde again. We've been swamped by calls from your friends and neighbors responding to our $500.00-per-family free exam offer. But, tired as we are, I'm still concerned we haven't heard from you, as my goal is for everyone in the area to enjoy excellent oral health in a happy dental home. As the enclosed article from Melinda Beeler's paper, *The Connection,* points out, **Not Having a Dental Examination Can KILL YOU!**

Most of us know oral cancer patients or victims. Thirty thousand Americans a year contract this disease and 8,000

133

of them die. **That's one American death per hour from oral cancer!** Everyone should have an annual oral cancer exam, but those who use tobacco and/or alcohol are **High-Risk Candidates.** If these letters do nothing else, at least be sure you and yours are checked for this deadly killer. An oral cancer examination is quick, painless and could save your life.

I'm sorry if talk of cancer frightens you. It's a word all of us dread. For too many the word "dentistry" is fearful, but **I'm here to tell you fearing dental care no longer makes sense**! I'll admit having dental work performed is less fun than eating ice cream, **BUT DENTISTRY DOESN'T HURT ANY MORE.**

Using gels to numb the gums before shots, combined with free laughing gas, has allowed our office to become famous for **gentle, comfortable, predictable and profound anesthesia.** (That's the title of an article I had published in one of America's most-read dental journals.) With laughing gas, **your kids don't need shots to fill baby teeth**, and they won't feel a thing, except a pleasant, floaty feeling.

Cable TV hooked to Virtual Reality glasses is something you have to experience to believe! It really helps distract kids and grownups alike during dental care, making time seem to fly by, as well as blocking sounds of the drill.

FREE GIANT SAGA, special play area, stickers, toys, activity books, free milk shakes and French-fry coupons make our office a place kids bring their friends to experience. We have an "adult toy box" too (just in case a grownup is ever well-behaved). Everyone is invited to help themselves to our **free health and refreshment bar** featuring coffee, tea, soft drinks, juice, fruit and muffins—even fresh-baked home-made bread!

The real key to comfortable dental care is our staff. Relax in our office and find the care you need—no more, no less—among warm, friendly, gentle people who treat every patient as members of their family. We can't offer these $500.00 free exams much longer. We hope you'll call toll-free 1-800-742-WILD to make an appointment.

Sincerely,

The Staff of John A. Wilde, D.D.S. P.C.

P.S. If you're just not certain about our generous offer and wish to stop by, say hello, tour our office and get to know us, we'd be happy to offer you our **free dental health kit**.

Different testimonials and a copy of an article I wrote about oral cancer, previously published in the Warsaw local paper, were included with this mailing.

Forth Warsaw Letter

"FINAL OFFER"

Dear Neighbor,

Our supply of **free dental health kits** and time available to offer our **$500.00 free dental examinations** are almost exhausted. It's been fun meeting your friends and neighbors, but the response has been so tremendous, **I doubt we'll ever be able to make an offer like this again!** Still, our goal is for everyone in this area to find a happy dental home, and I wanted to make one last effort to improve the oral health of you and yours.

Consider what you've learned about **oral cancer, gum disease, the modern wonder of modern cosmetic dental care and the advances that have made treatment so comfortable.** We are holding our offer open for **ONE MORE WEEK**. You still have a chance to SAVE **pain**, SAVE **expense**, SAVE **health**, SAVE **appearance** and SAVE **self-esteem**. But you must call 1-800-742-WILD today to make your no cost, no-obligation, free examination appointment. We hope to hear from you soon, and wish you the very best. This is truly a once-in-a-lifetime opportunity!

Sincerely,

The Staff of John A. Wilde, D.D.S., P.C.

P.S. A warranty, such as the sample enclosed, is given to every patient I treat. I know of no other dental office that demonstrates such absolute faith in the quality of their care.

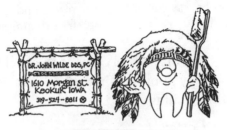

LIMITED WARRANTY CROWN OR BRIDGE

People always ask us how long should this last? In our office we strive for perfection and satisfaction. Which is why we are happy to provide you this warranty, something no other office is offering. Let us remember in today's technology almost everything we have learned is on the preventive side. Instead of going to the dentist every few years for "Drill, Bill and Fill," let's try preventative dentistry. If you spend 4 minutes in the morning and 4 minutes in the evening brushing, flossing and doing any other special treatments your dentist and hygienist have recommended and let your dentist of hygienist professionally clean your teeth, check for decay, apply a fluoride treatment, or apply sealants, you can prevent most all disease. This is why all of our warranties must be null and void if we don't see you for your regular 6-month check-ups. With 6-month check-ups your teeth and gums are winners!

1. FOR A PERIOD OF 3 YEARS FROM THE DATE OF SERVICE, WE WILL REFUND THE COST OF A CROWN OR BRIDGE DUE TO BREAKAGE, MISFIT, OR DECAY AT NO COST TO THE PATIENT.*

2. THIS WARRANTY IS NULL AND VOID IF THE PATIENT DOES NOT MAINTAIN HIS/HER 6-MONTH CONTINUING CARE CLEANING APPOINTMENTS.

*GOLD AND PORCELAIN CROWNS ARE THE SAME FOR PRACTICALLY ALL CASES EXCEPT THAT PORCELAIN CAN CHIP. APPROXIMATELY 1 OUT OF EVERY 100 PORCELAIN CROWNS WILL CHIP AND NEED REPLACING. THIS WILL NEVER HAPPEN WITH GOLD CROWNS. IF YOUR PORCELAIN CROWN CHIPS IN THE FIRST 3 YEARS WE WILL REPLACE IT FOR FREE. HOWEVER, IF IT CHIPS AFTER THE 3-YEAR PERIOD IT WOULD COST YOU THE REGULAR FEE FOR A NEW CROWN. THIS SHOULD BE TAKEN IN CONSIDERATION WHEN CHOOSING BETWEEN A PORCELAIN OR A GOLD CROWN.

I'd like to confess this warranty was stolen verbatim from the excellent work of my friend, Dr. Howard Farran, boy-wonder, dental genius, writer, speaker, now even a personal fitness expert . . . a man for all seasons!! (Although, come to think of it, Howard lives in Arizona, where they have but one season! At least Howard is a man for one season.)

We have different warranties for every type of major dental procedure we perform. The warranty is handed to the patient as the treatment plan is being discussed, not after treatment is complete, as I believe this concrete expression of our confidence and character significantly increases case acceptance.

I stand behind my treatment, and always have—warranty or no—and will refund or re-treat any care with which a patient is unhappy. If you share a similar commitment to accepting nothing short of the best you can provide, why not take advantage of your professionalism and fairness by offering a warranty for your work?

Here is one example of the page of testimonial(s) we sent with each of the four letters. Now, my mother raised no fools. This letter is clearly the pick of the litter. (That's Iowa-speak for best.) I was moved to tears when I first read this. It was written by a delightful lady after we crowned her remaining six lower anterior teeth, then fabricated a precision lower partial and upper denture.

How I envy this wonderful lady her writing ability! I'd like to send this letter with every mailing—I'd like to have it blown up and put on a billboard downtown—but we used a fresh testimonial page with each of the four letters. (Most testimonials were much shorter than the following masterpiece, so three or four were included—whatever fit well on a single page.)

> "*Very* few face the prospect of visiting their dentist joyfully, especially when the appointment was created to take care of dental problems. My experience, however, with the office of my dentist, Dr. John Wilde, has changed all of that.
> Presented with my mouthful of dental challenges, Dr. Wilde and his staff rose to the occasion. During each visit, I was made to feel like I was visiting with an old friend, while

within my mouth, five root canals were performed, an entire set of bottom caps were created and positioned into place, as well as additional preventative and recreative procedures were followed. Even when faced with extraction of a tooth, a procedure generally referred to a specialist, Dr. Wilde, and his associate, Dr. Long, painlessly removed the tooth.

As an older woman, on my own, I appreciate those who sincerely are looking out for my best interest. As my dentist, Dr. Wilde only prescribes treatments that are necessary. If there are other, more costly procedures, that could provide some benefit, I am given the option to choose, without any pressure. If I am not completely certain, there is always a chance to think and consider. My comfort and ease remain top priority, not only with my dentist, but also with every member of his staff.

The greatest gift I have been given, however, is not Dr. Wilde's excellent dental care: it is the tremendous human compassion that is extended in every encounter. In our high gloss, high pressure world, it is easy for people to be herded rather than helped, processed rather than sensitively touched. By his gracious and humble manner, my life has been enriched. Yes, I have greater dental health than I have had for years, but more importantly, I have been encouraged to expect the best out of life.

Dentist visits no longer are faced with fear, but with the knowledge that I will leave the office benefited, orally and emotionally. For that experience, I am sincerely grateful."

(No! This lovely patient was not my mother!)

The Real Scoop on Welcome Wagon

Years ago we had a very negative experience with Welcome Wagon (henceforth WW). We discovered their representative was not visiting people whose names we were given and billed for—just turning them in to WW headquarters and being paid for client contacts she never made. We also had a difficult time getting our membership fee refunded when we requested to withdraw from the WW organization, due to their representative's behavior. (WW no longer charges a membership fee to join. Participants are billed from $2.50 to $2.80 per family visit, varying by choices an office makes when they enroll.)

I didn't believe anything would ever get me involved with WW again (Fool me once, shame on you. Fool me twice, shame on me!) until one of my staff told me about meeting their new representative. Betsy said, "This lady is REALLY good . . . You have to meet her!" I began to hear a lot of well-done WW advertisements on the local radio, and Betsy wouldn't leave me alone, so one evening after work I reluctantly met the new WW representative. To my amazement, I signed a contract with this young lady that evening.

The new representative of WW, Ms. Lynda Betts, is a delight to be around—a real presence. Our relationship has been very positive in the four-plus years she has been our WW lady.

Our office has had both extremes of experience—from very poor to very positive—with WW. I'd like to explain exactly what we've discovered during these varied affiliations. Partially due to our first negative experience, we've been extremely careful and cautious, measuring and evaluating WW results more closely than anyone with a healthy psyche should. I've also worked diligently to create a letter and offer to be given out by the WW representative that fulfills all of the previously listed requirements for PR in our office.

What follows is the letter that Lynda distributes to each family during her WW visits:

WELCOME WAGON

PLEASE ACCEPT THIS ORAL HEALTH OFFER THAT COULD BE WORTH OVER $500 TO YOUR FAMILY!!

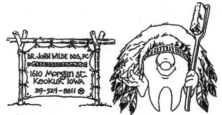

Congratulations on your move, from three dentists—two lifetime Keokuk residents and a third who has been here 23

139

years. All three doctors, and our staff of 10, wish to extend our welcome to the area and tell you **we love it here!**

Keokuk is a friendly, good-neighbor community. We'd like to prove that contention by offering every member of your family a **FREE DENTAL HEALTH EXAMINATION** that includes bitewing x-rays, blood pressure check, oral cancer examination (quick, easy, painless, and could save your life), and a cosmetic evaluation.

A complimentary oral health kit that contains an excellent toothbrush, floss, toothpaste, pen and magnet will be given to each new patient. If you don't need an exam right now, drop by our office, say hello and shake hands. Help yourself to tea, coffee, a cold drink, muffin or fruit from our patient health and refreshment bar. We'll be happy to give you the oral health kit as a housewarming gift.

Our office has a special love for children, so be sure to bring yours along to play our giant Saga machine, experience our special play area, and select a toy, sticker, and coloring book. We'd love to show you around as we're proud of our newly redecorated office featuring the finest in modern equipment and most friendly people in Keokuk.

We are a busy office and can only set aside a limited amount of time for these "welcome neighbor" free examinations. Please call **319-524-8811** or **1-800-742-WILD** to schedule your appointment and avoid being placed on our waiting list.

We look forward to meeting you and having you join our 4,723 (and growing) happy patient family!

Our little Indian logo is included on the official letter, as it is on every item that leaves our office. We present the items of the oral health kit inside a coffee mug with our office number and address printed on it, filled with sugarless candy and tied with a colorful ribbon. I doubt many people discard this nice mug, and since we purchase by the hundreds, our cost is only about a dollar per mug. (We order mugs from Logo Motion, 1-800-753-4182.)

We also send mugs and notes to thank patients who refer others to us, and to all who complete suggested treatment. A candy-filled mug and note of thanks—delivered to the patient's work-place, if they are employed outside the home, so as many people as possible notice the thoughtful gift—results in many calls and cards of gratitude to our office. I'd guess it also leaves our patient's coworkers wondering why their dentist never does anything nice like this.

We try to indicate a high-tech (finest in modern equipment) and high-touch (most friendly people in Keokuk) atmosphere in the letter. I feel people today demand technical excellence, but still want and need warm personal relationships.

Note our 800 number. Keokuk is located on the intersection of Iowa, Illinois and Missouri, so we receive a lot of long distance calls. Our office is the only one in our area offering a toll-free number. I can't prove it's worth the expense, but I know people can be funny about phone bills. I've had several patients spend thousands restoring their mouths, then send us a postcard indicating they were having trouble!!

What follows is a short article I wrote at the request of WW to appear in their national newsletter. I include it mostly to brag about my "national writing exposure," but also to clarify some additional considerations concerning WW.

Our Three Keys to Welcome Wagon Success
by John A. Wilde, D.D.S.

Our dental office has enjoyed a pleasant and profitable relationship with Welcome Wagon, and I'd like to take this opportunity to explain our system and document its performance.

The primary key to our success lies in the hands of our warm, sincere and caring Welcome Wagon representative, Ms. Lynda Betts. Lynda is a valued representative of our office team of whom we are justifiably proud.

Lynda is assisted in her efforts by our decision to offer a free dental examination and bitewing x-rays to anyone who takes advantage of our coupon offer. This is a $38 value, and I believe, the second key to our excellent response.

After we receive the names of the people Ms. Betts has contacted on our behalf, a 20-plus-year member of our staff with outstanding phone skills—Ms. Carol May—calls each potential client who has not yet scheduled his or her complimentary exam and greets them. She offers to make an appointment for a visit to our office, and also explains we exist to serve them any time they might have an oral health-related question or concern. This additional out-reaching—our personal and unusual show of commitment and concern—is our third success key.

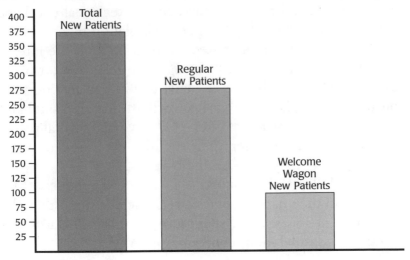

What remuneration have we received for our investment and labors? As the accompanying graph shows, our office's non-Welcome Wagon new patients for last year totaled 276. Of the 272 names we were given by Lynda, 35.6% scheduled oral examinations with our office. Thus Welcome Wagon added 98 patients to yield an annual total of 374 new patients—a **26% increase**.

What business wouldn't like to enhance their new clients by 26% based on one simple strategy? But, the value of these exams can't be quantified accurately in dollars or percentages. Of course, we provide for the immediate dental needs of these patients, but . . . how many apples come from one seed?

How many additional patients are referred by these pleased customers, and for how many years or decades will we serve them? How widely does our name become circulated throughout our community based on this Welcome Wagon exposure? What amount of goodwill and positive enhancement of our office reputation is created by our show of concern? I'm delighted to state that it will take decades to harvest all the sweet fruits of our efforts!

After I met Lynda and committed to WW, we invited her back for a tour of the office, to meet and visit with each of our staff and absorb the office atmosphere while we cared for patients. Lynda is active in community theater, singing and church work, including frequent appearances on a local religious television channel. We offered to lighten her teeth, free of charge, and she graciously accepted this care. Ms. Betts is grateful for this valuable service and her dazzling smile now also represents and recommends our office.

In short, we did everything we could to make Lynda one of our team, aware of, even committed to our office purpose. I believe this small investment in time and money has paid substantial dividends.

As the article states, the head of our office PR efforts calls all the WW names we are given. (Each WW client receives a complete monthly listing of everyone visited.) We welcome them to the area and offer to answer any questions they might have either about Keokuk, or our office. We also offer to schedule a free examination and bitewing appointment. You are observing our documented results, but I feel, even when someone doesn't immediately accept the free examination, we've made good use of an opportunity to establish our office as the most friendly and caring in the area.

Our Documented WW Results

After our first few months of working with WW we evaluated our results. Three categories of WW visits exist:

1. People moving to a new home,

2. Those just having a child (we also included special newborn and infant oral health instructions for these visits—when and how to brush your infant's teeth, warnings about baby bottle caries, when should your child first visit a dentist, etc.) and

3. Special occasions—weddings and major anniversaries, as 25 and 50 years.

Here are our office results by category for the first seven months we were with WW:

Patient moving .... called 272 ... 104 scheduled = 39%
Growing family ...... called 223 ..... 49 scheduled = 22%
Special Occasions .... called 28 .... 5 scheduled = 18%

In light of this data, we dropped all but patient moving from our description of whom we wanted Lynda to visit on our behalf. This reduced the staff's load of calling people unlikely to appoint, and the office out-of-pocket expense, as we pay a fee for every visit authorized by our agreement with WW.

During the same seven-month period we also examined the percentage of recommended treatment accepted. WW patients accepted 47% of suggested care as opposed to an 82% acceptance rate over the same period by non-WW patients.

If one's office is as busy as possible, I wouldn't bother with WW—or any other marketing activity. As it is, I feel we've received a positive return on investment, but this is a fairly expensive undertaking—at least by our frugal standards—and I'd urge anyone interested in WW to prepare one's offer carefully to give this program every chance of success, be certain follow-up calls are being made, then consistently and carefully monitor results, and adjust one's efforts as indicated.

Office Promotions

I'm going to use our no-cavity club as an illustration of the type of marketing activity we enjoy and believe to be valuable. As the PR calendar at the end of this chapter will attest, the no-cavity club is one of many such activities we routinely offer, including senior month, children's dental health month, coloring contests and many more. I choose to describe this particular event in detail as it may be our most effective practice enhancement vehicle, and accurately represents the general principles behind the great majority of our marketing efforts.

The No-Cavity Club

This undertaking fits our office description of an ideal marketing venture perfectly:

a) It's **simple** to do.

b) It's a lot of **fun** for staff, parents and especially our young patients.

c) The **cost is minimal**—four quality stuffed animals a year. (My wife purchases them at someplace like Wal-mart.)

d) The **impact** on our patients, practice and community is **significant**.

e) **It doesn't SEEM TO BE ADVERTISING.**

We have a HUGE STUFFED ANIMAL (don't save a few bucks here—go for maximum impact with the largest, most outrageous specimen you can buy!) sitting in our reception room with a sign around its neck stating, "**KIDS,** you can win me in the No-Cavity Club drawing!" Members of our club include:

1. All children who have perfect check-ups.

2. **Kids for whom we recommend treatment, after they have ALL their care completed.** Can you imagine kids pestering parents to get their dental work done so they can be included in the drawing? As mentioned in the clinical section, we use only N_2O—no shots—to restore primary teeth, so kids ENJOY their dental experience.

When kids "qualify as club members," they, their parents or our staff fill out a card stating the child's name and phone number, then drop it into our special no-cavity club drawing box (a shoe-box covered with shiny wrapping paper, with a rectangular hole cut in the top.)

Every three months we have a "drawing," to determine the stuffed critter's new owner. (This is usually rigged, as staff will have selected a child, for whatever reason, who they feel should have the animal. I've never won an argument with any woman, so I protest such injustice but mildly, as, like Pilate, I wash my hands of responsibility for this tainted contest!)

To this point we've had some fun and added energy and excitement to a mundane office. The next segment of our project leverages its impact dramatically. The name of each child entered in our contest is typed and a short note added to this list congratulating all the "no-cavity club winners" for their perfect mouths and stressing the importance of good oral health in children. The local paper sends a reporter who accepts our prepared list of names and our message, takes a picture of our winner, the stuffed animal (usually about the size of the kid) and one or two smiling staff members. (We select staff who don't resemble the stuffed animal too closely, to avoid confusion. I haven't been in a picture yet! I think the problem is with my ears.)

How do you get such items published in the paper without paying for an advertisement? By working at it. Newspapers are black holes that must be filled each day. Local news, like our contest, is free and of more interest than a generic news story purchased from a wire service. Photographs—especially ones of smiling kids with huge stuffed animals—grab reader attention and fill a lot of blank newspaper space.

Take time to develop a relationship with a local reporter. You or your staff may already know someone, or even have a newspaper staff member as a patient. Go out of your way to accommodate his or her schedule and do all you can—as preparing lists, typing copy, organizing people for the picture—to make the job simple.

This might not work for the *New York Times*, but smaller community papers, shoppers, even school papers are possible sources for such a venture and exist almost everywhere. We have an article, usually including a photograph, in our local paper concerning an office event almost every month.

The photo, along with our note of congratulations and all the kids' names, is published in the Big Wednesday Business Section of our local paper. Even children who don't win the animal get the thrill of seeing their name in the paper. How many of these articles do you think are clipped and hung on the refrigerator?

The contest is kept going constantly, and along with our world-class toy chest, GIANT SAGA MACHINE in the reception area, stickers, craft books, free milk-shake and French fry coupons, and our genuine enjoyment of these special little patients, it makes our office a very popular place for kids to visit, **bringing along their friends and parents**.

Our office has had articles featuring our virtual reality glasses, intra-oral camera system, new associate dentists or team members joining the office, continuing education courses taken, books I've had published, and many more appear in our local daily paper. I also wrote an oral health column for an area weekly paper for about two years (from which the oral cancer article included with the Warsaw letters came). People read these smaller papers carefully to discover information (and gossip) about their community, friends and neighbors.

My dear friend, Dr. Duane Schmidt, author of numerous exceptional dental books (available from PennWell Publishing—800-633-1681) and articles, is a successful dentist-entrepreneur, sole owner of an 8,000-square-foot, 30-plus staff office, and all-around good guy. He provides perhaps the ultimate illustration of charity that also proves highly effective for practice enhancement. Schmidty's office sees **several hundred new patients a MONTH**—more than enough reason to heed his wise counsel concerning marketing.

(Among his many accomplishments and credentials, Dr. Schmidt originated Doctors With a Heart—opening his office every Valentine's day to offer free care to anyone who shows up. This is now a national event, with health-care providers of every discipline participating.)

Dr. Schmidt invites everyone in the Cedar Rapids, Iowa, area to be his guest at his annual free Thanksgiving day dinner. (He believes no one should be alone on the holidays.) As does Schmidty with everything, he goes all out for this event, providing turkey with all the trimmings, including several choices of pie, roses for the ladies, and live music. This annual event has grown into the feeding of **THOUSANDS!** There is a great deal of news coverage before the event and local television stations make the festive dinner an annual stop.

As a result of Dr. Schmidt's efforts, thousands of people enjoy a delicious, nutritious Thanksgiving meal. Perhaps as important, these predominantly elderly guests spend a few hours in the company of other happy people—a true reason for thanks giving.

Schmidty makes no marketing pitch, passes out no coupons for a free examination. Near the end of the meal he stands, thanks all for coming, and invites them to return next year with a friend. I was deeply touched by experiencing this event. It's hard for me to imagine its impact on the community. Consider the warm light cast upon our profession by Doctors With a Heart and this generous Thanksgiving feast. I'd guess many hundreds of patients have called to make appointments in Dr. Schmidt's office, in part as a response to this splendid example of caring and sharing.

Like most effective marketing, Schmidty's Thanksgiving feast is a brilliant example of the genetic needs of all parties being met—the patient's for food and company; the office for goodwill that often results in new clients—within, even awarded by, the accepted parameters of society.

(Our family braved icy roads one year to drive the 120 miles north and assist in this blessed event by acting as volunteer food servers. The local television station aired a short interview with our youngest—then about five-year-old Rachel. In the course of their discussion, a youthful lady reporter asked Rachel if she liked Thanksgiving. Rachel replied, "No." The reporter asked why not, and with a look of penetrating anguish, Rachel replied, "Because the turkey has to die.")

I'm almost embarrassed to describe my charity efforts after expounding on Dr. Schmidt's prodigious and productive tour de force. (It must be obvious to every reader by now that I'm not one to allow embarrassment to stop me!) The following topic is not a pure marketing concept. It is a financially clever and sophisticated manner in which to make charitable donations. My family has chosen not to advertise or have our name linked to these local charity efforts, but one could easily use such projects as practice enhancement vehicles, to the betterment of all.

(I was recently asked to pose for a photo and accept a plaque identifying our family as the largest single contributor to a recent Big Brother/Big Sister fund-raiser. I declined with thanks, but such an opportunity is marvelous marketing, worth far more than the $500 donation Jo and I were pleased to make to the worthy effort.)

Support Charity the Smart Way

Dentistry is a profession of givers in a nation with a heritage of caring and helping. To buttress this contention, consider there are over 600,000 IRS-approved American charities. (And I seem to be on each one's mailing list!)

For decades I've tried to do my part, giving to carefully selected causes I felt to be of worth, trusting they were legitimate entities (being "taken" by two bogus charities of which I'm aware), dealing with increasingly more demanding record-keeping, hoping my gifts resulted in some good, although never able to witness that they did.

Wouldn't it be perfect to assist worthwhile charities, while an independent third party assures they are legitimate, to receive a major tax incentive in return for one's contribution, while all the bookkeeping, tax documentation, even mailing of checks is done for you? Too good to be true? I would have agreed, until I discovered charitable gift, or donor-advised funds.

How It Works

One may establish a charitable gift fund with various forms of assets—cash or securities—but once gifts are made to the fund, they are irrevocable. The contributed assets can be used for making grants to fund endowments, scholarships, or memorials. These funds often serve as an alternative to a private foundation because they are less costly to establish and easier to administer.

149

It is ideal to use stocks that have appreciated in value, and upon which one will owe significant taxes when they are sold, to fund the charitable account. Such equities can be sent directly to the fund, as allowing the fund to sell the stock assures there will be no confusion (or possible IRS challenges) regarding taxes. One deducts the full value of the shares contributed (not just their initial cost) from his or her taxes the year in which the gift is made.

The fund I've used assesses no loads or fees from one's donations. The only expenses are the normal fees charged to manage mutual funds that vary from 1% to .45%, based on one's choice of financial instruments in which to hold his or her contributions.

Once the fund is established, you select the charity and the timing of your gifts, then fill out and mail a simple form to the fund indicating the desired amount of your gift and the cause you wish to support. The fund verifies that you have selected an IRS-approved charity and sends them a check along with a letter identifying the patron, and explaining your gift (unless the donor chooses to remain anonymous). You receive statements that verify your giving according to the new, more stringent IRS standards.

For Example

Assume you purchased shares of stock some time ago for $2,500. While grateful that the equities have appreciated to be worth $10,000 today, you are unhappy to owe a capital gains tax on the $7,500 profit (28% capital gains tax rate x $7,500 profit = $2,100 of taxes due) if the securities are sold.

Rather than contributing after-tax dollars (money remaining after federal, state, local, FICA and Medicare taxes are paid), you decide to gift these stocks to charity. By so doing, you avoid the $2,100 capital gains tax and IN ADDITION, receive a tax deduction for the entire $10,000 face value of the stocks in the year you make the gift. The dollar value of the deduction depends on one's tax bracket, which could be as high as 38%, providing a $3,800 net tax savings to accompany the $2,100 capital gains tax savings. Not bad for an initial $2,500 investment!

Personal Value

Saving significant tax dollars and hassles on personal giving is wonderful, but the reason one contributes to charity is to help others. The money in the fund can be used to concentrate your giving and offer significant aid to charities and organizations of your choosing. Before establishing the fund, our family used a "shotgun" approach, firing little pellets of after-tax charitable dollars toward most who asked. With the fund we've chosen to focus our giving, like a high-powered rifle, to maximize its effect.

Jo and I decided to keep the money near home and support our financially challenged school district that has been jettisoning "non-essential" programs as a floundering ship does cargo. We established a fine arts department that has produced plays the past three years—the first theater our high school has enjoyed for over a decade.

We also instituted a writing program that involves everyone from elementary through high-school students. Annual writing contests are held, the winning works published in a local paper and every entry compiled in book form by a local printer for the students and parents to keep. Prizes—mainly consisting of gift certificates to a local bookstore and government savings bonds—are given to first, second and third place entries. Next year we plan to also support a middle school track and weight training program, both new to our system and struggling to begin.

Dentistry and the community in which we live have blessed our family financially. Reading the winning essays, watching students (many of them patients) perform in plays—none of which would have existed if not for our support—is a rewarding source of personal satisfaction I never received from dropping a check in the mail.

I present our experience only to illustrate possible uses of donor-advised funds. There are many worthy causes desperately seeking money on a local, national and international level. I be-

151

lieve you'll find the process of determining which causes you'll support to be a pleasant and interesting exercise.

While we make no effort to advertise our giving, in our small community there are few secrets and these projects reflect well on our office. I believe such endeavors enhance our bond with existing patients and may result in new patients seeking our care—a not unpleasant side-effect.

How to Begin

Fidelity was the first financial service company to sponsor a donor-advised fund, having begun operations in September of 1992. Similar funds are beginning to be offered by other firms (I imagine motivated by this fund's success), but Fidelity Investments Charitable Gift Fund is the company with whom I've dealt and the only one, to my knowledge, with any existing track record.

Opening a Charitable Gift Fund takes only a few minutes—about like opening a checking account. There is a minimum $10,000 initial contribution, but while you deduct the entire amount from your taxes the year the gift is made (subject to deduction limits set by the IRS), you can use these contributed dollars and the income they earn to fund your giving for as many years as you like—even after your death.

You have a choice of four pools of funds in which you can place your money. The growth pool, which we selected, has returned an average of 15.3% annually since its 1992 inception. While you receive no further deductions from these earnings, the income the fund creates is reinvested to generate more assets in your account, which are available to give to causes you select.

Please consult your tax adviser to see how this strategy can best work for you. You may reach Fidelity's Charitable Gift Fund by calling 1-800-682-4438 or faxing 1-617-476-7824. Ask for information on the Charitable Gift Fund and begin supporting charity, the smart way.

(The author has no interest in, nor receives any form of compensation from, Fidelity Investments—which is sort of a shame, now that I think about it. As a result of the previous article being published, I have been interviewed by *The Boston Globe* for a story on charitable giving, and *The Wall Street Journal* has requested permission to discuss the topic. This information has no relevance to you . . . I'm just bragging again.)

If charitable giving strained the definition of marketing, this next topic shatters it. The following article was published in our local paper, but I doubt we received any new patients because of it. (We did have one blessed soul stop by to contribute $10 to further our cause.)

I'm guilty here of expounding my personal beliefs. I'm no wise man, or someone who thinks he has all the answers. I do believe in a God, and that faith deeply affects my life. I also respect anyone's right to believe—or not believe—whatever they choose. (The Good Lord knows my beliefs and opinions have change repeatedly through the years, and the tears. This tendency to new personal understanding makes me open to accept almost any version of reality that is effective in guiding the life of another in a positive, joyous manner.) I hope you'll grant me similar tolerance as I express my beliefs.

I wish to state that I would never be, nor ever recommend anyone, be involved in a charity unless the organization and effort adds meaning to one's life. There are better, and more honest ways to enhance one's office than faking interest in worthy projects. But few don't believe in the spirit of Christmas, or have faith in children. Angel Tree is a project that is capable of helping children, parents and dentists achieve joy, and as such, I have included this discussion for the reader's consideration.

Dentists as Angels

Dentists as angels—doesn't that have a pleasant ring? A public relations dream for our oft-maligned profession! Unfortunately, dentists are more frequently linked to denizens of a fiery world the polar opposite of heaven. How then can a dentist and his or her staff earn their wings?

We must establish some background information before that question can be answered. After the fifth of my eight years of working my way through college, I was employed as a correctional officer (guard, hack or screw to inmates) at one of Iowa's two men's maximum security prisons. (If you're curious, I secured the job by telling prison officials I wasn't returning to college—lying through my teeth.)

My goal was to earn a few bucks to pay tuition and meager living expenses. I had no idea how that summer would change my life. I've been trying to improve the prison situation for the 29 years since I completed my guard duties. I've entered many penal institutions as part of Chuck Colson's Prison Fellowship group, taking part in two-day programs of education and Christian fellowship, and had inmate pen pals for almost 20 years. I can't forget the horror I witnessed within prison walls.

It's hardly news that crime is a major problem that extracts an escalating price from our society in terms of pain, suffering, lost dollars and decreased quality of life. Illegal behavior won't simply go away, and constructing more and larger prisons to house inmates isn't the answer, if for no other than purely financial reasons. Building prisons requires expenditures in the millions, and it costs taxpayers at least $20,000 annually to incarcerate each inmate. Prison populations are increasing rapidly, as is the financial burden of police, judicial and penal systems on society. A solution superior to the warehousing of prisoners is desperately needed.

Let's ignore the multifaceted cost of criminal activity and disregard the suffering, degradation and loss of those locked away. "Don't do the crime if you can't do the time," seems fair warning. Let's focus instead on the fate of some truly innocent victims—the children of those incarcerated. These kids are often forced to live in humiliation, confusion and poverty because of their parent's behavior. Of what transgression do they stand accused? I'd like to discuss a Prison Fellowship program dear to my heart called **Project Angel Tree.** By helping these infants I

154

feel we have a chance of improving their lives, and at the same time enhancing ourselves and society.

Our dental office has been an Angel Tree center for five years. In late summer we contact Prison Fellowship and complete the simple form telling them how many kids we can accept. The national Angel Tree list is compiled from incarcerated parents' requests that their children be remembered at Christmas. The children whose names we receive live in our immediate area. As soon as we receive the names of our "angels," we contact each child's guardian to be certain he or she approves of the gift-giving, and kids' clothing sizes and toy requests are recorded.

In December we place a banner over our office door proclaiming this place an official home of angels. The local paper is generous in coverage of our Christmas mission, their story and photos helping willing gift-givers find us. These volunteers, plus patients, our wonderful staff and local churches supply the presents.

Late one pre-Christmas afternoon we host a party in our reception room for the kids and parents. (We've met in church and hospital rooms too, when numbers of children and guardians overflowed our office space.) We provide pizza and soft drinks; the kids richly repay us by ripping off wrapping paper and delighting us with their joy and wonder at the clothes and toys inside—for many the only gift they'll receive—given in their imprisoned parent's name. The thrill of being remembered at Christmas by their often seldom-seen parent may be as meaningful as the present.

My church is also an Angel Tree center. In late November, a special tree is decorated with paper angels containing the name and gift descriptions (gender, age, clothing sizes, special toy requests) of each child. Volunteers select an angel, purchase a gift and return it to the church. Members of the congregation deliver the gifts to the kids' homes and personally share season's greetings. I feel it is ideal to be able to invite these people to join a caring church family and not abandon them after this seasonal act of giving.

In 1996 Project Angel Tree provided gifts for over 460,000 children nationwide . . . about four kids for every dentist in America!

I don't believe this effort will end criminal behavior, but I trust it will help. I know ignoring crime and its many victims isn't the solution to making our community and nation a safer place. Being involved in Angel Tree enhances the dental profession's image (and it needs help!), as well as brightly burnishing the reputation of the involved office, but I do this mostly because we are commanded to. Christ told us to be with those in prison. He also told us, Suffer the little children to come unto me, and forbid them not: for of such is the Kingdom of God.

I can't say with certainty what effect these gifts have on the kids. I can promise you an amazing amount of joy added to your holidays—frequently a time of depression and anguish—even among many free and affluent. Done with the right spirit, Angel Tree will bring your staff closer. While this isn't THE answer to the ills that plague our profession and society, it is one step in the right direction.

You may get further information about Angel Tree and Prison Fellowship's many other programs by writing Prison Fellowship, 1856 Old Reston Ave, Reston, Virginia, 20190 or calling 703-478-0100. There are a lot of kids living in your area hoping and praying for your help.

Patient Retainment

I must include the obligatory spiel, to the effect that when an office satisfies their patients' every wish and whim, they are rewarded by gobs of money being thrown their way, new patients are referred in herds and staff are downright inconvenienced by the perpetual adulation—if not outright worship—of the masses. No patient ever leaves such an office of behavioral wonder, even after moving off the continent, let alone to save a few bucks on some third-party insurance plan! (Want to have the most patients of any office in your area and be loved by all? WORK FOR FREE!)

Allow me to reiterate, the basic tenet of *Dentistry's Future* is to illustrate that through a more accurate perception of human nature, though it assumes many and varied guises, one's family, friends, staff and patients can be better understood at a deeper level of awareness. This discernment will allow one to fulfill needs even below the individual's level of conscious perception. For developing this ability one will be rewarded with success, wealth and joy.

(Take a moment to reflect on some past points we've developed. Has it occurred to you how powerful a tool the visceral understanding of the fear of rejection can be? And how one could choose to use this awareness to further his or her ends by more effectively serving others, making them feel accepted, thus decreasing painful anxiety? Or how awareness of the interplay between genetic and social forces sheds new light on many human dilemmas that before seemed confusing and contradictory?)

But even the most behaviorally aware can't control the actions of others—only guide them. For reasons of illness, lost jobs, personal tragedy, simple forgetfulness—patients will "fall through the cracks" of the most efficient office. For that reason, **CHART AUDIT**—the effort to restore failed relationships between patients and one's practice—is a perpetual task and also a valuable tool that helps achieve our office objectives.

Chart Audit

One must ask staff to face rejection when performing chart audit. Calling out-of-touch patients to encourage them to schedule an appointment means deliberately placing oneself in a position to be told "no." This negative response can be perceived, not just as a refusal of offered dental care, but as a denial of the person posing the oft-tremulous query. For this reason chart audit is always among the last jobs undertaken by hard-working dental team members. (Sort of the toilet scrubbing of dentistry—necessary but unpleasant.)

Collection calls used to pose a similar daunting behavioral barrier in our office until my wife assumed control of this delicate task many years ago. Our collection rate is always near 100%, with about $25,000 currently on our total accounts receivable— less than two weeks of production! Jo has real skills! Besides dealing with the fear of rejection, listening to people lie to one's face (ear?) while remaining perpetually calm and pleasant ain't easy!

There exist three essential ingredients for successful chart audit—one must have a leader, a team, and a clearly defined system. Let's consider the various facets of this perpetual process as implemented in our office.

1. Leader—The dentist provides the over-arching office vision and develops appropriate systems, but a single staff person must coordinate and monitor all chart audit efforts. This person is a champion—a prized jewel within the office—and should be acknowledged and rewarded as such. (Given public praise and private money.) This leader might emerge from the ranks of hygiene, the front office, even be a dentist. He or she must be someone who understands human behavior, possesses organizational ability, has excellent communication skills and works effectively with others.

2. Team—We'll detail possible team members when we consider the system during Step 4 of our examination.

3. Effective Dialogue—Before placing any calls, a chart audit person must carefully review the patient's record. Dialing numbers—calling patients cold—is a painful exercise in futility and doesn't portray one's office in the caring light one would desire. Specific facts, both personal and dental, are gleaned from the patient's record before any call is made.

We note personally meaningful events like special vacations, hobbies, birth of a child, pets, etc. in the permanent treatment record, as such information helps us to establish a deeper bond with the patient. It is pretty impressive to our clients when, six months or a year later, staff can remember such details. (Personally, I'm pretty impressed with myself when I can recall such facts as today's date, what I ate for my last meal, or my parents' phone number.) Often these personal insights help reestablish rapport with a patient out of contact with our office, demonstrating that we regard them as individuals, not just names with which to fill our schedule.

Armed with this personal and dental awareness, a typical call might begin, "Hi, Tom. This is Kathy from Dr. Wilde's office? **DR. WILDE ASKED ME TO CALL**. It's been 18 months since we checked your teeth. At that time we noted an area of possibly developing decay on the upper right, and **DR. WILDE IS CONCERNED**. Have you been experiencing any dental problems?"

The exact phrases, "Dr. Wilde asked me to call . . . he's concerned" work like magic! I'm uncertain why, but suspect patients respond to the idea of a busy dentist worrying about them. Technically, I'm not aware that Kathy is calling this patient at this precise moment. Generically, I am very concerned about any patient who has slipped away from regular care, having witnessed the dental disasters from such neglect countless times.

I would suggest a very precise dialogue be developed by one's team and role-played among staff until all are comfortable. Of course, each staff person should express her concern in her natural manner, but while form may vary, the CONTENT of each message should be similar, irrespective of who is making the call. (There does exist one best way to say anything, and this ideal must be identified and practiced.)

The clinical comment might have concerned bleeding gums, or reminding the patient of the terrible toothache he or she previously suffered and explaining we wouldn't want them to be forced to deal with excruciating pain like that ever again. (Reinforcing and deepening this experience is a powerful behavioral technique.) We'll also inquire if the patient has any questions or concerns. Perhaps he or she is fearful concerning some aspect of recommended care, feels we messed up the insurance in the past, or doesn't like the dentist's breath. (Hey—I use Scope all the time! And halitosis is better than no breath!

Although I will confess to an unsightly and burgeoning nasal hair bouquet. Perhaps injecting Nair?)

If problems can be identified, they can be corrected. If our chart audit caller has the necessary talent and training to allow patients to trust us and thus express their unhappiness, one has an invaluable opportunity to solve whatever is perceived to be the difficulty and assure the patient our office will make every effort to be certain this terrible event (it was terrible to the patient) doesn't happen again. (Need I add this concern and the proposed resolution are entered into the patient's permanent record?)

The staff members making these calls must be positive (to deal with rejection) and possess excellent people and phone skills. But, dentistry is a service business. Why would anyone hire a staff member that didn't fit this description?

If a patient advises us he is seeing another dentist, the staff person makes every effort to find a specific reason for this decision. Any concerns or comments are noted and this information clipped to the front of the record. **The record of each patient who leaves our office is placed on my desk.** I don't like this task, but the knowledge gained from studying why a patient chose to leave our care is necessary, vital to assimilate to allow our office to learn and improve. I review the problem, if any, and send a form letter thanking the patient for allowing us to be of service and assuring him he will be welcomed back into our happy dental family at any time. (I have way too much fear of rejection to personally call each patient and discuss why they're leaving our office—although I admire the hell out of dentists who possess such strength and courage!)

As mentioned in the course of our discussion on anesthetic, many patients do return to our practice, often after suffering pain in another office. Our patients begin to feel all dentists no longer hurt patients. I wish they were right, although I'd have to lower our fees if it were true.

4. The System—We require our entire front office team of three and the hygiene assistant to each make five chart audit calls per day. This is a target of *100 calls a week.* (Four staff x five days x five calls = 100.) We also have a monthly chart audit party where, from among the entire staff, five volunteers (we have five phone lines) spend from 5 to 7 p.m. doing nothing but making chart audit calls. (We close the office early to focus on this important mission.)

The office provides food: pizza, Chinese take-out—or Jo cooks. (My expanding girth is proof of my wife's culinary expertise!! You'd have to taste her Chucker (a game bird) Dijon on noodles to believe it!) We give prizes for first, second and third most patients scheduled—either cash or gifts that Jo selects. (My preference runs toward things like filleting knives, or similar objects not esteemed by the ladies of my office.) We do everything within our power to make this a fun contest, celebrating with every scheduled patient! Of course, all staff are paid for their time—even while dining.

This party gives the hygienist an opportunity to personally help fill her schedule. She is usually too busy to call patients during the day, but if the hygienist doesn't stay to support staff during this two hours a month, how can the doctor ask staff to be concerned about filling hygiene time? To tell a team member "it's your job to stay late" falls a bit short of behavioral excellence. We pay our hygienist based on her production, so a full schedule is important to her financial well-being. (We'll discuss this topic more thoroughly during Chapter 5—Expanded Hygiene.)

5. Monitors—Recall that measured behavior improves. We've had each chart audit participant record her daily calls on personal monitors, and also written the results on a team blackboard, left on display in the front office. Both systems work well, **as long as the dentist reviews and comments on each team member's chart and performance.** I place more emphasis on calls made, on effort over result, as I don't wish to add increased pressure to this already challenging task.

Take a deep breath and stretch. (If you think you're tired, you ought to try writing a book!) What follows is a CRITICAL

POINT. While a leader can and should delegate **authority**—for example, having others make chart audit calls—he or she must **never delegate responsibility**. This is a universal law, one example of which happens to be illustrated by chart audit. Staff have been granted the authority to make calls, but the dentist has the ultimate responsibility to be sure calls are being made and performed in a professional manner that represents the office in a positive light.

Tax work or personal finances are examples of two other critical areas where one may hire professional help and invest them with the authority to perform tasks, but must at all times keep a death grip on the fact that one must retain personal responsibility for the results. If this lesson is unclear, think it through. When you fail this test—and almost all of us have at times—certainly number me among the guilty—the resulting lessons are painful. In our current example, if one forfeits responsibility and doesn't monitor, encourage, insist on chart audit efforts being made, they will stop. The dentist will usually only realize this when he notices his hygienist is spending more time drinking coffee than treating patients.

We post the names of all who participated in the chart audit party and the prize-winners on the laboratory wall. This acknowledgement is another form of monitoring—of staff commitment to our purpose in this case. I usually thank each chart audit party participant for their support during our regular monthly staff meeting.

As we'll examine in Chapter 5, hygiene keeps meticulous personal monitors of open time, breaking it down into failed, cancelled and unscheduled minutes per day and per month. These statistics afford a clear idea of when chart audit emphasis becomes more critical. If we note even a slightly growing trend in open time, we can ask the staff to focus more energy on chart audit before a serious problem achieving a full schedule for hygiene occurs. It's a lot easier and more efficient to schedule a patient at their convenience during the next few weeks than it is to fill time open the day one is calling.

As with all PR, chart audit must be a continual effort. If one waits until open time is on the books, it will take weeks to organize this effort and even longer before one enjoys the results. Open time and lost production, once past, can never be regained.

Consider the effect of 10% unfilled time on the profitability of a typical office. Assuming a 65% overhead, a fully booked office has a 35% net. At 90% scheduled, net drops to 25%. This is a **28+% decrease in profit**, and to someone not watching closely—or not using effective monitors—a 10% decrease in busyness might not be apparent. (This would represent less than one hygiene opening per day in the average office.)

Substitute your overhead percentage and get an idea of how 10% open time affects your bottom line. How do you feel about absorbing a 28% pay cut for the same hours worked? Do you feel strongly enough to insist on a carefully monitored chart audit system for which you'll assume ultimate responsibility? Remember, a great deal of restorative care is diagnosed in hygiene, so enhanced hygiene performance benefits the entire office.

Even if no patients are scheduled, when skillfully done, chart audit provides a way for us to reach out to patients and express our concern and commitment to their dental health. Over the years we've witnessed hundreds of patients calling shortly after refusing a chart audit request to schedule an appointment. I suspect making patients aware of their lack of care causes them to start worrying. Worse things could happen! (Like an abscess developing into a cellulitis, or a bridge being destroyed before the patient is aware of trouble.)

Chart audit is a significant portion of our marketing effort. It's much easier to reactivate patients we've previously seen than to recruit new people. If this isn't true in your office, one needs to seriously evaluate office attitudes and procedures.

Public Relations Calendar

(Our PR leader dedicates a portion of every Wednesday to work on PR projects. It is critical that a specific time and place

be devoted to these important efforts, and that no staff or patient interruptions are tolerated during this sequestered period.
If one waits until everything else is completed to begin PR . . . it
never gets done!)

January 7 • Newspaper announcement of no-cavity club, place new
animal for next no-cavity club in reception room.

14 • Valentine coloring contest begins—snowflake.

21 • Make Welcome Wagon calls. Update main office bulletin board.

28 • Plan February preschool visits. Send mugs to patients
who referred and patients who completed all suggested
treatment.

February 2 • Visit Hawthorne School AM and PM—dental talk

4 • Children's Dental Health month projects implemented

11 • Judge Valentine coloring contest.

18 • Preschool tours, update bulletin board.

24 • Wellness clinic for George Washington School.

25 • Preschool tours of office—Welcome Wagon calls.

26 • Preschool tour at office.

March 4 • March Madness—Mad Hatters—Kids wear special
hats—take pictures.

11 • Mugs sent.

18 • Update patient pictures on bulletin board.

25 • Welcome Wagon calls.

31 • No-cavity club for quarter ends. Type notes, place new
animal in reception area.

April—Senior Smile month—alert all staff to take senior patients'
photo.

1 • Mug with sugar-free jelly beans mailed.

8 • No-cavity club announcement to newspaper—
schedule photo.

15 • Mail mugs for treatment completed, referrals.

22 • Update bulletin board, WW calls

May—Graduation Recognition month

6 • Senior smile winner selected. Gift certificate to restaurant ordered.

12 • Photo of Senior Smile winner, article in paper.

20 • Update bulletin board

27 • Welcome Wagon calls. Mugs sent.

June—Vacation Flossing—Most unique picture

3 • Start poster contest.

10 • Mail post card from your vacation contest.

17 • Update bulletin board.

24 • Draw for no-cavity club 2nd quarter—Mr Zoo animal.

Don't be concerned if every topic mentioned above isn't clear. The precise details of the implementation of our PR efforts are provided in *Freedom*. The purpose of reproducing part of our calendar here is to exhibit our organizational system. Each office should develop PR ideas consistent with its values and target patient population. We are constantly adjusting, refining, adding new topics to this calendar. Of course, Thanksgiving, Christmas and other special days are celebrated and our office decorated appropriately for the events.

REFOCUS THREE: CAN JOB = JOY?

By the glowing red numerals of your bedside clock, you see it's 3:37 a.m. You fell asleep the minute your exhausted head touched the pillow, but awakened moments ago with a pounding heart, in a sweat-soaked, blanket-twisted bed. You desperately need rest, as you face a full and demanding schedule tomorrow.

As you breathe deeply, making a deliberate effort to relax, you see unpaid bills—not sheep—jumping a fence. You hear the echo of the harsh words you shouted over your shoulder at your chairside as you exited the office after a stress-filled day. You visualize, with anguish, the less than ideal margins of a crown you seated anyway. You simply didn't have the time or strength to tell the patient it must be redone. You shift restlessly, your lower back aching, your stomach a bubbling cauldron of acid, your dry, pasty mouth tasting of swamp rot. Your spouse sighs, breathing deeply in the comfort of her sleep, as you shudder and wonder—dear God—why me?

Unfortunately, the nightmare scenario that began these thoughts doesn't require imagination for most dentists to experience—they've already been there—done that. At least, I doubt I'm the only one to ever awaken in pitch darkness, firmly in the grip of tension and fear! (Although addiction, and the guilt and mental disruption that accompanies it, moves this experience into a new dimension of horror I shudder even to recall.)

I had some challenging jobs as a kid, among them working in hayfields, at a sawmill, and as a janitor in a power plant. All these efforts had in common steaming heat, exhausting manual labor, dangerous conditions and low pay. Compared to these, shouldn't running a dental office be simple? One works in ideal temperatures, there is little heavy lifting, most of the day one is sitting down, and compensation sure beats what I was paid to harvest hay. What have dentists got to complain about?

But it is tough to run a dental office. The first step toward wellness is understanding that **business is difficult** . . . for everyone. Buddha's First Noble Truth, that life is pain, could as accurately have stated business life is pain. The lost health, failed relationships, even suicides and murders resulting from workplace stress exist for many who labor, not just dentists.

It's helpful to **acknowledge and accept this unpleasant truth—that managing a successful business is challenging to virtually everyone, even in industries not as technically demanding as dentistry**—and realize one isn't unique or alone, that some personal flaw or deficiency is not the cause of one's struggles, before going on.

If business is so hard, why have an occupation? Maybe one should move to a cave in the forest and seek the self-sufficient, idyllic, pastoral life? For me, the discipline and achievements available in work well done are an integral portion of personal joy. (Also, while I enjoy being outdoors, my family doesn't strike me as the bare-bones survival, cabin or cave type. Their definition of "roughing it" involves a night spent in a suite with only one color television. I love them anyway!)

Leisure time is wonderful, for a while, but I soon become restless (in large part due to my genetic mandate to acquire ever more). Even with no need of money, I require occupation(s) to afford the sense of accomplishment and pride my nature demands to be fulfilled.

(Today "work" consists mainly of writing, investing and managing my dental office. One good thing about fixing teeth— for me at least—is it makes any other task seem easy! I would like to candidly point out that, during the decade since Megan's injury, my unceasing quest has been, not for less work—that's just not me—but to **create maximum freedom in my life**. I'm pretty much there. People often ask, "What do you do if you aren't working?" My response is always, "Anything I wish!" Can you understand the joy in that statement, or—like so many others—does the idea of a life without firm daily structure puzzle or frighten you?)

I believe most people with the drive required to complete eight or more years of college need the rewards incumbent from a job well done. But, most dentists don't just work, they choose to labor with extreme diligence, almost constantly exposing themselves to incredible stress. Maybe this is self-serving, but I'm not aware of any other profession where intensely demanding work, to the degree dentistry routinely requires, occupies such a large segment of the typical business day.

By way of comparison, most physicians do few, if any, surgical procedures, and even the majority of surgeons spend a relatively small percentage of their day in the operating room. Combine technical difficulty, staff pressure, the fact dentists devote most of their office hours to caring for wide-awake, tense patients, laboring in the impossibly small, dark, moist and moving oral cavity, while simultaneously attempting to manage a successful business and deal with ever-increasing third-party and other external pressures—and a saint could develop insomnia!

Most dentists—at least those motivated enough to read books—in spite of the above-enumerated difficulties, labor mightily to make, not just the minimal money necessary to survive, but surplus, even abundant wealth. I believe many dentists feel one can work hard—even if engulfed in tension and misery—and that success enables them to afford the luxuries that (it seems) should create happiness, thus making one's job-related sacrifices meaningful, worthwhile.

Yet, it's hard to enjoy the fabulous vacations, when one is too tense and tired to relax. The home of one's dreams often is accompanied by the mortgage of one's nightmares. The luxury car is quiet, comfortable, shiny, a joy to drive, but are any of these material attainments worth all the long hours—irreplaceable segments of one's precious existence—of anguished labor? For what price is one wise to barter his or her strength, youth and health? **Trading misery at the office for joy later is a poor bargain**, at best. And it doesn't have to be that way!

Philosophers over the ages have agreed that humankind's every action is motivated by the belief that each behavioral choice one makes will eventually lead to joy. Consider Aristotle's famous wisdom, "For man, a reasoning, purposeful creature with a final endeavor in life, the supreme final end for the sake of which everything exists, is happiness." Unlike every other species—for good or ill—humans are able and willing to quest beyond basic survival and reproductive goals for the nebulous reward of joy.

Sadly, for many in the work-a-day world, even the greatest business and financial accomplishments, for which they labor and sacrifice greatly, leave them joyless. How have many, even among the ultra-successful and highly educated, missed the ultimate target of happiness, and how can this error be corrected to **achieve bliss in one's office**?

I was helped tremendously in the essential quest for joy on the job by the discovery of a brilliant, heart-warming book entitled *BUILDING THE HAPPINESS CENTERED BUSINESS*, written by an Australian dentist—my good friend—Dr. Paddi Lund. With a great deal of assistance from this very special book, and a modicum of my thought and experience, I'd like to examine the elusive goal of attaining a joyous office, without sacrificing financial well-being.

Before dealing with the office directly, I believe it is helpful to one's understanding to consider three essential segments of life. The demands of each must be fulfilled for one to experience the life of his or her dreams. These are:

1. GENETIC. One must be successful in accumulating enough of the basic necessities to allow survival and reproduction, to fulfill the inherent mandates of all life. One must feel these innate needs are being met through his or her job to be satiated and content.

2. SOCIAL OR CULTURAL. The fear of rejection has been discussed. To be satisfied in life one must be accepted by and comfortable within the culture he or she inhabits.

3. EGO, or SELF-IDENTITY. Successfully acquiring, being accepted by one's peers, yet failing to achieve joy is very possible—even common—when one fails to develop a positive sense of self. (The contemporary buzzword for such a predicament describes one as suffering from low self-esteem.)

All three of these primary needs must be satisfied for one to experience life to its fullest measure. I provide this thumbnail sketch here as this REFOCUS segment deals primarily with social and ego topics. Despite our focus for the moment, one must never lose track of genetic demands. Social acceptance, even cultural praise, fall short of happiness without accumulation (financial success in our culture, a sound hut and sufficient grain, fruit and meat in others) to a level that satiates one's innate quest and affords peace of mind.

Never forget there are three essential primary forces seeking gratification, whether one is aware of it or not. Failure to achieve in all three venues means settling for less than life has to offer—than it was intended to be—and thus being unable to achieve complete fulfillment.

The Foundation of Happiness Within Community

The bedrock of happiness within a culture is established by how people treat each other. The greatest impact doesn't result from confrontations or situations of urgent interaction. Due to the weight of sheer numbers, it is the mundane, every-day exchanges between individuals that exercise the most profound influence. Dr. Lund expresses this concept by stating, "Politeness oils the wheels of society." Consideration shown to others affirms the identity and dignity (ego sense) of those with whom one deals; thus it is the simple, everyday interchanges that most impact one's cultural acceptance.

These normal daily exchanges between people are called manners, and good manners within the office can take many forms. It may be as simple and basic as greeting each person by name the first time one sees them each day, or amiably and frequently saying please and thank you.

Humans share an innate need to be noticed. (That's why one is offended when he or she offers a casual greeting to an acquaintance on the street and it is not returned.) Such routine, seemingly meaningless exchanges control much of the tone of one's office and social environment. A wise leader never misses an opportunity to acknowledge another's existence—patient or staff—by looking him or her in the eye, smiling—perhaps even touching lightly—and speaking politely, using his or her name.

The essential ingredient to significantly enhance happiness in one's work environment is the awareness that **one needs to create a world replete with joy by his or her efforts**. One must understand that he or she can be only as happy as the people who surround one. That practicing good manners with every-one in all situations (but especially tension-filled moments) acknowledges others' existence, leads to reciprocal kindness, and thus joy is forthcoming for all.

The corollary—that non-polite behavior violates unspoken social covenants and destroys happiness, as in our example of a failure to return a simple greeting—is equally true and impor-tant.

Subgrouping

An essential portion of polite behavior is not gossiping, or talking behind another's back. In our office, at the beginning and end of every staff meeting, each team member commits, one at a time and out loud, to not subgroup. (**SUBGROUPING** is our expression for speaking in a negative manner behind a fellow staff member's back.) We individually promise twice, and verbally, as eliminating subgrouping is challenging to accom-plish, and because we realize polite, supportive behavior is an essential segment in our office and individual quest for joy. Subgrouping is the antithesis of Dr. Lund's "oil of society." It is a cancer that infects all who indulge and, if not eradicated, metas-tasizes to cause the demise of happiness within any group. The dentist must act as the leader, setting an example by NEVER

speaking in a negative manner about a staff member, or allowing any other teammate to speak negatively of another in the
doctor's presence.

Considering all the profound topics with which a successful modern dentist must be concerned, why waste time worrying
about the happiness of one's staff? Isn't that THEIR PROBLEM?
**If one desires his or her office to be the epitome of excellent
patient care, the people who work there must be happy.** Dentists seem to ignore this obvious truth, but no patient is fooled
by the most blinding smile and warm greeting, the most opu-
lent office decor, if the tension between teammates is as thick as
ocean fog. Being unfailingly polite and refusing to ever speak
unkindly of a fellow staff member are two huge steps toward
the attainment of happiness within the dental office.

Allow me to rephrase this central point: If one desires patients who respect and enjoy his or her office, are loyal and refer,
one must **treat staff as the dentist desires them to treat his or
her most important patients.** A wise team leader understands
such a focus to be vital—not just for team happiness—but to
facilitate providing excellent care in a pleasant office, essential
to the achievement of his or her own success and joy. (This certain sense that others' happiness directly affects one's joy is a
form of enlightened self-awareness of which few seem aware.)

Okay, pleasant, polite behavior seems possible enough on
the good days, but what happens when mistakes are inevitably
made? When undeniable errors occur, is one then justified in
reacting with anger?

Consider this: Do you treat your patients with outrage if
they disappoint you? Successful dentists don't, as they realize
satisfied, happy patients are vital to achieving their goals. Often,
hostility is reserved as a tool to control the less powerful. Do
you believe causing others pain can lead to your happiness? Is
emotional manipulation a technique consistent with the joy to
which you aspire? Do you believe abusing co-workers—for any
reason, under any situation, circumstance or condition—will help
you achieve your dreams?

(Some candor: Any doctor who allows even the slightest expression of displeasure with a teammate—someone he or she hired and trained—to be observed by patients or fellow workers, is perceived as a bully and jerk. I believe rightfully so, and would add such behavior indicates a lack of awareness bordering on self-destructive stupidity. I'm not speaking of throwing an instrument, but of allowing even the slightest tone of rebuke to enter one's voice. One can't help having feelings, and frustration is a common one in the demanding profession we have chosen. However, one can control his or her behavior, and masters consistently behave in a manner most in keeping with what is required to achieve his or her clearly defined goal.)

Blaming the System

Mistakes occur in every dental office. (If your office doesn't make any, then our office must be stabilizing the average by committing your share too!) Dr. Lund stresses, most errors—such as misfiled papers or lost lab work—are the fault of **system breakdowns**. Instead of seeking to affix blame, ***support your people and fix the system***. Accusing an individual robs the workplace of joy, and allows the defective system to continue creating havoc.

When problems arise, set aside a quiet time—as during the next regular staff meeting, or, perhaps at day's end—then one-on-one, behind closed doors, come together as teammates with a common goal to achieve an ideal solution. Avoid, at all cost, blaming and divisive accusation, as such strategies aren't effective and destroy delicate social accord.

There will occur days when all doesn't go as hoped and planned by the doctor. The value of a functioning team support system during these difficult times is beyond price or measure. One can't punish staff for less than ideal results and expect their help and understanding when things go wrong for the dentist. If the office leader has habitually "made people wrong," and created an atmosphere of strife and contention, it will be all staff can manage not to smile the next time a root fractures or the doctor can't get complete anesthesia!

174

People in glass dental offices (and staff see EVERYTHING) must ban stones completely. If one desires team support—especially on the tough days—one must unfailingly succor his or her co-workers, whatever the circumstances.

Let's further consider the essential nature of a joyous life with the assistance of additional perspective taken from ancient wisdom. Sophocles stated that, "Wisdom is the supreme part of happiness." **If one is happy, he or she has been wise!** Conversely, if one is unhappy, one has acted foolishly.

I spent a lot of years "being right" and "winning" conflicts, but, often at the expense of the ill will of others, and emotional and physical distress to myself. **Would you rather be happy or right?** Please afford this pivotal point your most serious consideration, as this is frequently the choice one is forced to make. If one engages in conflict, and triumphs, but isn't happy, one's behavior lacked wisdom.

Allow me to illustrate this point with a recent personal example. I've mentioned my happiness when son John moved back to the Keokuk area to practice law. We enjoy playing racquetball together. He is 27 years old and finished second nationally in 1997 power lifting competition—165-pound class. I'm old, slow, fat . . . but very competitive.

I almost allowed my competitiveness to destroy these times together, as I played with maximum intensity to win every possible point and lacked grace even in victory. Thank God I finally realized the idea was exercise, fun, and expressing mutual love—not just who got to 15 points first. My fixation on "winning" almost destroyed this wonderful experience with my son.

I still play as hard as I can, but am quick to applaud hustle or a nice shot on John's part. I simply made a decision that happiness was the primary goal . . . not triumph. (Although winning a contest fairly is certainly within my "rights.") The scores haven't changed—somehow I still manage to win a few more than I lose—but the pleasure of the game and our relationship has been greatly enhanced. The key was my realization that, even when I won games, I felt **unhappy**, and this emotion clearly showed I was failing to act with **wisdom.**

Recall Logan Pearsall Smith's guiding words, my motto: "There are two things to win at in life; first, to get what you want: and, after that, to enjoy it. Only the wisest of mankind achieves the second."

To a millionaire alcoholic, this seems a credo upon which to base a life—**to succeed and have the wisdom to enjoy it is my deliberate daily goal**. I hope some day to be wise. I already viscerally realize that without joy AND success, one's life is not fulfilled. I believe such twin lofty goals are impossible to achieve unless one is surrounded by happy people. For dentists these include family, staff, patients and friends.

Consider the ancient Hindu concept of **Karma**—a sort of cosmic cause and effect. Whatever one gives out to the world will eventually, unfailingly, return to him or her. Give out love and joy, and receive it in return. Give out anger and pain, and prepare to have it redound . . . whatsoever a man soweth, that shall he also reap. Often one is deluded into thinking he or she can cheat fate, as the results of both positive and negative actions are delayed. My carefully considered opinion is that nothing is more true—life returns to one, in equal measure, what he or she releases into the universe. By the manner in which you treat others, you determine what you will reap in your office, your life.

The Fate of the Happy Dental Office

But we've set as our ambitious goal the achievement of happiness, social acceptance and fulfilling genetic mandates. What financial effect does this other-focused, joy-as-a-goal outlook have on any business? Does concentrating on a system of happiness mean one will have to settle for a perpetually impecunious existence? What happens financially when one's attention is on people and not profit? Is it true that "nice guys finish last"?

Let me respond to this query in the somewhat rude, if Socratic fashion, of posing further questions. How do you react to a business—perhaps a restaurant or hotel—where the atmosphere is jovial, the staff obviously enjoying each other and their work, as they are unfailingly polite and pleasant? Do you think dental patients will avoid such a joyous place, preferring to search instead for an unhappy, tense, angry environment—where people want only to make money and get the hell out—from which to receive treatment?

As patients notice the comfortable, undeniable trust and respect that exists between dentist and staff—and such relationships can't be faked—their confidence in the office will quickly increase. More treatment is accepted in an atmosphere of high trust—low fear. Bills are not left unpaid to people one enjoys, admires and values. Indeed, most people will gladly pay a higher fee to participate in such an environment, even if the quality of service is perceived to be no different than in other practices. More patients are referred to enjoy a unique atmosphere of contentment in our frequently contentious world.

When you're happy in your office, the amount of money you make isn't as critical. You're not forced to frantically fixate on producing dollars to obtain objects or experiences to create happiness, as life is already filled with the pleasure of your workplace. But I must, in the spirit of fairness and candor, concisely state the obvious. An office replete with joy, if the doctor and staff continue to work and run it as a business, will prove far more successful and profitable than a place of stress and pain.

Can you comprehend the abject horror that results from a life dedicated to acquiring things? That includes no time for people and pleasure, as it's too consumed with the head-long pursuit of profit? Can you imagine an existence more frightening, more LONELY? This was Charles Dickens' message to humankind, delivered by his classic character, Ebenezer Scrooge. The moral of this story is universally understood, as within every human is a portion of old Ebenezer, tirelessly fulfilling his genetic mandate to acquire, but living a miserable, socially atrophied, unbalanced life.

To be fulfilled and happy, one must experience LOVE AT WORK. (Emotionally . . . not physically!) It is people, not things, that create joy. No level of financial gain can compensate for a lack of positive personal relationships within one's office. It is tragic how many have failed to understand this basic truth.

Focus on the creation of an office dedicated to joyfulness **FIRST**. No magic incantations, no pill, secret spell or expensive consultant will create joy. The process is obtainable without fee, available to all, and begins with an **awareness** of the essential need for joy and a **determination** to achieve it.

Learn to acknowledge individuals in a positive manner, and to forgo subgrouping forever. Support one's friends and team members, even—especially—when they're wrong. Everyone applauds when you excel, but who lifts you up, dusts you off and pats your back when you fail? That's what friends are for.

Don't wait for success to bring joy—*that's backward thinking*. Dentist and staff must come together to create an environment that deliberately focuses on and celebrates happiness. Everything one desires—success, wealth and joy—will flow from this blissful base.

Chapter Four

Business Systems

Hardly a week passes in which I'm not forced to interface with some plan, propaganda or scheme promoted as a vehicle to "save our profession." All the selfless folks out there, hard at work to rescue fee-for-service dentistry, **make me tired!** When people start claiming they are "only here to help," we in Iowa place hand over wallet . . . unless the offered source of assistance issues from some government entity. In such cases, we put both hands over our wallets, close our eyes, offer up a fervent prayer, and await the inevitable blow.

Relax and loosen the grip on your posterior. I'm not here to save you, the dental profession "as we know it," our nation, or anyone or anything else. But I believe my fervor for maximizing profitability has been established beyond question in virtually everything I've ever written.

As you know, I grew up hard-working, but poor. Money was—is—I suspect always will be—important to me, as is food to those who have experienced starvation. I make no apologies for this. When I fire a shell while I'm hunting, something I can eat was and is supposed to fall down—and bigger is indubitably better. When I work I'm supposed to make money, and Jo assures me more income is superior to less. So there can exist no misunderstandings, let me again state **I'M A NET-PROFIT GUY!**, pragmatic and proud of it.

One can enhance profit by increasing business, reducing expenses or some combination of the above. Which is most effective? ACHIEVING ALL THREE! **And developing specific, concise techniques to enhance one's ability to achieve maximum office profitability is what this chapter is all about.**

I'm a very active investor in individual stocks (to the tune of $1.85 million as this is written), as opposed to mutual funds that I only use for international equity investments. (Mutual holdings of $.25 million, as of this date.) When I discover a quality company that is growing profitably, and **is the low-cost producer in its field**, my broker is about to get a large buy order from her favorite customer, as I know the most efficient company within an industry is the least likely to fail, the most likely to prosper.

Permit a valuable side-bar. My broker is my daughter, Heather. Much as I dislike bragging about my children's accomplishments—we've never even sent a family Christmas letter!—I feel I must describe Heather's talents, purely for the benefit of my readers. The sacrifices authors (not to mention proud fathers) must make!

Heather completed her undergraduate business degree in **three years** with a 3.9-something GPA. She completed her master's in finance in one and a half years—although her grades declined to a 3.8-something. She is currently working on a Certified Financial Planner (CFP) degree, and her performance was rated number one in her brokerage firm (A.G. Edwards) training group for 1997.

The short version of this is you've never even heard of a broker with similar credentials. If you have any investment questions, call Heather Wilde at 319-524-5946 during normal business hours. Heather is **totally honest**, able to make the complex understandable, and, perhaps motivated by her dad's example, dedicated to serving others. (She makes no cold calls and has no investments she "pushes," but listens and reacts to each unique investor's situations and needs.) Don't worry—she's as beautiful as I am homely; as pleasant as I am irritable; as concise as I am verbose—doesn't look or act a thing like me!

Back to business systems. I'd like to think—although I have no way of knowing—that our office is the low-cost (NOT low-quality) producer of dentistry in our area. If we aren't, it's not from lack of perpetually trying on my part. (Although mere "trying" has never been deemed sufficient in my family. My father told us, "Steers try," if that bit of bovine wisdom translates beyond the Midwest. Guess I owe my pragmatism to my father.)

Ours is a higher-fee, higher-service and quality office, but I'm constantly reading, studying, analyzing data, going to courses, purchasing equipment and materials I'll never use personally, trying to enable my associate dentists to become a little more efficient.

Our office enjoys more than enough cash flow to invest in the most modern equipment and materials, but our team never has time to waste. (As befits a pragmatist, I purchase only implements I believe will enhance profitability. We have a nine-terminal computer system and five intraoral cameras, but I'm not a "new toy" or gadget guy, with sufficient lasers lying around to produce an office light show.)

Realizing TIME is everyone's most precious resource and firmly committing to use this perishable commodity wisely goes a long way toward making one more efficient. I'm horrified and amazed to see today's youth waste irreplaceable moments as if they had been granted eternity! Will Rogers advised investing in land as they ain't making any more of it. Know anyone with a functional time machine? Or a working fountain of youth?

Allow me to revisit this chapter's initial point. I'm not providing business suggestions to save dentistry—only advising how to employ and use systems that allow one to run a more efficient, profitable and happier office. (You'll just have to settle for that thin soup!)

But, are you curious as to how I believe dentistry as we know it can be "saved"? (I thought you might be.) Perhaps by selling air-abrasion and placing $90 comp-seals where there is no decay? (The hard part of "restoring" sound teeth is looking the patient in the eye—the clinical techniques seem simple enough. If you can handle the eye contact, or confidently explain what happens when this layer of plastic springs a leak, you're wasting time . . . get thee to a law school! For clarity's sake—and she undoubtedly deserves greater portions of my attention—allow me to state our office is very much pro-sealants and proud of the 20-some years we've placed them. And, while we are not ready to commit to air abrasion quite yet, the technology does show promise.)

Or maybe one can save the profession by enhancing one's ability to "present" the aforementioned $20,000 cases to the good, hard-working rural folks I see every day? I fear I lack the vision to explore such attractive options as these.

I think we "save dentistry" by becoming **business-people**—aware and concerned about overhead, profit and other similar pedestrian, tawdry, perhaps even to some demeaning details. **Learning to provide a valuable service at a competitive price is how every industry excels**, and it's past time dentistry joined the remainder of the business universe. I also contend that no national movement, organization, advertising campaign or legislation will rescue dentistry. Our salvation must occur **one office at a time!**

Dentists' self-created inadequacies have allowed the outside forces that threaten our existence to develop. If someone with no dental education or experience can enter the profession and run an office so efficiently that it puts mine out of business, he or she should!

Our profession has finally been "discovered" by those who trail money as fervently as my English springer spaniel follows the scent of a covey of quail. And neither entity—canine or (arguably) human—will abandon a promising trail. The time has arrived when dentists who "just don't like the business part" better start looking for a job working for someone who does.

I speak such heresy in the name of the **American free enterprise system,** that has made America's poor among the wealthier people in Earth's history, and for which I thank God! I'd suggest each of you do likewise, as history has frequently shown—and dentistry is threatening to provide another example—that those

182

who don't prize their freedom . . . forfeit it. (Reference pharmacy, optometry, most of modern medicine, mom and pop grocery stores—to mention a few examples of the last two decades.)

The fact that techniques for making one's business maximally profitable—those we are preparing to explore—also make it untouchable by any competition is mere serendipity. **(The most efficient, low-cost provider of a service in any industry need fear no competition.)**

Just because obtaining optimal profit for every office is also the best way to assure dentistry's future is no reason to cast aspersions, or accuse me of grandiose plans of dental redemption. Leave salvation to the great, creative minds within the profession, who happen to have expensive services and products to sell. (A bit catty—what?)

In the light of enhanced awareness, reconsider my query from this book's introduction: Was it ever acceptable—moral— for dentists to practice inefficiently and pass the cost of this ineptness on to the consumer? Isn't it each dentist's duty to offer the finest care he or she is able to provide, in the most proficient possible manner?

The Efficient Dental Office

How does one eliminate waste to create the businesslike, profitable dental office the competitive future demands? **To achieve this goal, precise, easily understood and consistently monitored systems must be established and regularly consulted concerning every facet of office behavior one wishes to maximize.**

Only meticulous measurements provide accurate feedback that allows optimal system refinement, and I consider my office—as is every business—to be a collection of systems. We have precisely detailed systems for EVERY clinical procedure, a system for collections, for new-patient processing, for inventory, etc.

Such a reductionistic analysis allows ideal development of each segment of the whole, but don't lose track of the big picture. Each system is a step on our journey to success, wealth and joy; thus one must be certain that every facet of one's endeavors is consistent with one's long-term values.

In and of itself, a single monitored particle of the system is without significance, yet all coalesce, as do tenuous rivulets and musical streams, to create a formidable river—the efficient and profitable modern dental office. In similar fashion, any system whose basis is inconsistent with values pollutes, fouls and diminishes one's total effort.

It is the dentist's—the business leader's—responsibility to provide the practice **vision** and design **monitors** to evaluate and accelerate progress toward the achievement of this maximally efficient and profitable modern dental facility. The systems employed to measure the journey to success must be in **writing** and **mandatory** for **all staff** to follow. (Allow me to reiterate this important truism, that **Measured Behavior Improves**.)

Each system must be constantly **evaluated and adjusted** to assure its employment enhances profitability, efficiency and joy within the office. (There exists little joy in inefficiency for me.) This concept seems clear enough, but fleshing out the details of this capsule summary is going to take some doing.

To assist in monitoring all systems, our office generates five legal-pad pages of internal monitors monthly to augment the seven pages of our accountant's profit and loss statement and the reams of data overload our office computer spews forth at every opportunity.

Computers are wonderful instruments of measurement, but also pose a threat. Information in excess, of questionable value, or that creates confusion, **hinders the positive effect careful monitoring provides.** (I used to have dreams of drowning under a wave of computer readouts . . . simultaneously asphyxiated and perplexed!)

Copies of our concise and meaningful internal data are disseminated and discussed with each team member during our monthly ½-day staff meetings. Many dentists are reluctant to share practice financial information with their teammates. After at least eight years of education, often going perilously into debt and struggling for years to make a practice solvent, they fear their staff might think they are making a profit!

I'm an American businessperson—not an employee of a socialist system—at least not yet! **As a proud capitalist, my duty is to make money.** This allows me to support my family, provide job security for my loyal staff, and pay onerous taxes, and insures I'll stay in business to provide care for the patients who honor me with their trust. Financial resources allow me to support worthy causes (as we'll examine in Chapter 8) and enjoy the freedom and choices that enhance my life's joy and meaning.

Perhaps wealth's greatest benefit is that its attainment provides a sense of accomplishment and fulfilled purpose that—at least to one burdened with my low self-esteem—is vital to positive feelings of self-worth, without which there can be no substantial joy. I appreciate the things having money allows me to purchase, but the abiding self-satisfaction forthcoming from awareness of employing my mind and energy to achieve success is more of a blessing than any possession or other experience I can envision.

I don't leave my Lexus at home and drive an old car to the office because I'm afraid people will think I make too much money, as I EARN WHAT I MAKE, FAIRLY AND HONESTLY. I gave more than equitable effort in return for what I received. To my mind, losing money or being unable to make a profit is something of which one should be ashamed—not making an honest income through hard and thoughtful labor.

Forgive the impassioned sermon, but I know the politically correct behavior of the day is to blend in, becoming one of the gang where everyone is "equal." Such behavior is currently defined as "fair" and mimicking this cant allows one to be deemed socially acceptable.

But it wasn't "fair" when I worked 100-hour weeks to finance and complete my education while others my age drove new cars, drank beer and played ball during their leisure time. Had I failed, no powerful agency was prepared to rescue me when I assumed the risk of entering private enterprise, as banks, savings and loans, Chrysler Corporation and now most of Asia have been rescued. None of the folks with whom I'm now supposed to be "fair" offered help on the difficult, lonely, often frightening pathway to achieving what I've earned in life.

I'm not bitter over achieving on my own, as being supported only by loved ones has made achievement even sweeter. I'll pay every penny of taxes I owe. (Which totaled well over $130,000 last year!) I gladly served two years in the armed forces, and have been involved in my church and community, attempting to assist those who indicate a willingness to put forth the effort required to help themselves. But I'll never feel guilty for enjoying the fruits of my determined effort to work as hard as I can to become all I'm capable of being.

Philosophy expounded, pep talk delivered, I realize sharing "private" information with staff will still remain difficult for some. It saddens me that our modern culture works to make one ashamed of any level of honestly achieved success. I wish I could appeal to all to consider the plight of our culture if individuals didn't possess the courage and willingness to sacrifice essential to establish any new business, and that rewards must be forthcoming for such behavior to occur. But I have little power to alter the prevailing mind-set.

But openly sharing office progress, and having the staff realize you're profitable, is a risk those who wish extraordinary results must take—another brave step toward achievement—as developing a synergistic team demands openness, candor and honesty. Maximizing one's office potential requires the dynamic energy of a group of minds and bodies working towards achieving a commonly held, clearly delineated goal.

Every member of our team is aware of and concerned with the office's financial health, as they understand their fiscal future is linked to the financial well-being of the practice. (Any of you old enough to remember fictional wealthy industrialist General Bullmoose from the Li'l Abner comics? His famous line was, "What's good for Bullmoose is good for America." Within my office, I'm Bullmoose—this is not an olfactory comparison—and what's good for me is good for my team.)

Anyway, staff total the office bank deposit every night. A dentist must be on hallucinogens if he or she thinks driving the muddy, rusting, old Ford to the office will convince employees, who deposit thousands in the practice's bank account each week, that the dentist is doing poorly. If you never show team members differently, they'll believe you keep 90% of the total deposits!

I hate it when I have to return to the topic. Is it just me, or are the digressions the best part of this effort? Maybe if I put brackets around the entire book? Anyway . . . this fiscal connection between office and employee well-being is immediate and precise in the case of dentists and hygienists who are paid in our office based on their production. (More on this subject when we deal with expanded hygiene and associate dentists in the following chapters.)

While the effect of profit and loss is delayed and indirect for other team members, I frequently point out it is upon the figures our soon-to-be-discussed monitors display that six-month salary adjustments are based.

I've raised fees and salaries every six months since President Carter's policies and 20% inflation convinced me such a philosophy was prudent. I didn't raise fees during my first three years in practice, until I came to understand that low fees are merely a reflection of low self-esteem. Modern dental care is expensive, even if the dentist would forfeit all profit. (If one cut his or her fees in half—and lost money—it would still be quite costly to save one tooth requiring endodontics, a post and crown.) Average dental-office overheads have increased by 1% a year for over a decade, and as with any business, **adjusting prices to reflect costs is mandatory, if the business entity hopes to remain viable.**

Our monitors include data on a year-to-date, year-to-year, monthly, and **hourly** basis. Such precise information allows one to spot trends early and work to enhance positives, while quickly rectifying negatives, thus maximizing potential.

I've never before written about monitors, yet our office has carefully measured performance for years. It is a topic I fully understand to be integral to success (recall our discussion of

187

consultants who for $30,000 fees tell one what and how to measure, then harass one into doing it?), but it is a daunting task to write about it, impossible to consider in an article, almost impossible in a chapter, worthy of a book all its own.

Thankfully, such a book—and an excellent one—does exist. *KNOWING THE NUMBERS: Gain and Retain Control of Your Practice* (henceforth *Numbers*) was published in 1989, and is available from PennWell publishing—1-800-752-9764. As with most works of timeless wisdom, *Numbers* has retained its value over the years. The authors, Joe Dunlap, D.D.S., and John Wagner, D.M.D., are men I'm proud and honored to call my friends. Both have played a significant role in whatever accomplishments I've been blessed to achieve.

Dr. John Wagner has a business background degree (unlike Heather's, I don't know his GPA), practiced dentistry for a number of years, and has been a full-time dental consultant for over a decade. He served my office well in the shadowy past, when my hair was still brown, during the transitional times when I first added an associate dentist to our expanding office menagerie. (And John didn't charge a crippling $30,000 to help guide our office to a more profitable future, but a fair and reasonable fee for his valuable services that rewarded his efforts and allowed our office to prosper—not merely survive—after a consultant's ministrations.)

Dr. John originally set up the in-house monitors for our office that I'll be describing in detail. Over the years we've modified these monitors annually, streamlining and refining as best suited our singular purpose. After years of gradual changes, I have no idea how much of John's origin work remains. If a section seems lucent and brilliant, that's undoubtedly John's influence. If you can't figure out what in hell I'm talking about—that's likely my modification.

Dr. Joe Dunlap is the consummate dental writer. He is the author of numerous PennWell book publications and past editor of *Dental Economics*, a mentor and hero to me. I've heard Joe lecture—he is a brimming fount of wisdom (which is, by its nature, a messy situation)—worthy of any dentist's attention.

188

Joe, as much as any other soul, encouraged and made possible my first book.

Beginning to write a book is a intimidating task that consumes hundreds of hours and the majority of one's mental energy for months. It's seldom undertaken by anyone with a lick of sense, a friend in the world . . . even a dog. (I have three dogs. Must be the friends and sense I lack.) Joe was gracious enough to review a very early, VERY rough draft of *Focus*, and his encouragement allowed a writer who had no idea what he was doing (me) to find the courage to begin what has become my joy, as it is Joe's . . . a usually harmless form of auto-stimulation involving playing with various combinations of the written word.

Joe's gracious letter concerning whether I should continue efforts with my manuscript informed me, "You have an illness for which the only cure is being published." Joe, I'm sorry to be contrary, but for once in your life you were mistaken. There is no cure!

Dr. John's monitors helped my practice become more responsive and profitable. The ultimate proof of their value is that a baker's dozen years later, they are still a centrally important portion of our business systems. Dissection, consideration and reflection on the meanings inherent in these various measurements will provide the bulk of this chapter.

Dr. Joe's encouragement has sentenced me to at least five hours, almost every morning, locked away in my basement study, typing with two fingers for lo, these many years. There seems to be no hope of pardon! Writing keeps me out of my wife's way . . . so at least somebody's happy! (Readers who don't know me might be concerned that Jo pines for my company during my self-imposed exile, but she's a courageous woman and has assured me I'm "an easy guy to get along without!")

Those of you serious about obtaining the most efficient, thus low-cost and high-profit office must call PennWell and obtain, study and implement the wisdom in *Numbers*.

Clinical Monitors

I suppose it's appropriate to once again confess to knowing next to nothing about clinical dentistry. (If confession is indeed good for the soul—mine must be healthy enough to run a marathon!) Fortunately, I have a friend whom I (and many others who actually know something about the subject) consider to be the world's leading authority on clinical efficiency, and he's written two excellent and timely books on the subject.

If one wants to hone his or her clinical skills to a razor's edge by eliminating all wasteful and frustrating inefficiency, he or she needs to order Dr. Ed Silker's fine book, *Building Your Million Dollar Solo Practice*. (Call 1-800-450-0091 to order or receive information on two books and a number of helpful items Dr. Ed makes available.)

Ed Silker is THE efficiency expert of the dental industry, and his writing mirrors his clinical technique—spare, concise and easily understood. (I know—my thought processes are as convoluted as an inflamed small bowel.) Along with precise instructions as to how one can refine literally every clinical technique, Ed will tell you how he moved to Deerwood, Minnesota (population 524!!), and built a million-dollar practice in a few years' time. I seriously doubt he can explain why he moved to Deerwood—but be fair—nobody could. I visited with him (thank God, over the phone) on a rare day when his office was a little slow . . . partially due to the minus 40-degree temperatures!!!

Dr. Silker practiced in Arizona—rumor has it he gave Howard Farran his first job. The fact these two great men found each other doesn't surprise me. First, there is no such thing as coincidence—and second, nothing Howard does surprises me!

Allow me to end this brief clinical section by forwarding the only discovery concerning equipment of my lengthy career: Sometimes, if a piece of equipment doesn't work at all, it's because nobody turned it on. **Check the switch and outlet**—it can save lots of frustration! You're welcome. One does what one can!

190

Monthly Office Monitors

I love people and the emotional possibilities of the written word. I find numbers dull and tedious. I took five years of high-school and college mathematics, getting good grades, apparently learning next to nothing. Numbers have always been difficult—a bit uncertain and intimidating to me.

While monitors may represent the epicenter of the "business part" many dentists avoid like a sexually transmitted disease, one must understand that in business—be it managing a dental practice or analyzing an investment opportunity—it is within these dry digits that the pulse and brain waves of any enterprise may be comprehended.

Recall that wise men have stated where one stumbles, there lies his or her treasure.

It is hard work to fathom, for most of us impossible to enjoy—despite my efforts to do everything possible to make the following information clear and interesting—the arid numbers of business. But it is **imperative to success** that one comprehend, implement and utilize these critical measures. Without success, one can't obtain wealth, and opportunities for joy are diminished.

The remainder of this chapter will review the five pages of monthly monitors we (the "we" here actually being Jo) generate internally. I'll explain the significance of key figures, gleaned and organized from incomprehensible mountains of data our computers spit forth, and demonstrate how we employ this data to spot trends and address them in a proactive manner. We'll use our un-doctored, actual 1997 monitors, with nothing changed to protect the innocent or guilty. My personal production figures will provide comic relief from the tension build-up and tedium inherent in statistical analysis.

I believe it correct and proper that Page 1 (see page 193) be entitled *Doctor's and Hygienist's Performance Monitors*. When one strips away the numerous facades that veil dental reality, what dentists and hygienists produce is what an office's performance consists of. If nothing is produced, neither the finest monitors—nor anything else—will make much difference!

It is undoubtedly no longer correct, proper, or appropriate that Dr. Wilde and his puny figures be the first presented. The high rank of yours truly is strictly a matter of historical precedent. (Said differently, we do it this way . . . because this is the way we do it, sort of like the government.)

Let's begin by considering Dr. Wilde's December of 1997—an excellent month in which to hunt!—the data from which is recorded directly below.

Line 2. Production	$4,519
Line 3. Days worked/hours	1 3/10—11
Line 4. Production per hour	$410
Line 5. NP, Adult/child—total patients	3-2 / 39

The top figure—$4,519—is my total production for the month!! (I was sorely tempted to analyze April and my $21,507 production total—if I could have formulated some plausible excuse to consider that month, other than personal shame.)

The column immediately below indicates I worked a total of 1 3/10 days, or 11 grueling hours for the month. (I swear it seemed more like 12!) Line 4 shows my production per hour to be $410. Line 5 reveals I saw three adult (A) and two child (C) new patients among the total of 39 people who had the misfortune to receive my tender ministrations that month.

If one reviews the top (production) column for my year, (Line 2) beginning with $15,341 produced in January, he or she will note that in July a precipitous drop from my previously demanding four- to five-day work months occurred. At that point I began to work about two days per month, my production dropping from the $15,000 range to around $7,000 per month.

This sea change was due to two factors:

1. An enhanced personal laziness beyond what was once considered rock bottom.

2. Dr. Joseph White—a recent graduate of the University of Iowa—began gracing our office with his significant presence during the later stages of June, 1997.

1997 Doctor's and Hygienist's Performance Monitors

#		Jan	Feb	March	April	May	June	July	Aug	Sept	Oct	Nov	Dec
1	**Dr. Wilde:**												
2	Production	15,341	11,209	18,324	21,507	13,548	14,159	6,065	6,974	7,569	14,754	6,074	4,519
3	Days wkd/Hrs	4/32	4.25/34	5/40	5.5/45	4.25/34	5/39	2/16	1.5/12	1.8/14.75	2.25/18	1.8/14+30	1.3/11
4	Prod/Hr	479	330	458	478	398	363	379	581	513	819	418	210
5	NP A-C/#pts	6-3/100	8-3/104	6-5/121	12-4/154	4-7/120	11-13/161	—/44	1-0/39	5-2/47	4-4/85	4-2/65	3-2/39
6	YTD Production	15,341	26,550	45,874	67,381	90,929	95,089	101,155	108,129	115,698	130,452	136,526	141,045
7	Days wkd/Hrs	4/32	8.25/66	13.25/106	18.75/151	23/185	25/224	30/240	31.5/252	33.3/267	35.5/285	27.3/299.5	38.6/310.5
8	Prod/Hr	479	402	433	446	437	425	421	429	433	457	455	454
9	NP/#pts	6-3/100	14-6/204	20-11/325	32-15/479	36-22/599	60-25/760	60-25/804	61-25/816	66-27/863	70-31/948	74-33/1013	77-35/1052
10	**Dr. Long:**												
11	Production	24,136	19,429	20,514	22,291	22,131	14,299	27,796	22,459	23,594	24,418	19,779	21,425
12	Days wkd/Hrs	15.5/122.5	1325/106	14.75/118	155/124.5	14/113	10/87	16/126	13.75/110	14.25/115	16.5/132.6	12.1/97.5	13.5/108+20
13	Prod/Hr	197	183	174	179	196	164	221	204	205	184	202	198
14	NP A-C/#pts	3-3/308	3-8/296	3-4/314	7-4/338	5-0/314	5-2/248	6-5/275	5-4/297	3-3/271	4-5/275	7-1/209	8-5/222
15	YTD Production	24,136	43,565	64,080	86,371	108,453	122,752	150,549	173,009	196,608	221,026	240,805	262,231
16	Days wkd/Hrs	15.5/122.5	28.75/228.5	43.5/346.5	59/471	73/584	83/671	99/797	112.75/907	127/1022	143.5/1154	155.6/1251	169.1/1359
17	Prod/Hr	197	190	185	183	186	183	189	191	192	191	192	192
18	NP/#pts	3-3/308	6-11/604	9-15/918	16-19/1256	21-19/1570	26-21/1818	32-26/2093	37-30/2390	40-33/2261	44-38/2536	51-40/2745	54-45/2967
19	**Dr. White:**												
20	Production						3,305	12,619	16,515	15,839	19,014	15,900	15,015
21	Days wkd/Hrs						6/34	10/82	12/95	11.8/94.5	13.8/111	9.1/73.6	8/64+25
22	Prod/Hr						97	137	154	158	161	170	177
23	NP A-C/#pts						1-0/56	6-8/168	9-15/208	5-4/187	13-6/194	4-0/131	9-4/128
24	YTD Production						3,305	15,925	32,441	48,280	67,294	83,194	98,209
25	Days wkd/Hrs						6/34	16/116	28/211	40.25/305.5	54/416.5	63.1/489	71/553.5
26	Prod/Hr						97	137	154	158	161	170	177
27	NP/#pts						1/56	7-8/224	16-23/432	21-27/619	34-33/813	38-33/944	47-37/1072
28	**Melissa** Prod	13,904	13,13,537	14,481	13,774	14,490	14,422	11,650	15,749	13,793	15,750	12,118	12,266
29	Days wkd/Hrs	15.75/125.5	14.5/117	14.75/118	16.5/131	15.75/126	13/105	12/96	15.5/123	15.25/122	16.75/134	14/113	11.5/91.6
30	Prod/Hr	111	116	123	105	115	137	121	128	113	129	107	133
31	#pts	208	178	219	210	205	201	177	224	212	229	184	178
32	YTD Production	13,904	27,441	41,922	55,696	70,187	84,609	96,259	112,008	125,802	141,552	153,670	165,936
33	Days wkd/Hrs	15.75/125.5	30.25/242.5	45/360.5	61.5/491.5	77.25/617.5	90.35/722.5	102.25/818.5	117.75/941.5	133/1063.5	150/1198	164/1311.5	175.5/1403
34	Prod/Hr	111	111	116	113	114	117	117	119	118	118	117	118
35	#pts	208	386	605	815	1020	1221	1398	1622	1834	2063	2247	2425

Joe really wants to fix teeth—I don't. In numerous situations, he's already better at it than I am, so this arrangement—him working, me not—made everyone happy!

Line 6. Year to Date (YTD) Production	$141,045
Line 7. Days worked / Hours	38 2/3/ 310.5
Line 8. Production per hour	$454
Line 9. New patients, Adult, Child/total pts.	77-35 / 1052

The second column of four figures (Lines 6 - 9) delineates my running (in December, crawling) totals of the afore-reported four statistics for the year. For all of 1997 I produced $141,045 working 38 2/3 days, or 310.5 hours. My average production per hour for the year was $454. I saw 77 adult new patients and 35 children as new patients among the 1,052 hardy souls forced to endure my breath at close range.

I consider production per hour to be THE critical production statistic. Days worked per month vary by calendar days in the month, vacations, weather, illness, attitude, etc. Average hourly production figures allow a much more accurate depiction of clinical performance. This said, my 1997 variation, from a low of $330 per hour in February, to a high of $819 in October, means little. I work so few days that a couple of big cases—or lack of same—greatly distort my numbers.

A more precise image of my production prowess, or lack of same, will be gained from observing the running production per hour totals (Line 8), where short-term factors eventually even out. The only trend visible in my hourly average production running total is a gradual hourly increase beginning when I reduce my time to two days per month (July's $421 increasing monthly to a $454 final total). Guess the extra two days off per month left me fresher!

In short, my varied levels of interest and enthusiasm make detection of any trends (except perhaps apathy) from my personal data unlikely. (I suddenly realize the only justification for keeping track of my production at all is to embarrass me and make my associates and readers feel good about themselves. Reason enough!)

For Dr. Lowell Long, my friend and trusted right hand (and often my left, too), 1997 marked his tenth year in our office. Allow this paean: Lowell does a wonderful job clinically. He is hard-working, conscientious, dependable, dedicated, great with patients, gentle, respected and loved by staff, and always does his best. He is a real asset to our office!

Lowell's numbers (lines 10 - 18) aren't much help in illustrating the importance of this data, however. His figures are pretty stable, showing neither real growth, nor significant decline. His production stays in the $20,000 to $24,000 range, except during June when productivity declined, as Dr. Long enjoyed a well-deserved and overdue vacation.

Lowell seems content—or at least voices no discontent—at this steadiness. He enjoys clinical dentistry, insists his days not be damaged by over-scheduling and the resultant stress created, and exhibits little interest in the business aspect of the profession. This works out well, as I like business, and have but slight interest in the clinical aspect at this point in my existence. I wish Jo and I were as compatible!

Let's continue down the page (lines 19 - 27) to our "baby dentist," Dr. White, to observe how these individual production figures can assist in the analysis of our office. Joe's production per hour went from $97 in June to $232 per hour in December, with steady growth in between! An upward trend would be expected as a recent graduate learned to utilize two operatories effectively, worked with a skilled chairside (thanks, Amanda!), and refined his clinical technique.

What one wouldn't expect is an hourly production average of $232—significantly higher than the ADA statistics for all dentists—seven months after graduation! But Joe White is a motivated, exceptionally talented young dentist.

HOWEVER, total production, as well as **days and hours worked per month, peaked in October**, at $19,014 and 13.8; days declining to 9 and 8 in November and December respectively. Here is a sign of SIGNIFICANT TROUBLE—of declining dollars due to a decreasing patient load—as Joe would prefer to work a minimum of 16 days per month.

Our team began to address this problem in November. Joe saw 19 new patients in October—seemingly more than enough to allow his production to expand in the following month. Our staff reviewed data concerning new-patient exams performed by all dentists for the previous three months. We discovered John's examinations resulted in significantly higher accepted treatment levels than examinations provided by our other dentists, so the office began an effort to schedule me to perform more new-patient examinations.

(I do new-patient exams and removable prosthodontics only since January, 1998. It took a little while to reach the decision that my time would be most valuable doing examinations, then to adjust our scheduling and have these changes reflect in the monitors, but the modifications are now firmly established and I saw 9 new patients during one day in early January.)

As must a proactive leader, I initiated several candid, one-on-one, closed-door meetings with staff and discovered Joe sometimes ran significantly behind schedule. My response was to immediately ask him to re-time all of his procedures and to stress the vital importance of timeliness in private practice.

Staff also indicated anesthetic was perhaps not given as gently, and sometimes was not as profound, as would be ideal. Joe and I discussed techniques for gentle, predictable and profound anesthetic. I explained in very candid fashion that working on patients who weren't comfortable was absolutely forbidden in our office. If Joe wasn't able to obtain complete anesthesia, he needed to stop treatment and refer the patient to someone (Dr. Long or possibly an appropriate specialist) who could. As embarrassing and frustrating as postponed treatment would prove, it is superior to losing that patient, their family and all future referrals after causing them pain.

I also sent Joe to the first of a series of excellent orthodontic courses provided by Dr. Skip Truit as my guest. (The expense is a good investment in Joe and our office.) Joe has already begun to take over some orthopedic cases, which should enhance his production immediately.

During this autumn period the previously discussed Warsaw letters were sent, the resulting $17,000 of diagnosed care helping quickly boost Joe's schedule in early 1998.

Joe and I had several private meetings to discuss problems and consider possible solutions. These conversations concluded with the entire staff meeting one night after work to discuss nothing but Dr. White and what he and his teammates could do to enhance productivity and patient satisfaction. An agenda was prepared by the staff who led the meeting. (I was present at the staff's request, trying hard to just shut up and listen for once.) A productive hour of discussion and brainstorming followed.

Staff support is essential for any dentist to succeed, but even more imperative for a young dentist. With every associate we've added, in some form or manner, patients will ask staff, "Is he good? Is she gentle?" Even the slightest hesitation to either query by team members means patients won't be scheduling with the new dentist.

Will all of these efforts produce the desired effect of enhancing Joe's performance? Despite the exertion and energy put forth, the results ultimately depend on Dr. White. Our patients won't tolerate being kept waiting, or suffering any discomfort during care. Neither will such occurrences be acceptable to our team of professionals who pride themselves on our office's outstanding care. Despite Joe's superb clinical skills, if he can't become behaviorally adept, and demonstrate by his actions a clear understanding of the human dynamics woven throughout this book, he will fail in our office.

As I write these words, our annual all-day staff meeting is a few weeks away. We close the office for this event and rent a local hotel meeting room (NOT BEDROOM) to avoid all possible distractions and interruptions. Salaries are paid to all but dentists, and snacks and lunch provided by the office.

This is a day in which all staff may relax, free of time constraints and ringing phones, and consider our office purpose as individuals and as a group. It is a time devoted to clarifying vision, communication, and team understanding. I'm confident a great deal of our discussion will focus on the critical issue of helping Dr. Joe enhance his career.

The point I wish to make concerning our monitors is that, as illustrated in the case of Dr. White, our team knew not only that his production was down—the least sophisticated monitors should provide that data—but that the cause of the problem was in our office's inability to consistently schedule a full day of patients for Joe. We didn't have to examine clinical skills, or discuss ways to enhance productivity. Joe's monitors (hourly production figures) showed he excelled in these areas. Focusing effort on these strengths would have wasted time, frustrated everyone involved, and meant we'd misdiagnosed—and thus failed to address—the true cause of our problem.

Instead, guided by precise data from the monitors we've just examined, our team could concentrate its effort on ways in which Dr. White could provide a more satisfactory service to please patients who received his care, then enhancing case acceptance and referrals.

It's hard to adequately explain to one who's not experienced similar monitors the power inherent within such precise information and how it allows one to accurately and certainly diagnose and confront the precise problem facing his or her office. Being certain we are correct concerning the nature of our problem by action based on factual information, rather than "educated guesses," lends focus, confidence and power to our corrective efforts. As we persevere in our exertions, future monitors illustrate precisely the status of our progress.

Whatever one's system of monitors, a level of data required to expeditiously identify trends, and thus enable a motivated team to influence them toward the preferred outcome, must be perpetually forthcoming.

Hygiene Monitors

We'll be discussing hygiene at length in Chapter 5, but let's take a brief look at the data before us. Examine the column of average production per hour under year to date (Line 34)—the running average—and you'll see a steady increase from $111 per hour in January to $118 per hour in December—a 6.3% rate of growth. The average monthly production for the year is slightly below $14,000. In addition to this direct production, hygiene, assisted by their two intraoral cameras, schedules a great deal of the dentist's clinical procedure.

Suffice it to state that I consider hygiene to be the bedrock upon which our office is founded. This department is very profitable, (details in Chapter 5) and our hygiene people assume major responsibility for the excellent periodontal health of our patients (the basis of any dental practice that claims to be preventive oriented). Because they treat most patients more frequently than the dentist—routinely scheduling three-, four- and six-month recalls as part of our soft-tissue management program—hygiene people are essential to establishing a bond between our office and patients.

I've worked with seven hygienists, employing the first one ever to provide care for patients in Keokuk, Iowa, and have never been without one for more than a few weeks at any time during my career. I'm a big fan and supporter of the hygiene profession—both of the fine people it is comprised of, and the valuable service they provide—but I've also suffered through relationships with hygienists that were unpleasant . . . to be as kind as possible.

Ms. Melissa Lannery, our current hygienist of almost three years, drives 70 miles one-way to work in our office—rain, snow, sleet, ice or even on the occasional nice Midwestern day. Melissa embodies the rare combination of displaying clinical excellence in all she does and being a true behavioral adept (Melissa would say she likes people—same thing), a wonderful person who, in a completely professional manner, enhances the success and joy in our office every day. We've nicknamed her "Sunshine." (By way of comparison, on my best days, I may possess one of these positive traits . . . but then I didn't have many "best days." I'd guess I have a few nicknames in the office too, but none have ever been repeated within range of my hearing.)

Perhaps some of you can relate to my experience. I've had relationships with past hygienists in which being informed they wished to speak with me after office hours made me break out in an icy sweat. They were perpetually dissatisfied, always wanted more, and were not part of the team—I believe because they felt above other staff. I tolerated them, at the cost of my dignity and self-respect (I'm lucky to be encumbered by but scant quantities of either of these virtues) because—and this may shock you—despite my exhaustive efforts, it's a little hard to recruit hygienists to Keokuk, Iowa.

Here seems an opportunity for me to advise my long-suffering, loyal readers how to establish an ideal relationship with their hygienist that is mutually profitable and enhances the success and joy of the entire office. I don't have a clue, other than to advise you to hire someone as wonderful as our Melissa. We've discussed how one can't change the basic values an employee brings to one's office, but how one must create a hiring process that identifies people with beliefs similar to one's own. (As is usually the case, Melissa was the sole applicant for our hygiene opening . . . which made her selection an even easier choice.)

Don't be deceived by this short discussion of hygiene. The following chapter is totally devoted to the subject. I know offices exist without a hygienist, and am fully aware of the difficulties inherent in establishing a successful, pleasant hygiene operation; yet I see no way to achieve success, wealth or joy without a powerful contribution from one's hygiene department. I believe a profitable, relationship-building hygiene department to be essential to the success of virtually every dental office of the future.

A Philosophy of Numbers

A quintessential factor with all monitors—I guess as is true for virtually every facet of practice success—is the attitude of the dentist. For monitors to work their legerdemain, guiding an office to efficiency and profitability, the office leader must recognize these numbers as the vital signs of his or her practice's health, and study them as devoutly as one hopes a physician will consider one's own vitals when he or she offers care.

I believe the majority of dentists do little more than glance even at the most simple of accountant's monthly profit and loss (henceforth P and L) statements. Dentists too frequently tend to measure the practice's health by what's left in the checkbook after the bills are paid. I've called my accountant, on average, once a month to ask questions or discuss data on my P and L and related business and/or tax topics for 20 years. (In contemporary America, taxes are by far the biggest single expense of the average household, consuming more income than housing, food, transportation and clothing combined!! And you don't ask your tax specialist questions!!?)

My accountant (Mr. Ed Whitham) frequently informs me he seldom gets a call from any of his doctor clients (and professional practices are his special interest). Ed also volunteered that his job would be easier if every client checked his or her figures as carefully as do I, because fewer errors could go unheeded. (Ed may say that just to be kind, as, despite his unfailing graciousness, I do feel somewhat guilty for bothering him so frequently.)

I sense the need for another pithy pep talk. A leader must continually reinforce his or her vision, be it of an office or in a book. Repetition is essential to assure critical messages are understood and implemented. One doesn't tell his family he loves them once, then trust they'll always remember!

I understand dentists aren't trained as accountants, and all these numbers are boring and a little intimidating. Remember the information contained within these sparse digits has the potential to expand one's office's profitability tremendously by identifying strengths and allowing further growth in these areas, while highlighting weaknesses that DEMAND ONE'S ATTENTION.

The numbers may prove wearisome, but few excel in any endeavor by doing only the things they like. If that were possible, I'd exercise with the television remote and only eat ice cream! PLEASE WORK HARD and stay focused to visualize how having access to such office data will help one's practice thrive.

Operating Matrix page 2

The top five lines of this second page restate total production for the month by each provider, and add the percentage of total office production each provider's contribution for that month represents. (As an example, as seen on Line 2, my $4,519 effort in December was a CRITICAL 10% of the total office production.)

While these numbers have already been reported, scattered about on Page 1, we bring them together here to allow for a more concise comparison of each provider's monthly production.

The two columns directly below these top four show This Year's (TY)—Line 6—total office monthly production compared to Last Year's (LY)—Line 7—total office monthly production. If one studies this line for the complete year, he or she will note only in February and May did 1997 production fail to surpass 1996. This is a good thing! This trend of 1997 being superior to 1996 increased after July when Dr. White became productive. (Or perhaps getting Dr. Wilde out of the office proved to be the critical ingredient.)

Suppose a dentist/entrepreneur studied his or her monitors and noted that production per month was tending downward from the previous year. By referring to production per hour (on Page 1), one could instantly determine if he or she were working fewer hours, or if the decline was due to decreased hourly efficiency. Fewer hours could be indicative of a declining patient base, as was the case for our office with Dr. Joe. If so, prompt action to reactivate existing patients (as chart audit) and/or enhance new patients (perhaps launching a direct mail campaign?) could be initiated.

Or the monitors may reflect the dentist's desire to work fewer hours. Even then, this laziness may be reconsidered after a candid look at the effect of sloth (finally, an area where I do possess expertise!) on office profitability.

If the hypothetical problem involved a decline in hourly production—something I'd be alarmed to see—the staff could discuss possible causes such as:

1997 Operating Matrix page 2

		Jan	%	Feb	%	March	%	April	%	May	%	June	%	July	%	Aug	%	Sept	%	Oct	%	Nov	%	Dec	%
1	**Production:**																								
2	John	15,341	29	11,209	25	18,324	35	21,507	37	13,548	27	14,159	31	6,066	11	6,974	9	7,569	12	14,754	19	6,074	11	4,519	10
3	Lowell	24,136	45	19,430	44	20,515	38	22,291	39	22,132	44	14,299	31	27,796	48	22,459	37	23,599	38	24,418	33	19,779	36	21,426	39
4	Joseph											3,306	7	12,619	21	16,515	28	13,793	23	19,014	26	15,900	30	15,015	28
5	Melissa	13,904	26	13,538	31	14,481	27	13,773	24	14,490	29	14,422	31	11,650	20	15,749	26	15,839	27	15,705	22	12,118	22	12,266	23
6	TY	53,381		44,177		53,320		57,571		49,681		46,187		57,599		61,698		60,800		73,937		53,866		53,228	
7	LY	51,199		45,791		50,365		53,894		52,385		39,411		56,520		49,768		48,838		54,365		47,229		44,854	
8	YTD John	15,341		26,550	30	44,874	30	66,381	32	79,929	31	94,088	31	100,154	27	107,128	25	114,697	24	130,452	24	136,526	22	141,045	21
9	Lowell	24,136		43,566	42	64,081	42	86,372	41	108,504	41	122,804	40	150,600	42	173,060	41	196,659	41	221,026	41	240,805	39	262,231	39
10	Joseph											3,306	1	15,925	4	32,441	8	46,234	9	67,244	11	83,194	13	98,209	15
11	Melissa	13,904		27,442	28	41,923	28	55,696	27	70,186	27	84,608	28	96,258	27	112,007	26	127,846	26	141,552	26	153,670	26	165,936	25
12	TY	53,381		97,558		150,853		208,424		258,106		304,293		361,892		423,591		485,436		559,373		613,218		666,446	
13	LY	51,199		96,990		147,355		201,250		253,635		293,046		349,566		399,334		448,172		502,537		549,766		594,620	
14	**Collections:**																								
15	John	15,875	103	11,253	100	16,245	89	18,372	85	16,087	119	15,372	109	10,155	167	7,348	95	8,183	108	13,770	93	9,556	157	5,902	130
16	Lowell	22,210	92	20,691	106	21,894	107	22,033	99	23,180	105	20,238	141	21,185	76	22,184	99	27,678	117	25,007	102	18,454	93	23,332	109
17	Joseph											1,485	45	9,203	73	10,999	67	13,577	98	17,462	92	16,831	138	15,422	103
18	Melissa	12,283	88	12,451	92	14,291	92	13,863	101	13,760	95	15,589	108	13,185	113	14,552	92	13,938	87	21,036	133	12,438	78	13,885	113
19	unassign	(4,644)		(2,867)		(3,453)		(5,424)		(3,348)		(2,868)		(4,691)		(3,674)		(5,099)		(7,781)		(6,773)		7,501	
20	TY	50,369		44,343		52,432		54,270		53,028		52,685		53,730		55,085		63,376		71,157		53,845		61,346	
21	LY	48,689		49,075		41,401		50,311		58,999		44,129		42,699		45,082		42,546		50,167		50,922		42,093	
22	YTD John	15,875		27,129	102	43,375	97	61,748	93	77,836	97	93,208	99	103,364	103	110,712	90	118,895	103	132,665	101	142,221	104	148,123	105
23	Lowell	22,210		42,902	98	64,797	101	86,831	101	110,011	101	130,249	108	151,435	101	173,620	100	201,298	102	226,305	102	244,759	101	268,091	102
24	Joseph											1,485	.5	9,203	58	20,203	54	33,780	73	51,242	76	68,073	85	83,495	85
25	Melissa	12,283		24,735	90	39,026	90	52,889	95	66,650	95	82,239	97	95,424	99	109,977	98	123,915	96	144,951	102	157,389	100	171,274	103
26	TY	50,367		94,766		147,198		201,468		254,497		307,181		360,911		415,996		479,372		550,529		604,374		665,720	
27	LY	48,689		97,764		139,166		189,476		248,476		292,605		335,304		380,386		422,932		473,099		524,021		566,114	
28	**C/P:**																								
29	TY	94		101		98		94		106		114		94		89		104		96		100		115	
30	LY	95		107		82		93		117		110		91		110		97		98		95		102	
31	YTD	94		97		98		97		99		101		100		99		99		98		98		100	

1. Personal phone calls taken by the dentist during scheduled treatment time. (I accept calls only from other doctors—never personal calls, even from family—unless there is an emergency. In the rare times when I'm in the office, my total focus is on providing the best possible, most efficient care of which I'm capable. This has been the case since the first day my office opened.)

2. Poor scheduling, perhaps with too many small appointments clogging the appointment book and not enough emphasis placed on longer, more productive and profitable procedures. (I block from 9 to 12 a.m. for major procedures, as this is the time during which I'm most effective. It's a little scary to realize I define myself as optimally competent only nine hours per month!)

3. Or, 99% of the time the correct answer to explain declining hourly production, a loss of focus due to **leadership failure**. The dentist hasn't been **responsible** for the team's success and perhaps ignored holes in the schedule, did not begin the day with a positive team meeting, displayed a fecal attitude in general, was "not feeling well" (had my share and yours of those days of malaise when I drank), etc.

Whatever the diagnosis—and frequently multiple factors are involved—**the power of monitors** lies within their ability to demonstrate to everyone on the team, with indisputable facts, that a problem exists. Careful monitor analysis can help identify the basic reason for the problem (such as reduced work hours, or lower hourly production) and thus help correctly focus the entire team's attention and effort on the clearly delineated difficulty.

In short, by employing accurate monitors, not only is the office leader made aware of trends more quickly, but he or she is able to document the existence of a concern and factually illustrate the problem to the entire team. (Assume production has declined in hygiene. Can you see the advantage of stating, "Last month our hourly production averaged 15% below the same month a year ago" versus, "We don't seem as busy.")?

Dealing with mutually accepted facts also shifts the tenor of the discussion away from personalities and blame to a shared and clearly defined problem. Dealing with a common objective can enhance team unity as the difficulty is addressed and solved by the group working as a unit with a common, greater-than-self purpose. (Remember, our focus is on fixing systems, not blaming people.)

If only fragments of the monitors are shared with staff when it is convenient for the dentist to reveal them, the results of this data won't be nearly as profound, as to the staff who are never allowed to study and understand the monitors, meager examples will seem numbers extracted from thin air. Even if information is presented in a manner that makes its meaning clear—as difficult as this task would be—one would have to be concerned with the credibility such fragmented data would be given by team members.

Also, it takes hours to prepare monitors, and while I've never personally created them, I can't believe the compilation of this data is the highlight of a busy staff person's day. **The dentist must personally evaluate, then demonstrate the usefulness of monitors with the entire team if he or she wishes them accurately kept.**

(To make things even tougher for Jo, I insist monitors be prepared, at the latest, during the first week of the following month, as any delay in receiving this data reduces the effectiveness and potential impact of this information.)

The next four columns (lines 8 - 11) give a running total of each provider's production for the year, again including percentages. (For example, study December, 1997, for Melissa—Line 11.) With one provider and lower fees, this department accounted for $165,936, or 25% of total office production.) Comparing this data to the previous year's percentages (available from our 1996 monitors) will clearly identify a provider whose productivity is either growing quickly, or decreasing in relation to the rest of the office.

The following two columns (Lines 12 and 13) complete the production segment of our monitors by comparing this year's

(TY) total production ($666,446) to last year's (LY) total production ($594,620).

I realize these numbers seem puny to you million-dollar producers. I'm making no effort to appear as anything other than what I am—a small-town dentist with a bread-and-butter, mediocre practice who is (refreshingly?) candid to the point of embarrassment. (If not foolishness!)

But please consider the fact that from this humble practice, by age 40, I was free of all debt and had $1 million in the bank—sufficient money for my family of six, and our simple needs, that I never needed to work again. (I grow and shoot most of our food—just need a little lard and salt once in a while!) Once again, my goal is not to produce $1 million through grinding effort and long hours—but to achieve financial independence (freedom!) and JOY. Whether one is consciously aware or not, I suspect these to be the goals of most individuals.

I trust my achievement of financial freedom, after only 13 years in private practice, and after paying 100% of education and practice opening expense, will create hope and inspiration for dentists like myself who feel they lack the skill, drive, personality or extraordinary talent to achieve the levels of success that "big shots" within the profession glibly discuss. I believe my data prove fiscal liberty is possible for the average dentist willing to work smart and hard.

And while I'm being candid, my W-2 income from the practice of dentistry alone for 1997 (not including books, investments or any source of revenue but dental office profit) was $224,000. My monitors show I treated patients 38 2/3 days, or 310.5 hours, so **HOURLY NET** was **$721** or **$5,793 NET per day.**

Once again, please understand I feel my candor to be necessary to allow each reader to honestly evaluate my words and discover what true value may exist within them that has the capability to change their life. I know some are offended by open, honest discussions of money. Their umbrage is a gamble I'm willing to assume. If this book doesn't help readers advance and enhance their lives, I've wasted potential hunting time—not something on which I'd like to reflect—as life is indeed short.

Some minor embarrassment or criticism of my openness is a small price to risk for such a worthy goal.

Reflect on your personal dental hero, mentor, guru: he or she with the practice you most admire, whose books you've read, tapes you've seen, for whom you've traveled long miles to bask in reflected brilliance. How much factual knowledge is available about their practice, let alone their personal finances? Do you possess any documentation proving they have achieved that which they encourage you to attempt, or are you left with nothing more substantial than glowing, but generalized statements of success? How much do they currently practice, or when did they retire? If you are to trust them, to PAY FOR THEIR ADVICE, don't you **deserve** to have answers to these questions?

Forgive these possibly defensive, definitely impassioned assertions. I guess you know I don't consider myself a shining example of perfection, but as I've written, lectured and traveled, I've come to meet and know many of those within the profession I've admired from afar, and have been amazed and horrified at the truth I've seen—so different from the impressions I'd absorbed.

Our $666,446 production (Line 12) was a 12% increase from the $594,620 (Line 13) total of 1996. This seems positive, but my net profit declined due to the sharp decrease in my personal production (I have to pay the associate's additional salary when he produces dentistry instead of me) and the distractions and disruptions of adding a new provider that historically take six months, at least in our office, to assimilate. (The fiscal effects of adding an additional dentist will be more thoroughly demonstrated in the collection portion that immediately follows.)

I'm a little concerned that in 1997—which proved to be a devil of a year—our office produced 666. I'll make the sign of the cross to ward off evil spirits, but I'm glad the numbers didn't start with 333, despite any possible occult ramifications.

Collections

The first column of four under collections (Page 2, Lines 15 - 18) states monthly dollar totals collected per provider and the percentage of total production for that month that this dollars-collected figure represents. (For example, in December of 1997—on line 15—Dr. Wilde collected $5,902, or 130% of his paltry $4,519 of production.)

Consider Dr. White's collection percentages (Line 17) of 138% in November and 103% in December. Good news?! Maybe. **When production declines, collection PERCENTAGE often increases,** as one is always collecting a portion of past production. (Again on Line 17, Joseph's October production was $19,014, while November production dropped to $15,900 and December fell to $15,015.)

So increased collection with increased production is always positive. Increased collection percentage with decreased production totals gives the illusion of fine collections—but don't be deceived. Lower collected total dollars follow lower production as surely as a calf follows its mother.

(Kindly ignore Line 19, marked "Unassigned." This means nothing to us—merely an idiosyncrasy our computer insists on stating that we record so our totals balance.)

The following two columns (Lines 20 and 21) compare this year's (TY) collection per month to last year's (LY) collections for the same month in terms of total dollars. As was the case with production, only in February and May were 1997 total collected dollars less than for the same month of 1996.

The following four columns (Lines 22 - 25) list running monthly collection data for the year by provider in total dollars and percent of production collected. Note (Line 24, December) that Dr. White collected 85% of his total production for his months in our office (while I paid 100% of his overhead expense). Recall the last two months of 1997 Joe's collections were in excess of 100%, indicating the approximate six months it takes a new dentist to get collections on track has elapsed, and both Joe's and my net should improve in future months as a result of this event of passage.

This roughly six-month delayed cash flow represents a major portion of what I meant when I mentioned the disruption adding a new provider causes to my net. It's not Joe's fault, and nothing is wrong (although with my first associate this six-month decline in collected dollars, juxtaposed with the sharp increase in overhead from more care being provided, scared the hell out of me!) It takes time for revenue flow to stabilize, and assuming the same effective office financial systems the senior dentist has employed are followed for new dentists, no permanent reduction in collections should occur.

I made the **terrible error of paying my first associate based on production**, reasoning (and thinking is always where I get in trouble) since our office historically collected around 100%, and my experienced staff remained in charge of financial arrangements, paying on production should be no problem.

Consider the situation of a new graduate with two hours open on his or her schedule and only a meager toothache patient on the horizon requiring care. In our scenario, this emergency patient has never previously been treated in our office. She has an abscessed lower right molar that will require an endo, post and core, and crown to retain.

The associate has the choice of performing the pulpotomy and scheduling a complete examination—as should always be the case with any new patient presenting with an emergency in an efficiently run office—or saying, "Your tooth needs a root canal and crown. I can do all that today, if you like."

The associate would be paid around $300 for this effort, about 10 times the compensation he or she would earn from the pulpotomy. In providing the definitive care, he or she would also be productive—earning and learning. That's a lot of temptation for anyone—let alone a neophyte dentist who may be deeply in debt—to resist. If the patient never pays—or drops dead when she gets the bill—the practice owner is out the roughly $300 in salary plus all overhead expense. In short, paying an associate dentist based on production creates pressure not conducive to a long-term relationship, a profitable practice or a good night's sleep for the office owner.

The next two columns (Lines 26 and 27) are total office dollars collected in a running total for this year and the preceding year. (In 1997 our office collected a total of $665,720, while in 1996 total collected dollars were $566,114. I'm glad to have the **666** altered, but would rather it had been elevated to 667 or greater.)

The following two columns (Lines 29 and 30) of this page record the collection percentage of production for each month of the current year (December 1997 collection was 115% of that month's production) and previous year (December 1996 collections were 103% of that month's production).

One might be reflecting, "it's hard to produce or collect over the holidays! How did they manage 115% and 103% collections in December?" To tell the unvarnished truth, I haven't a clue, but feel free to call Jo—the office number is 319-524-8811 and she's almost always there—and ask her to reveal her secrets.

The final column of the page (Line 31) is the major key to fiscal health—the running total percentage of collection for the year. (If one scans ahead to December, 1997, one will note our office collected 100% of dollars produced.)

I suppose to be thorough, I need to explain how we use this data. The significance of collection figures is one can't pay bills or purchase 12-gauge shotgun shells with production—only with dollars one collects. If one accepts lower collection rates due to looser office payment policies, he or she will produce more, as people can "afford" care they don't pay for, but while one works harder to perform more dentistry, the office will **NET LESS.**

An additional "benefit" of inefficient collections is one has the joy of collecting overdue money that builds staff character and makes them appreciate almost any other job in the office.

Despite forfeiting all this potential fun, our office works hard to collect 100% of production, and usually does. Care to examine how?

Collection Policies

Collection policy is another area in which I possess little documentable expertise. (What a surprise!) I'll describe what our office does, and detail our results, but resources are available that offer greater wisdom than I possess concerning the nuances of collections. I can't suggest one definitive foundation of collection information, either in the form of a book or mentor/guru. Our office policies have evolved piecemeal, by implementing guidance from a plethora of sources over the decades. Our office does have **one collection "secret." We are constantly aware of and working on collections as a team**. (I realize diligent, consistent, hard work is not the kind of "secret" one hopes will be revealed.)

Office collection policy must be a portion of the **dentist's vision**. Collections are too integral to office success to allow anyone but the doctor—he or she who assumes **final responsibility**—to be in charge of establishing policy, despite fear and trepidation generated when considering the always emotional issue of money. (I believe dentists don't wish to deal with money matters, not because this topic is beneath their dignity—most can't afford this much dignity—but simply because of our old buddy, the ancient and innate fear of rejection.)

Our office annually achieves approximately 100% collections, as will be displayed in a moment when our monitors reveal a total accounts receivable, accumulated since 1974, of $32,391 as of 1 January, 1998.

Keeping accounts receivable at around two weeks of production requires constant staff effort and unrelenting dentist attention. Pages 4 and 5 of our monitors are reviewed with front-office staff only during our regular monthly front-office meeting. (Each month we hold a dentists' meeting, a full staff meeting, a hygiene meeting and a front-office meeting. Only I am privileged to be included in all. Staff meetings are discussed at length in Chapter 8 of *Focus*.)

As the office leader, I never let a month pass without a discussion of collection policy and monitors, be the news bad or good. (I assure you, it's all right to thank staff when things go well. Contrary to what most dentists appear to believe, one's team won't quit working if you say something nice!)

Our office payment policy includes an offer of a 5% discount on work paid for on or before the day treatment is rendered. An 8% discount is awarded if ALL suggested care is paid for in advance of treatment. (This is powerful! For a $3,000 ortho or restorative case, this is a $240 savings that will motivate many to raise the money before care begins. These prepaid people seldom fail appointments and, I believe, follow our instructions more faithfully.) We also offer senior citizens (age 62 and above) a 10% discount if care is paid any time (either day of or lump sum in advance) before treatment is provided.

Don't enter into the policy of offering discounts lightly. A 10% discount in an office with a 70% overhead means forfeiting **33% of one's NET!** If one can collect around 100% without discounting, that is ideal. It is my *unproven assumption* that our discounts not only enhance collections, but result in more treatment being accepted. Our office has higher fees for our area (considering rural Iowa fee schedules, that may be akin to saying one smells good . . . for a skunk!) thus increased profit margin, which allows more room for discounts.

Our office accepts credit cards, and we've worked with Norwest and two different purely dental credit-card organizations over the years. Perhaps these options are presented by our office without much sophistication or enthusiasm. Whatever the reason, in Keokuk, these methods of finance are not of much value. (Maybe a case a year is financed through either source.)

The Keokuk area is predominantly composed of middle-class to blue-collar citizens. We have no great poverty, and few truly wealthy families. People in our area are hard-working fiscal conservatives who tend to pay their bills and avoid debt. It's much more common for people to save six months before starting ortho to take advantage of the cash discount, rather than going into debt, paying interest to some third party and having the illusion of receiving a discount.

Personally, I'm glad our patients show such fiscal restraint and wisdom. We may forfeit an occasional incident of impulsive, emotional case and debt acceptance, but I prefer clients to exhibit a strong sense of financial responsibility, as from this sound basis they can be stable users of my services over the long haul. I also sleep better not worrying that care accepted from our office in the emotion of a moment resulted in financial distress for our patients. (I see salesmanship must be added to the already ponderous list of skills I lack.)

Every year I can recall, little old Iowa finishes first or second in national school testing scores. Perhaps the citizens of this sometimes ignored, disdained, fly-over state are smart enough to avoid the sucking morass of debt so common among the "sophisticated" (defined in Iowa as changing underwear daily) areas of this wealthy land? When I opened our office in 1974, many patients didn't have checking accounts! Today many don't have, or won't use, credit cards.

Our office charges 1½ percent monthly interest on accounts due, and has since going to a computer billing system around 10 years ago. (I can't imagine calculating interest by hand, unless one has only two patients who owe money.) I believe charging interest gets our accounts paid, right along with other BUSINESSES. It's pleasant—downright heartwarming—to believe one's loving, loyal and appreciative patients will pay the dental bill with no interest charges before credit-card and other interest-charging debt. If one has that belief, I'd suggest cutting back on one's medication.

An essential for 100% collections: ALWAYS perform a complete examination, including written treatment plan, and have precise, documented financial arrangements recorded in one's computer or on a ledger, before anything other than emergency care is rendered. Occasionally one of our office providers violates this policy—for what he or she considers a good reason—and we are always sorry!

We perform a credit check using a computer modem connected to one of the national credit company systems on every new patient. It takes about one minute to complete, costs $6.27 per enquiry, and allows us to present financial policy based on the individual's past credit history—not our mood that day, how busy we've been, or how long since we've been stuck with a large, uncollectible bill.

Though I recommend credit checks highly—identifying one deadbeat can pay for years of credit-check services—I insist each dentist consult a local attorney to determine what types of credit checks, and under what circumstances they are allowed, in his or her area. Five or six large national companies exist, as well as some local or regional credit bureaus, with whom one can work. One's office does NOT need to be computerized to employ credit-checking services.

Based on this credit check, and/or our office's history with patients of record, we rate EVERY client as an A, B, or C credit patient. This rating is entered into the computer and is printed next to the patient's name on every provider's daily schedule— helpful if discussions of future care arise chairside.

Policies for A credit patients basically consist of whatever works for them. These are individuals who our past dealings, or their credit record, indicate will meet their financial obligations in a timely manner.

B credit patients have good, but not outstanding, financial histories. This means we require more money in advance and very specific collection plans.

C patients have already proven they don't pay their bills. Extending credit is an exercise in futility, and thus C patients are either cash or no-charge treatment, based on the dentist's discretion. (Each provider in our office has complete authority to treat any patient at no charge for whatever reason they wish— friend, family, replacing failed care, or their honest perception of dental need without possible patient resources. On the other hand, the patients we assume will pay, I expect to collect from.)

Modern credit companies condense all information into one number that reflects the credit-worthiness of that family. The companies provide guidelines to help interpret this final figure, so understanding credit ratings is no longer an art, but a fairly concise science.

Many offices treat everyone as an A credit risk, until accounts receivable escalate to the point of threatening the office's existence. Then the dentist often decides to address out-of-control accounts receivable by treating everyone as a C credit risk, offending and driving off the best patients.(You've just been treated to a condensed version of a fairly typical dental management conclusion that reflects many dentists' customary tendency

214

to be blown by any breeze, reacting to situations rather than making carefully thought-out, proactive, values-based decisions.)

Our office attempts to do the **fair thing** and establish financial relationships with each patient as his or her past behavior demonstrates they deserve to be treated. Fair isn't treating all the same, but rather in a manner consistent with their unique financial history. Isn't fairness all one can expect from life?

Caring for a patient and not being paid creates stress, frustration and ill feelings in one's office, but also in the community as this deadbeat expounds on his or her perception of the flaws of your office—such as expecting payment. (Remember the old saw about a denture never being comfortable until it's paid for?)

One is much better off to go hunting and not treat someone, than to provide care and not be paid. (Hunting doesn't require as great an out-of-pocket expense as providing uncompensated dental care, is good exercise, fun, returns one to fresh air and the splendor of nature all are genetically programmed to love, can provide untainted meat—free of society's ubiquitous chemicals—and reduces stress. Those who argue fixing teeth is more fun will need to provide their own list of benefits to buttress such reckless contentions!)

For ANY PATIENT NOT PAYING CASH, all mutually agreed upon financial arrangements are recorded in the computer, and a "pink card" (a postcard-sized piece of paper that is pink) is filled out by the staff member who established precise credit arrangements immediately after the examination appointment. This card details all financial commitments made, such as how much is to be paid and when. The card of a typical B patient might note he or she will pay $500 before treatment begins, and the remainder in $100 payments due on the first of each month.

We also have Truth In Lending forms signed if we extend credit in excess of three months, as required by federal law—but we seldom plan to extend credit for this long a period.

The pink cards are filed with the ONE PERSON IN OUR OFFICE RESPONSIBLE FOR FOLLOWING UP ON CREDIT ARRANGEMENTS (my long-suffering wife, Jo). She checks these agreements monthly, calls any who fall out of financial commitment **immediately** (if the agreement states payment will be by the first, and no money has arrived, a call should be made by the seventh.) She doesn't hesitate to use her judgement to postpone future care (that's right—she cancels their next appointment!) if agreements aren't being honored. (Such line-of-fire decisions must ALWAYS BE BACKED BY THE DENTIST, even if he or she disagrees, as failure to support your teammate even once means this hard call will never be made again.)

Jo's superb at collections, understanding, from painful past experience, that only perpetual monitoring keeps this already onerous task from becoming a nightmare, and possessing the afore-mentioned and rare ability to be lied to directly and remain pleasant. Jo understands fully that **collections are about maintaining relationships with our patients—not just money.** People who owe money don't receive needed care and don't refer—often leaving our office to find another dentist who will extend credit.

(Our credit checks routinely show multiple health-care providers, sometimes including several dentists, already owed by our potential C patients. When we insist on cash, these patients usually go to another office, where they will receive credit!)

Making collection calls can trigger enormous fear of rejection. (I've never made one—wimp that I am! How about you, doctor?) I believe it's essential that one person make every call, or confusion results, as, even with clear notes describing every past interaction, one can never be completely certain if what the patient tells the caller concerning previously arranged financial conditions made by another team member is accurate.

Jo goes by the pseudonym of Phoebe when dealing with collection matters. (I have no idea how the name was selected. Perhaps Phoebe is the Greek goddess of collections?) I assume the additional identity adds to Jo's comfort level, and all our team understands any call for Phoebe deals with collection concerns. (If someone will do a great job on collections, she may call herself Cat Woman or Queen Elizabeth, for all I care. Whatever works!)

A wise business owner nurtures and supports the brave souls responsible for collections in the office, as their efforts are essential to the practice's well-being and one skilled in this emotional arena is as rare as he or she is precious.

One way to support this valuable team member is for the dentist to **NEVER DISCUSS FINANCES WITH ANY PATIENT**. Making up collection policy chairside as one goes along, no matter how noble or logical one's motivation, creates chaos for those who have to attempt to remember all these special situations and deal with them weeks later.

I've seen hunting dogs refuse to point after several missed shots. (I said I liked to hunt—not that I could hit anything.) Failure to support collection policy can result in a similar diminished performance. Collections is hardly a job to which anyone looks forward. This makes it even more imperative for the office leader to constantly **support** and **monitor** collection effort **BEFORE** serious cash flow problems develop.

Operating Matrix

(see next page) The first half of Page 3 is subtitled PATIENTS, and deals with data focusing on documentation of patient visit patterns.

The first two columns (Lines 2 and 3) display the total number of patients seen each month by all providers combined, This Year (TY) and Last Year (LY). Note the number of patient visits in our office for 1997 has increased from 1996, especially after Dr. Joe joined our ranks. The decline in patients seen during November and December in both 1996 and 1997 is due to the practice closing for several normal working days during the holidays. (And the epicenter of hunting seasons—I'm hunting deer, turkey, quail, pheasants, squirrel, rabbits and ducks—even a few doves and woodcock—during these two blessed months. I'd hunt something else, if there was anything else around here to hunt.)

The next column (Lines 4 and 5) begins the critical study of **new-patient flow—the life's blood of every dental office.** (Data

Operating Matrix

#	Item	Jan	Feb	Mar	Apr	May	June	July	Aug	Sept	Oct	Nov	Dec
1	**Patients**												
2	Total TY	616	578	654	702	639	666	664	768	732	783	589	567
3	Total LY	624	588	566	711	595	565	679	686	613	684	588	525
4	New Pts A	9 (2ww)	12(1ww)	9(3ww)	19(4ww)	9(3ww)	17(4ww)	15(3ww)	12(2ww)	21(3ww)	15(2war)	20(1ww)	
5	New Pts C	6	11	9	9	7	15(5ww)	13	19(2ww)	9	15(1ww)	3	11(1ww)
6	Total TY	15(2ww)	23(1ww)	18(4ww)	28(4ww)	16(3ww)	32(9ww)	25(1ww)	34(5ww)	22(2ww)	36	18	31(2ww)
7	Total LY	24(3ww)	35(5ww)	38(12ww)	24(7ww)	29(6ww)	50(7ww)	27(6ww)	24(5ww)	24(1ww)	16(2ww)	24(1ww)	24(1ww)
8	YTD TY	15(2ww)	38(3ww)	56(7ww)	84(11ww)	100(14ww)	132(32ww)	157(24ww)	191(29ww)	213(31ww)	249(34ww)	267(34ww)	298(36ww)
9	YTD LY	24(3ww)	59(8ww)	97(20ww)	128(29ww)	152(36ww)	191(42ww)	241(49ww)	268(55ww)	292(60ww)	316(61ww)	332(63ww)	356(64ww)
10	**Production/Hr**												
11	TY	$191	$173	$193	$191	$182	$176	$180	$174	$183	$187	$180	$183
12	LY	$182	$198	$204	$186	$180	$168	$182	$169	$188	$171	$173	$190
13	Dr Howe TY	280	256	276	301	273	262	320	354	345	396	298	275
14	Dr Howe LY	300	272	263	318	290 3/4	235	311	295	258.75	318	272.5	236
15	A/R	32,818.32	33,134	32,987	37,607	34,404	28,214.51	32,375.86	38,907	36,638.19	39,105	32,611	32,391.28
16	A/R TY												
17	A/R LY	28,980.75	25,816.20	34,956	38,747	30,938	27,233	31,069	26,022	27,728	28,587	31,064	29,664

on new patients occupy lines 4 - 9.) We differentiate between adult (A) and child (C) new patients due to the normally varied level of treatment needs—although orthopedics and orthodontics tends to even this customary disparity. We also identify new patients received as a result of Welcome Wagon (WW) and our recent Warsaw letter patients. Neither is charged for exams and bitewing x-rays, and recall that WW patients don't accept treatment at nearly the same level as our non-WW patients, so their value is less. (Warsaw folks accepted care at approximately our regular patient rate.)

Note, as have we, the steady decline in WW new patients (illustrated in these monitors in December on Lines 8 and 9) from over 100, to 64 to 36. We are redoubling our phone efforts and reevaluating our WW status in light of this trend. Three possible explanations jump to mind:

1. We've failed to be conscientious with our follow-up phone calls. (Kathy, the head of our PR efforts, assures me she is emphasizing these calls and reviewing old lists to discover possible WW people we failed to contact.)

2. Fewer people are moving into our area. Trends in real estate activity definitely cycle based on national and local economic conditions.

3. Our WW representative may have lost some of her enthusiasm and is making fewer visits. (Our office receives a monthly listing of calls made by our charming WW lady, and the numbers have declined significantly.) We have no control over our WW representative's effort, other than to drop WW participation. (Of course, we are only billed per visit made.)

I suspect a combination of these three, and probably also three additional factors at which I can't even guess, has led to our deteriorating results, but we'll be focused in the future and evaluate the WW situation carefully. Were this data not included in our monitors, I'd have no awareness of the WW reality unless an alert staff member notified me.

Lines 8 and 9 are running totals of new-patient flow comparing 1997 to 1996. This comparison explains why our marketing chapter is so long! If one considers December on Lines 8 and 9, he or she will note that in 1996 we saw 356 new patients (64 from WW, or 292 non-WW people). In 1997 this total dropped to 298 new patients, of which 36 were WW (or 262 non-WW new patients).

This decrease of 30 new patients (292-262 = 30), not including WW, is a major concern to me. By April of 1997 (we had declined from 97 new patients seen by March of 1996, to 56 in March of 1997), I had already become concerned and begun to activate many of the efforts documented in the marketing segment of this book.

Note that in the final five months of 1997, our new-patient flow was 26 ABOVE 1996 totals, but I won't feel secure until our 1998 total of non-WW new patients rings in around 300. At least until then, I'll continue to emphasize service in our staff meetings and search for new methods to market our office that fit my parameters of acceptable practice promotion.

Let's consider our office's specific reaction in 1997 to our common concerns about declining new-patient flow. As I write these words (February 1998) we have focused on each team member's enhancing his or her efforts to personally refer new patients. As with every other facet of an outstanding office, the attraction of new patients must be a project that involves all staff. During our regular full staff meeting, we award a cash bonus—a fresh, crisp $20 bill per patient—to any team member who referred a patient to our office, after that individual completes a new-patient examination. We include a liberal dollop of praise for this team member's demonstration of his or her faith in our office.

Our office is also very involved with preschool and school visits. I feel children's visits to our office, even more than oral health lectures we give within the classroom, are a tremendous service to dentistry!

Preschool visits are a lot of fun. We give each child a ride in our "magic chair," sometimes with two or three kids simultaneously seated in the chair. We show them our "straw" (small suction) and how it can drink all by itself; the little gun that shoots air and water; give them each a "kiss" from our suction, show each child his or her teeth in our little mirror (no explorer—scary and dangerous), and generally have a great time showing off. (There's usually one crier, but these kids cry everywhere, not just in your office. Don't be concerned.)

We print each of our guests' names on a certificate that we sign proclaiming he or she visited our office. (These proclamations are printed on colorful paper, and often end up on the family's refrigerator, serving as a nice ad for our practice.) We also give every child a toothbrush (complete with our office name, logo and phone number), a coupon for free malt or fries from a local fast-food place, plus a toy and sticker from our collection.

Visiting our office in the company of their teacher and friends makes this a fun event, not a threatening one, and we do everything within our power to make this (often) first dental experience a positive, if not downright joyful and exciting occurrence!

Over the years, I've witnessed many kids who have made visits to our or other area offices hop in our chair, thrilled to have their first dental examination, and proud to explain what they already know about the light, chair and mirror. This wonderful start to a lifelong dental relationship seems critically important to me, and if this worthy effort enhances our community reputation and stimulates new-patient flow, such benefits are merely frosting on the delicious cake of serving our area's children on behalf of the dental community.

The final half of our third page is subtitled PRODUCTION PER HOUR.

The first two columns (Lines 11 and 12) compare 1996 and 1997 figures for total production of all office health-care providers (dentists and hygienist) divided by total number of hours in which all providers treated patients. This is a measure of the collective office ability to work smarter—not harder. The higher the average hourly production, the more efficient—

smart—our group has been. (Recall, individual providers' hourly production is listed on Page 1.)

I can see no trend comparing these two years. If one took the time to total these figures (I did), 1997 hourly production for total office providers is approximately 1% above 1996 figure. Not too impressive in light of a 5% to 6% annual fee increase.

The following two columns (Lines 13 and 14) compare total health care providers' hours worked each month for the last two years. Here one can note many more hours worked per month in 1997. Dr. Joe's 1997 production per hour averages $177, versus my $454, so the poor guy has to work longer hours to keep abreast of our past production levels.

No great significance is apparent within Lines 11 - 14 in our office at this time. Dr. Joe's longer hours and lower average production balance Dr. John's decreasing hours and higher production. In past years we've noted both increasing and declining overall efficiency and referred to the individual monitors to identify the precise reason for either trend.

The last two columns on this page (Lines 15 and 17) are running totals of accounts receivable for this year (TY) and last year (LY). The final two pages of our monitors deal with collections, but Pages 4 and 5 are shared ONLY with the three members of our front-office team during our monthly front-office meeting, as I don't feel other team members need or wish to be aware of this detailed level of collection data. I insist ALL staff—no matter what their job description—be aware of accounts receivable, so include this important information on the bottom of Page 3.

Note that for the two years displayed, accounts receivable varied from a low of $25,816 (February, 1996) to a high of $39,105 (this peak, during October, 1997, occurring, not coincidentally, five months after Dr. Joe joined us). Many ideas and philosophies exist concerning accounts receivable. Let me posit two points:

1. As stated, patients who owe one's office money don't like you, don't schedule care and don't refer. Reflect on one's

personal experience concerning money owed. **Debt damages relationships.** No matter how excellent the care provided, one's office is fortunate if it isn't slandered by debtors. Howard Farran refers to "dental over-production," by which he means situations where dentists provide care without assurance money can be collected. The cost of collections is high in terms of real dollars spent, frustration for team and ill-will generated among (often ex-) patients.

2. I'd rather have my money in the bank than on the books, as it's a hell of a lot easier to pay bills with it there, and I'm confident in my ability to make money work for me. (More on investing in Chapter 8.)

I've read that high accounts receivable will "carry" one through a bad time, as when illness or disaster closes the office. Maybe. Again, I'm no expert on receivables, but I've got more faith in my bank balance supporting my family than I do in patients paying past due accounts, if I'm ill or the office has been destroyed.

The value of money owed declines each day the debt remains unpaid. According to the ADA publication, *Successful Valuation of a Dental Practice* (p. 23), accounts receivable at 60 to 90 days past due are worth 50 - 74% on the dollar, while after 90 days their value declines to 0 - 50%. There seems to me a definite trend of people growing more reluctant to pay their bills as time after treatment lengthens. But then, I'm growing old and cynical . . . well into my curmudgeonhood.

Collections

(see next page) Allow me to reiterate that these final two pages are discussed between myself and our dynamic and experienced front-office trio only. I feel an apology is owed to faithful readers concerning the final two pages of our monitors. There are few lessons I can extract from this data . . . and it's all Jo's fault.

She is the driving force behind our office collection policy. When one suffers the abuse inherent in calling those who owe

Collections

		Jan	Feb	March	April	May	June	July	Aug	Sept	Oct	Nov	Dec
1	A/R	32,818	33,134	34,956	37,607	34,404	28,214	32,275	38,907	36,638.19	39,109	32,611	32,391
2	Production	53,381	44,166	53,295	57,571	49,681	46,187	57,599	61,698	60,800	73,937	53,845	53,228
3	Collections	50,369	44,343	52,432	54,276	53,028	52,685	53,730	55,085	63,376	71,757	57,192	58,526
4	C/P	94%	101%	98%	94%	107%	114%	94%	89%	104%	96%	106%	110%
5	# Coll ltrs	66	88	93	106	76	119	86		106	104	90	
6	# Statements	292	309	312	319	322	309	303	362	330	322	312	311
7	#Calls	30	23	20	28	28	17	30	32	18	14	29	8
8	#NA				1				2	5	2	9	5
9	Amt called about	11,028	13,905	10,566	14,723	11,863	8,981	6,911	10,929	9,791	8,455	18,350	12,273
10	Amt Paid	3,992	5,823	4,253	4,540	4,939	3,093	2,119	2,367	3,234	1,847	4,305	4,132
11	% Pd (called about)	36%	42%	40%	31%	42%	34%	31%	22%	33%	27%	23%	34%
12	% Pd of total	8%	13%	8%	8%	9%	6%	4%	4%	5%	3%	8%	7%
13	New Amt	1,314	2,033	1,888	3,491	944	1,708	826	3,317	1,060	1,418	2,483	312
14	Old Amt	9,714	11,882	8,678	11,232	10,919	7,272	6,086	7,612	8,731	7,037	15,867	11,961
15	Amt Kci Br							111	445		164		367
16	Amt Pd												
17	Amt to Sm Claim				122								
18	Amt Pd												
19	Amt to NACC												
20	Amt Pd											1,011	
21	Amt Written Off	146		122	122		111	945		164			

money—as Jo has for years—one makes EVERY POSSIBLE EFFORT TO KEEP COLLECTION CALLS UNDER CONTROL. Jo gives inspired talks to the team every few months on collection efforts if she sees the slightest problems developing, such as a failure to complete pink cards on EVERY account being granted credit, or improper financial arrangements allowed, especially with C patients. (C means cash or no charge, remember?)

If our office had $100,000 on the books—and we did, not long after our first associate joined us—these two pages would make more interesting reading! (We began using a form of our current monitors in the year I first added an associate. During those traumatic $100,000 days I was forced to review these pages in the bathroom . . . draw your own conclusions.) As is, I'll do my best to point out the few lessons that can be extracted from our data, and illustrate hypothetical situations where particular information will prove advantageous in an office in need of more dynamic collection activity.

A written, concise collection policy, clearly understood and followed by each staff member (**especially dentists**) is essential to our quest (success, wealth and happiness). My low confrontation tolerance makes delegation easy—I've never asked for money from patients in my life! (Sure, my $454 per hour productive time is too important to spend discussing finances, but, again in all candor, my active fear of rejection is a much more significant contributing factor.)

The more directly the doctor is involved in collections, the better for the financial health of the office, as long as the dentist possesses the discipline to ALWAYS follow the fiscal policy he or she has established to guide the practice. I limit my involvement to two areas:

1. I NEVER discuss finances with any patient. When patients ask about money matters I smile and reply, "Ms. Impecunious, we have an agreement in our office. I don't interfere in financial arrangements and the ladies in front don't fix teeth." This usually gets me off the hook in a polite manner,

and is abetted by the fact I can't even remember our fees (they change every six months), let alone explain or fill out an insurance form. (A complete lack of skills in many areas simplifies, thus enhances my life. I enthusiastically recommend selective ignorance to everyone!)

2. I review these fiscal monitors in great detail **with my staff EVERY MONTH**. Clearly, I have delegated the **authority** to staff to deal with money matters, but I **retain full responsibility** to see it is being done exactly as this facet of the office vision I've developed (our collection policy) dictates.

Always keep in mind, accounts receivable are primarily about patient relationships. High accounts due means many patients are out of contact with one's office. On to the data.

The first column (Lines 1 - 4) repeats accounts receivable, production, collection and collection percentage for each month of the current year. This data is scattered throughout the first three pages, but is reproduced here in tandem to facilitate our front-office meeting discussion of these topics without requiring us to flip through five full pages of figures to ferret out these basic collection totals. We've discussed this data previously, so let's move on to the unique segments of these two pages.

The following two columns (Lines 5 and 6) reflect our collection labors via the mail.

Line 5. Number of collections letters (# coll. ltrs)

These are letters sent to patients who owe money **in excess of 30 days**. Our computer automatically prints a letter even if $1 is overdue, so the total number of letters generated isn't too significant. (We manually review these letters and discard ones with minuscule balances. Our expense in billing such small amounts makes them cost-inefficient to send, and receiving a bill for a few dollars tends to irritate patients.)

But, the trend in number of letters sent informs us of the total number of accounts past due. If our collection letters jumped to 150 (note they ranged between 66 and 119 in 1997), I'd become very concerned our collection efforts were deficient and press my staff for an explanation.

Line 6. Statements mailed

This states the total number of people who owe us money and are sent a regular monthly statement. The total includes overdue accounts. Again, the trend is the key. If we see a sharp increase in statements, and we have a corresponding increase in production, I'm not concerned. (This was the case in August, where statements mailed ballooned to 362, with production of $61,700, after Dr. White had contributed his efforts to our cause for a quarter.)

However, if number of statements sent increases without an increase in production, it may indicate our financial arrangements and/or over-the-counter collections are weak and these vital efforts need clarification and/or reinforcement from the boss. (We make a deliberate, determined effort to collect small balances over the counter, to avoid expensive, time-consuming billing.)

Collection Calls

The next eight columns (Lines 7 - 14) deal with our phone collection efforts. The sheer amount of this recorded data is a lucent statement as to how important follow-up collections calls are. No relationships are built, no questions answered, no compassion shown by repeated collections letters that grow perpetually more harsh in tone and/or bright in hue. A staff member, skilled with people and aware of her mission (re-establishing relationships) can provide all the above-listed benefits as a caring ambassador of one's office concerning the delicate, personal and emotional matter of money owed.

There is a risk inherent in having the practice owner's family member in charge of overdue patient accounts. This is their money too, and they might be too aggressive and strident in collection efforts, perhaps taking non-payment personally, thus driving patients from the office.

I've overheard Jo's collection calls many times. Her focus is always to inquire if the patient is having a problem or needs assistance, as we are puzzled by his or her lateness in paying and fear some trouble—which we'd be delighted to help solve—

may have occurred. Jo has an excellent voice and manner, and seemingly infinite patience for this difficult task.

(Our office will accept virtually ANY EFFORT on the patient's part to pay. If "times are tough" and they send $10 per month, as long as the sawbuck comes every month, we'll make no calls or other collection efforts. Even if payment is a few dollars per month, we consider these patients to be keeping their commitment. I'm not suggesting this is the proper way in which collections should be handled; that is an issue of personal values. I had little money for the first 30 years of my life, and Jo and I may be too empathetic concerning such trying times to be optimally effective in the competitive collection industry.)

Line 7. Calls

The first column dealing with collection calls records how many such phone contacts were made that month. Here our office made a mistake that allows me to demonstrate how our monitors function! Note how September and October calls made declined? (September—18, October—14, then up to 29 in November.) Jo was very busy training Dr. White, and two additional new staff added with him, concerning front-office policy and especially how to use the computers that are integral to every task done in our office. Despite the special needs of this time, the day stubbornly refused to expand beyond 24 hours, and Jo's collection efforts faltered! (There is no system of which I'm aware, where decreased efforts don't lead to declining results. This is why monitors and the active participation of the dentist are essential.) This slip will be more apparent as we continue to review the phone collection data.

Line 8. NA

The NA column is collection calls placed where no one answered, and is Jo's idea. This means nothing to me, but documents her efforts. If someone is willing to face rejection and call about money, they can monitor their navel lint, for all I care.

Line 9. Amount called about

This is the total balance owed on all accounts reached by phone. (Note in November, when emphasis shifted from training to collections, this amount increased to $18,350, as efforts were made to compensate for lower called-about amounts during the previous two months.)

Our monitors allowed us to spot this trend in declining phone collection calls quickly. We realized Jo was too involved in the **urgent** task of training—that had to be done—and had momentarily lost sight of the **important** task of collecting money. It's nicer to discover this fact from monitors, rather then when one can't pay the bills! In response to this realization, we crafted a plan to involve other senior staff in training, freeing sufficient time for Jo to complete needed collection duties in November.

Stephen R. Covey, author of the seminal book, *The Seven Habits of Highly Effective People*, which I've read, underlined, taken notes on and read again, goes into great detail concerning how urgent tasks—like answering the phone—are completed often at the expense of important tasks, as thanking a team member for a job well done, thus reinforcing positive behavior. (In our example training was urgent, collections important.) *Habits* also elegantly explores the relationship personal values play in achievement.

If you've read this book, read it again. If you haven't read *Habits*, pick it up immediately—despite its 1989 publishing date, it's still in EVERY bookstore—and dive in as soon as you finish this tome. You're in for a real treat. It's inspirational brain candy!

Line 10. Amount paid

This records the total dollars paid on accounts called about that month. (In December of 1997, $4,132 was paid from a total of $12,273 overdue accounts called about.) Don't be short-sighted regarding this data. At first glance it may appear the dollars collected are not that significant. What can't be measured is how many patient questions were answered, future payment arrangements agreed upon, and positive feelings about our caring office restored.

While I can't overstate the critical, but intangible, nature of relationship-building within collection call efforts, a quick perusal of the total dollars collected as the result of calls for the year reveals (Line 10, Page 5) $44,648 brought in from these efforts. Since I've paid overhead already, whether money is collected or not, this means **$44,648 was added to my net** during 1997 as a result of collection calls. How many concepts have you recently considered with the potential to add $44,648 to your NET?

Line 11. Percentage of called about production paid

This column states what percent of the total dollars called about was paid. (The $4,132 collected in December was 34% of the $12,273 called about.) Page 5, Line 11 lists this column as a running percent for the year and is more informative.

Line 12. Percent of total production

This lists what percent of total office collections for the month the payments on called-upon accounts made. (In December, our $4,132 collected from past due accounts reached by phone was 7% of total collected dollars, and elevated December's collection percentage to 110%.)

Line 13. New Amount

This illustrates the amount of receivables called about that has been turned over (via our pink cards) for these calls for the first time this month.

Line 14. Old Amount

This is the dollar total called about that had been in the phone collection program previous to this month. Again, consider the $15,867 of old amount called about in November—double the preceding two months—as an indication of slippage in our system. (If one reviews all the data within our monitors carefully, there will always be MULTIPLE SIGNS indicating a developing problem. This deliberate redundancy acts as a safety measure to assure no trends remain undetected.)

If the new amount increases one must be concerned that our credit policies aren't being firmly adhered to—specifically not extending credit to C accounts. It could also indicate less effective efforts to collect money over the counter . . . always our preferred collection method.

If the old amount increases—and recall the longer money is overdue, the less its value—one's entire collection policy should be scrutinized.

One of the major frustrations of three decades of dental practice is the necessity of repeatedly solving the same problems. Handling money is a delicate, often unpleasant task. Even experienced staff with excellent skills will slip regarding collection policy and effort if not monitored and encouraged by the office leader.

Collection Efforts Made Outside the Office

Unfortunately (for the reader's experience, but not for my fiscal health), we had little activity in collection efforts made outside our office during 1997. Since we collected 100% in-office, this is a good thing.

Forgive my redundancy concerning this crucial point: It is critical that money be collected as soon as possible, as numerous studies have proven the longer a debt is owed, the less its probability of payment. This ever-declining value of debt is part of the reason precise and effective collection systems are a must for every successful business. (More so in our ever more competitive service industry, as dentists can't repossess their products!)

A totally cash practice, offering no credit, may seem ideal, if the loss of treatment acceptance and patients occasioned from such a strict policy can be tolerated. The following statement may be nothing more than a manifestation of my insecurity; however, I can't imagine an all-cash practice surviving in Keokuk, where every other dentist in the area extends credit, seemingly without examining credit-worthiness.

Every office should possess a clearly defined, understood and incorporated policy for debt due for 30 days or less. Our policy consists of our A, B, and C credit ratings and subsequent possible credit arrangements based on each patient's status; making efforts to maximize over-the-counter collections; plus sending a statement by the 28th of each month. Establishing a specific monthly target date by which statements are mailed, that is recorded on the office calendar, is vital.

Years ago, as a solo dentist without monitors, I discovered, long after the fact, that our office totally skipped sending statements one month! Are you certain this has never happened in your office? Without monitors, how would you know? Do you think the staff will tell, or patients call your home to complain about not being billed?

A definite policy should also exist if debt exceeds 30 days. In our office the computer generates a different letter for past-due accounts, and **most critically,** the first call is made from our pink slips as close as possible to the day after our patient has violated his or her financial agreement. Calls are continued each month accounts remain overdue, and the details of each conversation recorded in our computer records. We have differing letters mailed to accounts overdue 30, 60 and 90 days. I invested significant time and thought into crafting each of these past-due messages. I wish I could believe these carefully worded missives made the slightest difference.

At 120 days, the process of turning accounts over to an outside collection party begins in our office. One's staff must understand, accept and support this policy.

Great care must be taken when the possibility of resorting to outside collection efforts is discussed with one's patients. This is the LAST THING we wish to happen, as it almost always means a permanent end to patient relationships. (We will see clients whom we've turned over for collection if they pay in advance of care. But had they the ability to pay in advance—or even in arrears—we'd not have turned them over.)

Also, federal statutes are in place to prevent harassment of debtors. To suggest one will turn a party over to an outside collection agency and not act on this statement in a timely manner places the dentist in potential legal difficulties. Federal laws to protect debtors have real teeth in the form of fines and penalties. Outside-the-office collection efforts must be implemented with knowledge, discipline and concern.

Here are the three sources of outside collection efforts utilized by our office:

Lines 15 and 16. Our local Keokuk Credit Bureau is used for small amounts of debt, approximately $100 or below. The credit bureau keeps 50% of what they collect, and years ago, when we were forced to resort to outside collections frequently (before Jo took over), our monitors showed we'd eventually receive about 25% of money turned over to the credit bureau. This would be acceptable, if WE HAD ZERO OVERHEAD! (Line 15 indicates dollars turned over—Amt K. Cr. Br. Line 16 records amount paid—Amt. PD.)

Lines 17 and 18. Over the years, Small Claims Court has proven to be our most effective outside-the-office collection tool. The law and procedure for small claims vary from state to state, so check your situation. For example, in Illinois a corporation must be represented by an attorney to appear in small claims court, the resultant expense virtually destroying any value of this potential collection aid for our professional corporation's small accounts. (Claims court would still be viable for large debts, but thank God, we aren't brain-dead enough to get taken for thousands, and there are maximum dollar limits to claims allowed to be adjudicated in the small claims venue.)

In Iowa, as of this writing at least, one simply fills out a form, and pays a fee (currently $30) to have a claim brought before the court of small claims. We also have to pay the sheriff's costs of serving papers on the debtor, this tariff varying from $16 to $30 based on mileage to the person's home. Both these fees become part of our total claim against the debtor. A judge hears these cases, but no attorneys are required to be present.

To the best of my knowledge, our office has never failed to receive a judgement against the debtor. However, this is not the same as receiving the money! Although the judge orders the debt paid, the debtor still might not comply. If the debtor is employed, one can garnishee wages based on this claim, receiving a percentage of the debtor's every paycheck as set by law. This is a path we've chosen not to follow for many years—but again, this choice is mainly a measure of my insecurity, despite my desire to present this as compassion.

ʿLet me clarify one point. I don't use "insecurity" in a pejorative manner. Risking rejection by one's community and peers to collect a few more dollars can be a painful experience, depending on the individual's values and situation. I'd give serious consideration to the possible effects of vigorous collection policies before acting. Are they consistent with joy? Each case should be evaluated based on its particular circumstances. For example, I'd tend to treat a business owner with a home on the golf course in a different manner than a family of six with no phone.)

Often we win a decision, and still aren't paid . . . until four years later, or whenever the patient wishes to secure a loan, perhaps to purchase a car or home. Then our judgement, waiting patiently on the legal record, must be settled before the loan can be processed.

Investigate the law in your state. Some are friendly to those seeking honest bill payment, some not. However, even under the best of conditions, it is advantageous to keep tight control over in-office collections and have no need to engage any of these outside agencies. (Each is time-consuming and stress-producing.) No outside collection techniques can help our ultimate quest of restoring relationships. **These agents are to collections what an extraction is to dentistry—an unpleasant last resort.**

Lines 19 and 20. NACC is a national collection agency we have used in the past. (It's been a few years since we've turned anything over to them.) These are collection pros and play hardball. A number of national agencies exist, but I'm (thank God!) no expert here. Perhaps your accountant or lawyer can be of service if you have a significant amount of long overdue accounts to clean up.

If one considers employing a professional collection agency, carefully review their literature, and schedule an interview with a representative of the firm to determine if their collection tactics are consistent with one's values. Remember, they will be acting as an extension of one's practice.

The final column of this page (Line 21) is the total amount turned over for collection per month to each of these three parties. (Once money is turned over for third party collections, we write it off our books, re-entering the money as collections if we are paid.) If one's accounts receivable are high, I'd expect to see steady activity here to ensure staff are complying with office collection policies as regards steps to be taken based on debt outstanding over 120 days.

I've had staff who, despite being competent with collections, were uncomfortable concerning these outside collection agencies. I needed to carefully monitor to be certain this final step in our collection system was properly utilized. I suspect, if employees have past or present personal problems with money, it may be emotionally difficult for them to "turn someone over."

Collections YTD

(see next page) This data is identical to that recorded on Page 4, only presented in a running total format, rather than broken down by months. As we've already witnessed, observing running totals can facilitate one's ability to spot trends.

The first four columns (Lines 1 - 4) accounts receivable, (placed first for the benefit of our front-office staff's focused attention), production, collection and collection percentage— represent the **basic vital signs of a business**. Though you are already aware of these figures, it's convenient to have such critical barometers concisely bunched to provide a quick but succinct overview of office financial status.

Key figures on Page 5 include the percentage paid on amounts called about (Line 11) and percentage paid of total production (Line 12) recorded under the phone collection data. (For 1997 these final totals were 32% and 7%, respectively.) I retain the year-end final monitors indefinitely. (I am able to discard monthly monitors due to our running totals, keeping only Jo's original work sheets as records.) By comparing only these two collection totals with previous years, one can quickly estimate the effectiveness and effort dedicated to collection calls.

Collections YTD

	Jan	Feb	March	April	May	June	July	August	Sept	Oct	Nov	Dec
1 A/R	32,818	33,134	34,956	37,607	34,404	28,214	32,275	38,907	36,638	39,105	32,611	32,391
2 Productions	53,381	97,547	150,842	208,424	258,106	304,293	361,892	423,591	485,436	559,373	613,218	666,446
3 Collections	50,369	94,712	147,144	201,468	254,497	307,182	360,912	415,997	479,372	550,529	607,721	666,247
4 C/P	94%	97%	98%	97%	99%	101%	99.7%	98%	98%	98%	100%	100%
5 # Coll Ltrs	66	154	247	353	429	548	634	666	772	876	966	
6 # Statements	292	601	913	1232	1554	1863	2166	2528	2858	3180	3492	3803
7 # Calls	30	53	73	101	129	146	176	208	226	240	269	277
8 #NA				1	1					2	9	5
9 Amt Called About	11,028	24,934	35,500	50,224	62,087	71,068	77,979	88,909	98,700	107,155	125,505	137,778
10 Amt Pd	3,992	9,816	14,070	18,610	23,550	26,643	28,762	31,130	34,364	36,211	40,516	44,648
11 % Pd (Called About)	36%	39%	40%	37%	38%	38%	37%	35%	34%	34%	32%	32%
12 % Pd of Total	8%	10%	10%	9%	9%	9%	8%	7%	7%	7%	7%	7%
13 New Amt	1,314	3,347	5,235	8,726	9,670	11,379	12,205	15,522	16,582	18,000	20,483	20,795
14 Old Amt	9,714	21,596	30,275	41,508	52,427	59,699	65,785	73,398	82,129	89,166	105,033	118,811
15 Amt K Cu B							111	556		720		367
16 Amt Pd												
17 Amt In Cl				122	122						1,011	
18 Amt Pd												
19 Amt to NACC												
20 Amt Pd												
21 Amt NACC												
22 Amt Pd												
23 Amt Written Off		146	268	268		379	936					

Again, our office, sporting 100% collections, offers little to critique. If an office's collection percentage decreases, one should see an increase in these calling figures (indicating greater exertion), as more money is on the books to pursue. If calling efficiency numbers decline, one must determine if insufficient effort is being made, as was the case when our Page 4 monitors indicated fewer calls (our predicament when Jo was training staff), or if the calls are being completed and the communication skills and/or attitude of the collection caller is the difficulty.

In collection calls, as in all areas of business, monitors help specifically identify the **cause of the problem**, and allow one to take appropriate and prompt action to correct whatever obstacle exists.

Perhaps the person making collection calls hates the job and just goes through the motions. Make every effort to replace her at this task, as if she continues in a job she detests, the office collections and patient relations will suffer until she either leaves or is fired.

Studying books, attending courses and role-playing can refine the skills of an employee with a good attitude toward collections—one who believes bills and obligations should be honored.

Team support from all staff concerning collection duties is essential. Our office policy stipulates the person who made poor or non-existent financial arrangements is personally required to follow up on the client and report collection progress during staff meetings. **There exists no force as efficient in modifying behavior as being held responsible for the outcome of one's decisions**. If accountability is abdicated, it is unlikely that learning will occur or behavior change.

I prefer to think of this policy as educational, while the staff sees it as punitive. The truth lies somewhere in the middle. As a self-proclaimed pragmatist, I can assure all that if consistently implemented, this tactic works!

(This may be the single most critical concept concerning raising responsible children. To paraphrase my colorful father,

"If you shit in your own nest, you can damn well expect to clean it up.")

Being rewarded by the office leader, both in salary and emotional support, for collection efforts well done, is also essential. I determine raises every six months, based on my perception of each team member's effort and value. The same salary adjustment is seldom made for any two team members.

Allow me to reiterate the essential warning to NEVER fail to back the collection specialist's judgement, as if a patient convinces the dentist to buckle and not support the policy he or she set, the office monetary system has been euthanized. A single instance of non-support might cause damage that will never be repaired.

The last column of Page 5 indicates we turned $936.20 over to outside collections for the year and received NOTHING IN PAYMENT. We could probably do somewhat better . . . but I'm an easy-going guy. At 100% collections, I don't have much to say to my staff except "great going, gang!"

Collection Summary

Our computer system allows us to instantly check production or collection for the year, month or day with nothing more than a few seconds and keystrokes.

The scheduled production for each dentist and hygienist for that date is penciled at the top of each day sheet (the computer printout of the daily schedule of patients to be seen by each provider), along with the total office collection percentage for the month to date. (As an example, my schedule might display $2,432 and 99%, as my scheduled production for that day and the office collection percentage for the month to date.)

I mention collection percent—be it good or bad—at most morning huddles. Collections are a TEAM EFFORT, starting with the dentist, but including every employee. All need to be aware of the office collection situation and do what is needed to support this critical business effort. As I have been known to mention, I can't pay salary unless patients pay me.

In our morning clearing, the front might caution the providers to do no more than palliative treatment on a scheduled emergency patient until firm financial arrangements are established. The computer may have already identified this person with a C credit rating printed next to his or her name on the schedule. The front may have asked this patient to bring a predetermined cash payment, required before care begins, based on a credit check or past fiscal history within our office.

I'm going to say this once more, as I know how often staff are betrayed by their doctor, and the teeth-grinding rage this bequeaths. The dentist and chairside MUST SUPPORT THIS FRONT-OFFICE REQUEST, or one's system has been damaged, and the front-office person embarrassed by lack of support for the policy the doctor installed and ordered followed. After such a treachery, long-term problems within the office team concerning the REAL collection policy (based not on what has been said or written, but what has been done) will just be beginning.

It is not acceptable for the dentist to provide care until all financial and insurance questions have been answered and written fiscal arrangements established for each patient's needed care. As we've discussed, our office is willing to relieve pain, even if no money is available, and every provider in our office has complete autonomy to provide free care if, in their judgement, it is warranted. Also, A-rated patients with years of outstanding payment history might occasionally prove an exception to our customary financial arrangements. This is not a violation of policy, as we are merely treating these outstanding patients in a manner their past payment history has shown to be appropriate.

Do we lose patients because of our rigid credit policy? You bet! All the ones who don't pay their bills. (You guys and gals can have them!) It's cheaper and easier on my aging body and mind to have a cup of coffee and read an exciting dental book than to expand overhead, add frustration and assume legal risks and obligations providing care for which one has no realistic chance of being paid.

Possible Additional Monitors

What additional monitors might an office employ? Analyze anything that is important and which one wishes to improve within one's practice. We've measured new patients on a daily basis, listing the month to date total on the top of every provider's day sheet. We've had separate monitors to track units of crown and bridge treatment, and in hygiene for the number of Rotadent toothbrushes and tooth-lightening cases presented and accepted.

There is a finite limit to the time, energy and interest one can ask a busy team to expend on monitors. **Don't go nuts here!** Carefully develop a system designed for your office's specific needs. A set pattern of how and when this data will be reviewed must also be established. Perhaps key figures are reviewed at the morning huddle, and others at regular staff meetings.

There may exist excellent offices that don't have positive morning huddles or regular staff meetings, but I've never experienced one. If a dentist doesn't begin each day with a positive, informative staff meeting, and doesn't hold regularly scheduled staff meetings, I seriously question his or her commitment to success and excellence.

MOST VITAL is the leader's awareness that these figures are his or her compass and road map to a chosen level of success, needing only effort and time to allow one to achieve the life of his or her dreams.

I apologize if this chapter was as challenging to read as it was to write. I hope you agree the information may have been long, tedious, and dry . . . but **NECESSARY TO THE ATTAINMENT OF OUR THREE-HEADED GOAL.** An entire book on monitors is needed, but I sure won't be writing it! (My thanks again to Drs. Dunlap and Wagner for their excellent work.)

I repeat, I'm no expert on monitors and collections, but I hope our results (100% collections isn't too embarrassing) lend credence to our policies. The next step to implement depends on one's needs. Let's consider collections as an example. If one's accounts receivable are in excess of six weeks of production, **one's office is in crisis.** Identify, from among the many available, a dedicated source of help on collections and office efficiency and employ these services. Vow to never allow such a mess to develop again, and remain diligent in your efforts to correct this practice weakness.

If one's accounts are in the two to six weeks of production range, the information just reviewed, accompanied by enhanced emphasis from the office leader, and involving one's entire team, may be sufficient to return one to his or her accounts receivable goal. (If one offers discounts for pre-payment, one's accounts receivable should remain around 100%, as pre-paying speeds collection rate, thus increasing collection percentage.)

If one's accounts are at or below two weeks, and production is good, he or she is already fully aware that collections and office monitors are a constant area of focused attention within the successful, modern dental practice. Congratulations!

REFOCUS FOUR: OF THINGS THAT GO BUMP IN THE NIGHT

It's after 5 p.m., it's been a tough day, and it ain't over yet. This sharply curved, mesial-buccal root of number 14 is showing you no mercy, despite the late hour and your fatigue. You silently vow to NEVER AGAIN allow molar endo to be scheduled late in the afternoon, then feel the number 35 file fracture and sweat simultaneously begin to trickle down your rib-cage.

This is not your most satisfied patient. You had trouble achieving profound anesthesia. Despite using N_2O, topical, and "the pad," Mr. Timorous screamed when you numbed the palate! Images of angry confrontations, legal summonses, public disgrace and financial ruin assault your weary brain. You stare, transfixed in horror, into the access opening of the tooth, down which chances of your promising future seem to flee. Heart pounding, pulse racing, your body is telling you with all its might to run for freedom.

Reliving this horrifying scenario—to which, in some form or another, all dentists have fallen prey—leaves one suffering hormonal surges of emotion, tasting the bitter, metallic dregs of dread in the nether regions of one's throat. The trigger might be a letter from an attorney, a call from the IRS, someone merely whispering the initials O.S.H.A.—whatever one's current "terror de jour." The physical and emotional waves that break over one during such times are sensations all would like to avoid. What if we could? What would one do—where would one be, if one had no fear?

243

Intriguing question, topical and timely as we enter the brave new world of the next millennium. Also, one for which I can provide an almost certain answer: DEAD. Stepped in front of a car, fell off a cliff, was bitten by a poisonous snake, murdered by a jealous spouse, contracted AIDS.

Fear—much as pain—is an **essential ingredient of well-being and success.** Its critical job is to alert one of impending danger, thus allowing one to protect himself or herself. This is the reason natural selection has favored the apprehension resulting from confrontation throughout the ages, unwilling to relax this protective reflex, even in the relative safety of modern life. Time may prove the sagacity of this decision that condemns humans to continue living in fear in this always uncertain world.

Yet, granted its protective function, fear causes much of modern humankind's anguish. Few escape its painful grip, and for many anxiety drastically diminishes their health, emotional state, and quality of life. Confusing, isn't it? You see, *fear is the parent of both courage and cowardice.* And like rain, fear comes to all: the just and unjust. One determines—by one's actions, one's decisions—with which child, courage or cowardice, one chooses to live.

Uncontrolled fear paralyzes and isolates. It robs one of flexibility and choices, creating shame that renders one unable to seek help. The message of out-of-control **fear** is Forget Everything And Run. Mindless panic—the offspring of fear out of control—can ensue, one's imagination running wild, leaping like mountain goats to ever more dizzying images of disaster. Thus unchecked, **fear** becomes Fantasied Experiences Appearing Real. One's entire existence can become dominated by chimeras of impending disaster—most of which will never occur—but can drain one's strength, immobilize one into a state of inactivity and control one's life by consuming one's thoughts, energy and time.

Granted, fear is a necessary, important part of human existence, its presence enhancing the odds of one's well-being, even survival. While only the foolish would wish for a fearless life, many long for relief from the agony—the sleepless nights, emotional turmoil, ulcerated stomach lining, flayed-nerve pain, cancer-inciting damage—that chronic fear inflicts. Definite decisions, patterns, mechanisms can be implemented that allow one to put fear to productive and healthy use, while controlling the painful, debilitating side-effects that damage mind and body.

The Constructive Use of Fear

By employing the four-step formula that follows, one can tame the savage beast of fear, make of its fierce energy an invaluable resource and ally, while retaining the benefit of its protective function. The ability to wisely employ such a ubiquitous and puissant force can enhance professional success and personal joy.

Step One: Name one's fear

Unfettered fear can result in mindless panic, incapacitating one, like a deer captured in headlights, at the precise moment when decisive action is most critical. Once named, a fear becomes merely a problem to be solved, no longer an overwhelming presence, beyond one's power to influence. Emerson told us, "Fear always springs from ignorance." The act of naming allows one to begin to understand and thus **establish control**. If one simply waits, hoping fear will leave of its own accord, one's trepidation grows in might.

In our opening scenario, the problem is a simple mechanical one—a fractured endodontic file. After a moment's reflection, one realizes a broken reamer is seldom listed as the cause of death on a coroner's report. One's fear now defined, and thus brought under some control, one's mind can begin to function, searching for possible remedies.

Step Two: Focus ahead

The difficulty named, one can peer into the future to see possible benefits that might redound from dealing with the now defined PROBLEM. Often fear leaves one overwhelmed by feelings of the moment. By future-focusing, one's current situation receives some perspective, and one becomes energized by the possible benefits that can be perceived. By looking beyond the immediate dilemma, **Hope**—the fuel by which problems are resolved—is created.

Don't become crushed between the anvil of yesterday's regrets and the hammer of tomorrow's fear. Focus on what one can do NOW—in the marvelous gift of the present moment—the only time in which anyone may act. Fear is an emotion of vague tomorrows, strength is of the lucent today. Remember the admonition of Henry Ford—that obstacles are what one sees when he or she looks away from the goal—and fix one's unwavering vision on solutions. **Hope's child is courage!**

What possible benefits could the current conundrum bequeath? Every dentist who treats abscessed teeth must learn to deal with the rare, but unavoidable fractured instrument. It has simply become your time to learn, and in this new knowledge, to grow.

Step Three: Accept personal responsibility

Step three is not an area in which modern American society excels, but to grow, one must quit blaming others. Remember, **fixing the blame doesn't fix the problem**. One must accept responsibility if one is ever to gain control of one's current situation, of one's professional well-being, of one's life. Being personally accountable for a problem means one is empowered to achieve a solution. Helpless victims have no such abilities . . . no such hope.

It does no good to think that the instrument might have arrived from the manufacturer defective, that the assistant should have noted the wear and discarded it, that if the patient had opened wider—as you'd asked and pleaded—this could have been avoided. True or false, none of these factors change reality. As the doctor treating this patient, the responsibility for achieving the best possible outcome is yours—no matter what the circumstances.

The seed of hope planted, one's calming mind must center on a single issue: What am I to do now? Only with such concentration will one be able to take the final step in his or her battle with fear.

Step Four: Take action

One attacks fear with action. Sophocles advised, "Heaven ne'er helps the man who will not act." (Dad told me the Lord helps those who help themselves.) Fear assaults those who are weak, and constructs a prison from which action has the power to free you.

Wishful thinking is waiting, helplessly, powerlessly hoping something will happen. Positive thinking is believing and working toward an ideal result. **Cowardice is a reaction; courage is an action—a deliberate choice**. People are neither inherently brave nor weak. Courage levels vary by the situation and emotional state one is in, but each brave choice implemented increases the likelihood of further courageous decisions. It is the pattern of behavioral choices that occur throughout one's lifetime—something over which each has control—that makes you a victim of fear or its master.

Thus understood and accepted, fear becomes a teacher, as one is able to search for the meaning inherent within anxiety. Courage and wisdom make apprehension merely the warning of an impending challenge from which one who is prepared may grow.

The coward in us screams, "Fill the tooth and hope for the best. Maybe no one will ever know." In courage, you stop for an x-ray. (And take a few deep, cleansing, calming breaths—as I know of no magic, no level of understanding—able to make fear pleasant.) You see the file fractured near the apex and decide it is best left as is. Completing the fill, you sit the patient up, put a hand on his shoulder, look him squarely in the eye, and forthrightly explain the situation.

You tell Mr. T. it is likely no problem will ever result from this sterile piece of stainless steel lodged in the root. As an honest, if not perfect dentist, you want him to be aware of the situation. You'll continue to monitor healing in the area, proceeding as the situation dictates. The fact of the fractured file and the explanation you shared with your patient are noted in the record.

Let's consider another, more typical, everyday dental scenario—the fear of presenting complete treatment—the horse upon which the fate of every dental office rides. (Or substitute any other personally relevant form of confrontation that entails the possible "death sentence" of rejection and expulsion from the tribe. Universal truths are applicable in every situation.) In such a case, how might one best proceed in light of this new understanding?

1. Name one's fear

Here fear's name is "rejection" and its mechanism is now understood. One's thought might run: "If I tell this new patient what she requires to restore optimal oral health, she might think I'm greedy—only after her money—and repeat this opinion to others. She hasn't had anything other then emergency care and patchwork dentistry for years. How can I hope to change the patterns of a lifetime?"

Those who have studied this work, or human behavior in general, will respond to this internal dialogue thinking, "Wait a minute. I sense my old nemesis . . . the fear of rejection. I've spent a lifetime suffering and under-achieving due to this innate anxiety. I'll listen to fear's counsel, and I'll proceed with appropriate caution, but I no longer allow this emotion to control my decisions and behavior."

2. Focus ahead

Consider the fruits of courage—the joy for team, patient and dentists when an unhealthy, unstable mouth is restored to a state of maximum health, comfort and beauty that may last a lifetime. The dentist will enjoy the well-earned financial success such worthy efforts create, as well as the patient's gratitude and the self-satisfaction of a job well done that is the foundation for lasting happiness.

The patient avoids fractured and lost teeth, the endodontic and periodontal complication that, if existing problems continue unchecked, will destroy the patient's dentition. Her health, longevity, self-confidence and quality of life are all enhanced. Isn't achieving this happy ending the reason you are a dentist?

3. *Accept personal responsibility*

As the trained and licensed expert of dental health care in whom this patient sought to place her trust, it is one's **moral and legal responsibility** to act in a fiduciary capacity in a manner consistent with the patient's self-interest. This is your patient, doctor. There is no one else upon whom this mantle of responsibility and opportunity may be draped.

Dentists are educators and behavioral experts, not merely highly skilled technicians. One's duty is not fulfilled by blurting out a diagnosis. Draw upon your training, experience, and understanding of the human psyche. Use questions to skillfully explore and help clarify each patient's oral health values and desires. It is the health care provider's obligation to develop the behavioral excellence required to allow him or her to enter each patient's understanding and assist in the co-development of a plan to achieve ideal oral health.

Suggesting unneeded care is unethical, immoral and illegal. Such over-treatment might result in short-term monetary gain, but is a formula for long-term disaster that includes, among its many bitter fruits, loss of self-respect. Yet, it takes very few years in this demanding profession to realize that inferior-quality, patchwork dental care, is part of the problem—not the solution. Despite trepidation concerning the risk of rejection, one must fully understand his or her obligation to offer all the care one's training, the dental profession and the legal community deem proper.

4. *Take action*

Read this book and other dental and behavioral texts to maximize one's people skills. Strive for clinical excellence in all you do. Help the patient through a dental-health values clarification—not with lectures and pamphlets—but by asking value-exposing questions, using an intraoral camera and/or a hand-held mirror to deftly educate.

Finally, when one has done all he or she can, accept the patient's decision, if consistent with one's values (I'd be comfortable with any type of restoration, but would refuse to treat any patient who demanded extraction of restorable teeth), and act with clarity and peace of mind.

Fear isn't pleasant, even for the bravest. But it is a vital and inescapable portion of life. With right understanding, one can comprehend fear as a friend and guide. One can sense within its icy grasp the seeds of growth and strength. One can greet fear as the emotion that, when wisely employed to one's advantage, is capable of leading one from the shuddering dark of night to the power and beauty of a sun-filled day.

Chapter Five

Profitable Hygiene

I wish every reader's understanding to be pristine when it comes to the main theme of this chapter, dedicated to dental hygiene. My slogan is shamelessly borrowed from the great minds that devised the campaign strategy resulting in President Clinton's winning his first election. Altered for our purpose, it states unequivocally, "It's all about **PROFIT**, stupid."

As is my wont, we'll drift all over the place, but this book is dedicated to helping others reach their maximum potential within the modern dental world (this achievement being foundational to the attainment of our three-headed goal—success, wealth and joy). Don't let my verbiage ever distract from the central premise of this chapter: **No modern office can achieve its optimal potential without having a highly PROFITABLE hygiene department!! NONE!!!**

There will certainly be no clinical portion to this discussion. I last applied scaler to tooth over 20 years ago, and I was no good at it then. I'm more familiar with Gracie Allen than I am with Gracie Curettes. (My grandparents told me about George Burns and Gracie.) None of the associates ever employed in our office has had any interest in, or demonstrated ability for, performing prophys. No type of periodontal surgery has been offered in our office for 20 years. All forms of soft tissue management are assigned to the capable hands of our hygienist.

Dental hygiene exemplifies great potential juxtaposed with enormous conflict and distress. **In no other area of our profession is the typical dentist's lack of business acumen more glaringly apparent, or a viable option to enhance fiscal return more available.** Hygiene represents a rich vein of ore over which most dental offices camp unaware, not even attempting to sift nuggets with their fingers from the fecund dust below their feet.

I speak with dentists frequently concerning a variety of matters (too damn few of which involve hunting). No topic generates more emotion than the subject of hygiene. The complaints and concerns I most often hear include:

Dentists' Concerns with Hygiene

1. Hygiene loses money

A dear friend of mine went through an extensive one-day course where his entire office numbers were analyzed to the most minute level. His office employs five hygienists. This dental entrepreneur extraordinaire was horrified to find he was **losing approximately $5 per prophy!** That's a bite, when one's staff performs around 40 prophys a day, or 200 per week!

Mercifully, most dentists don't have sufficient patients or staff to allow them to lose money at that level. As a matter of fact, few even know with certainty if their office makes a profit, or suffers a loss, from hygiene. If the hygienist's production is greater than his or her salary, is one doing okay? Sure . . . unless the hygienist is treating patients IN YOUR OFFICE, and thus there exists significant other overhead expense with which one must cope. But let's reserve a discussion concerning the calculation of overhead and profit in hygiene for a bit later.

At this juncture, suffice it to say many dentists consider hygiene as a money-losing, time-eating, pain-in-the-rump, necessary-evil segment of their practice.

2. Hygienists' attitudes can be less than ideal

In a great deal of our nation, hygienists are in short supply, thus great demand. This is sure as hell true in small rural communities of the Midwest, and has been FOREVER! I personally know of excellent offices—thank the Good Lord, not mine—who have spent YEARS in efforts to replace their hygienist. We'll consider recruiting hygienists shortly, but allow me to note that it's been a decade since my most diligent search efforts were able to attract more than one potential hygienist employee.

I believe this supply/demand relationship can create a conundrum, where the potential hygienist-employee is, in fact, the boss. I've often interviewed hygienists who had multiple job offers already on the table, while he or she was the only applicant our office had been able to attract. Such an inverse and confusing relationship—where employees have more leverage than the potential employer—can cause stress for all involved.

I've mentioned how being summoned to my office by our hygienist at the end of the day used to occasion violent shakes and cold sweats. It didn't matter what she wanted—and past hygienists have been quite inventive concerning wants, and as insatiable in their demands as a satyr—I knew I had little choice but to force a smile and agree with the requirement of the moment.

I pay all salaries and it is my name on the office door, but in the small portion of the planet where I reside, if push comes to shove, no matter the hygienist's skills or attitude, both of us know the hygienist could be working in another office the following week, while I'd be fortunate to replace her in a month! (Please recall our current wonderful hygienist, Melissa, aka "Sunshine," is a joy and blessing to our office. I consider her to be the epitome of professionalism and am frequently embarrassed by how short of her lofty standards in attitude and ability I fall.)

When dentists discuss hygiene, I hear expressions such as "prima donna" he or she acts like they are too good for the rest of the team, won't make an effort to fit in, is self-centered . . . you get the idea.

3. Hygiene is perceived as a disrupter of the day and drag on dentist's production

Performing hygiene recare examinations is not listed among the top 5,000 favorite pastimes of the average dentist. Lengthy, complex, demanding treatment is frequently forced to be interrupted because of hygiene checks, and if the examination is not done promptly, the dentist must often face the gimlet-eyed gaze of a behind-schedule-and-not-happy-about-it hygienist. (Brrrr!)

All realize this is not the hygienist's fault, as his or her professionalism, office policy and patient needs demand timeliness. But it's tiring to run this circuit of recall checks every day, and the frustration of being forced to interrupt treatment, seemingly at the worst possible moment, combined with the fact that one need not have an MBA to realize the examinations one abandoned his or her eight-veneer case three times to perform are nowhere near as profitable as fine restorative dental care, results in a mental state for many dentists far to the left of Nirvana.

4. Hygiene is seen as a disproportionate drain on staff effort and cause of office stress

Keeping a hygiene schedule full requires a great deal of staff time. Many dentists wonder if this energy would not be more wisely invested in public relations, checking on insurance questions, or any other activity resulting in maximizing the dentist's production. Assisting hygiene patients at the end of their treatment adds stress to the front desk, crowds the reception room and generally pushes the office toward unpleasant overload, all for the reward of a seemingly minor, if not negative, remuneration.

Other concerns exist, but I think one can grasp the idea inherent within these basic four that many dentists are frustrated and concerned with the status of hygiene as it exists in many modern dental offices. Most dentists realize that, within our profession's current 70% overhead world, they can't afford to reduce time devoted to restorative care to personally perform the low-production task of cleaning teeth. Dentists and patients desperately need the valuable services of hygienists, despite the above-listed negative factors.

Hygiene's Concerns with Dentistry

Don't believe for a second, doctor, that the frustration concerning hygiene is a one-way street, or one may be run over by traffic headed in the opposite direction.

I read PennWell Publishing's *RDH Magazine* carefully each month. The editor, Mark Hartley, is a fine professional, excellent writer, and a friend. I've written for his publication several times. I receive *RDH*, as I like to remain abreast of what's happening in the world of hygiene.

I believe most dentists would be amazed by the controversy, unrest and naked anger displayed toward dentists and the dental profession in many of this fine magazine's articles. There is a very vocal segment (I have no idea of their numbers, but the pointed rhetoric is powerful and perpetual) who consider organized dentistry as the enemy and are dedicated and determined to struggle valiantly to "throw off the shackles of dentist oppression," and enhance the autonomy of the hygiene profession.

I'm a vocal proponent of hygiene, and the valuable, honorable and skilled members of this profession, but I'm obviously not whom they would choose to be their spokesperson. Given my lack of access to hygiene's inner circle, my perception of their complaint is that being controlled by dental boards and dentists stifles opportunities to independently define their profession and truncates growth potential. I believe many feel that a number of dentists perceive hygienists as their enemies. After what I witnessed at my alma mater, I would be inclined to concur with these sentiments.

When the University of Iowa College of Dentistry began efforts to discontinue the hygiene department a few years ago, I wrote a letter to all 1,400 Iowa dentists urging them to act to save this venerable and excellent program. Around 15 responded expressing concern and a willingness to help. (I blame this anemic result on typical dental apathy and short-sightedness . . . although it may have been due to a crappy letter.)

I spoke to the dean of the Dental College, the associate dean of the University of Iowa, an aide to the governor, among others,

255

and read transcripts of the three-member tribunal that reached the decision to recommend closure. I expressed my shock and concern to everyone who would listen that a fine program, producing badly needed talent, was to be discontinued. When the program was cancelled, it left the state of Iowa with two associate schools graduating approximately 30 hygienists per year to provide for the needs of 1,400 dentists.

I was appalled at what seemed, to my un-jaundiced eye, a political hatchet job, where the more powerful dental profession chose to destroy the weaker hygiene department. I heard whispered reasons for the close so personal and offensive I won't repeat them—and as most readers can attest by now, little offends me. (Or as Jo says, "All my taste is in my mouth.")

In summary, a very real problem exists within the dentist-hygienist relationship, at least on the macro level. (I know of many individual situations, similar to our office, where the relationship between hygienist and dentist working together is one of mutual respect and affection . . . generally, it's hoped, confined to a platonic level). As to hygienist's sense of persecution, it has been said one isn't paranoid if they really are after you.

I've read articles from both dentists and hygienists concerning the cause and possible solutions to this raw interface that damages and embarrasses both professions. There are many suggestions extant to ameliorate these problems, ranging from establishing more hygiene schools to group psychotherapy of the Rodney King, "Can't we all just get along?" school of thought. Most of the proposed solutions contain some merit, but are merely hacking at the leaves of the dilemma. As this chapter progresses, I will advance a bold proposal to the profession that strikes to the root of the conundrum.

Keep my contention—that the basic cause of the dentist-versus-hygienist conflict is fiscal—in the forefront of one's awareness as we proceed. As we discuss optimizing hygiene, evaluate what portion of existing distress results from financial disappointments of hygienists and dentists. **The ultimate solution to a financially based problem lies not in identifying clever ways to slice the existing asset pie to everyone's satisfaction,** but to establish a system that makes abundant revenue (bigger pie) available to all parties.

By law in most states, the dentist is the business owner, so it is incumbent upon the doctor to devise a plan to enhance hygiene income and improve relationships of all parties involved. (To eliminate confusion, if one's name appears on the door and the bottom line of the paychecks, like it or not, he or she is the responsible party.)

Answers will be forthcoming from sound business principles and increased awareness that both dentist's and hygienist's times are rare and valuable commodities. Any effort or expense that serves to enhance the productivity of these providers represent a positive and valuable investment.

If a system can be established that:

1. is extraordinarily profitable for dental practices,

2. ends the hygienist shortage instantly,

3. allows hygienists to be significantly better compensated, and also enhances their working environment,

4. while providing superior care for every patient—we'll have established a rare and difficult accomplishment, a win/win/win/win scenario. Such an enlightened office, basking in the glow of this triumphant achievement, will enjoy the serenity bequeathed by a mind-set of mutual abundance, not divisive scarcity.

This describes the dentist-hygienist universe in which I choose to reside. Please allow the thoughts that follow to serve as my personal invitation for all to join me. The necessary ticket is an understanding and implementing of the concept of *expanded hygiene*.

The Mechanism of Expanded Hygiene

(Chapter 14 of *Focus* is devoted to expanded hygiene, but this discussion takes advantage of an additional five years of experience and contemplation to examine the issue in much greater depth.)

Let's observe expanded hygiene in action. As our hygienist is treating her first patient of the day in Room 1, her assistant seats the next hygiene patient in the second room the chairside has previously prepared.

The hygiene assistant exposes any already dentist diagnosed x-rays (I review each patient's record before the day begins, noting any needed x-rays on the day sheet), helps the patient review and update his medical history (this updated medical history is initialed and dated by the patient), takes a blood pressure reading if indicated, and makes certain the patient is comfortable while spending a few moments establishing rapport and answering questions.

When the hygienist completes her portion of care for the first patient, she shifts to the second room where the next patient awaits. All instrumentation and equipment is ready, and she can immediately wash her hands, don gloves and begin performing therapy.

The assistant moves to the first room where she notifies the dentist through our intercom system that "the patient in Room 1 is ready for his **first check**." She then polishes, flosses, and administers topical fluoride (if law allows in your state). She reviews oral hygiene and demonstrates any dental health aids, (flossing instructions, bridge cleaners, electric brushes) the hygienist or dentist has recommended. If the dentist has still not arrived when these tasks are completed, the hygiene assistant returns to the intercom to announce, "Doctor, Mr. Businessman is ready in Room 1 for his **second check**." This is the dentist's notification that it's past time to perform this examination. (Don't you wish one always had two chances to get things right in life?)

Having two rooms available for strictly hygiene use means NEVER HAVING TO DELAY THE EXPENSIVE TALENT THAT IS THE HYGIENIST BY REQUIRING HIM OR HER TO WAIT FOR THE DENTIST TO SHOW UP TO COMPLETE THE EXAMINATION. It also means never forcing the hygienist to interrupt care to allow an exam, resulting in the hygienist's running behind schedule. It also blesses the dentist with a 20- to 30-minute window of time—the hygiene assistant is totally interruptible—in which to perform examinations. It's a lot more convenient to take a break in restorative care sometime within the next 30 minutes, than within the next three.

The hygiene assistant charts and takes notes during the dentist's examination, allowing the hygienist to continue the care for which he or she is highly compensated and uniquely qualified, in the tranquility of the adjacent room. The examination completed, the assistant appoints the patient for his next recare visit (on one of our five treatment room computers), escorts him to the front office, then returns to the operatory, sterilizes instruments and prepares the room for the following patient, when the cycle begins anew.

I'd strongly suggest hygiene personnel schedule recare themselves, as fewer people involved in any system means decreasing chances of errors occurring. The hygienist can also allocate precisely the time needed for the ideal treatment of every unique patient, based on anxiety, plaque and tartar build-up, root sensitivity and including 10 minutes to chat with Ms. Hussy, if one accepts the inevitable fate that one indeed will be chatting, whether the time is scheduled or not.

Also, if paid on commission—a suggestion I recommend and will more fully elucidate in a moment—the hygienist's compensation will depend on each patient's understanding and committing to diagnosed and recommended periodontal treatment. This fiscal reality enhances the tendency for the advantages of preventive care to be fully addressed and stressed by the hygiene team with every patient, as the hygienist's salary is directly affected by his or her ability to gain patient treatment acceptance. (Sound familiar, doctor?)

On the **FIRST DAY** our office switched to compensation based on percentage of production our hygiene revenue **increased 25%** and has never faltered. One can argue it is an employee's duty to work as hard as possible, regardless of the level of compensation. The Soviet Union vigorously examined this philosophy of labor without chance of enhanced personal gain, without notable success.

It used to bug me to see my highly compensated hygienist enjoying a cup of coffee during "open time," still being paid her hourly salary. Now I'm happy to provide the coffee, but I'm not paying for her time as she sips.

I've heard concerns that a hygienist won't perform his or her job as thoroughly—will rush, miss areas of debris, cause patients pain—if compensated by percentage. If the dentist checks each patient, as required by law, he or she should note any areas of calculus that survived the cleaning. A skilled staff should hear and repeat any complaints of roughness, even if the dentist is not directly informed by patients. And I believe hygienists will understand that doing everything within their power to promote the office and establish long-term, positive patient relationships is in their best interests, as they won't be paid to treat patients who don't return for care.

In all candor, I've employed associate dentists who were deficient in skill and/or motivation, and whose work has been suspect. Despite discussed interpersonal problems, I have never experienced a lack of professionalism, skill or dedication from any hygienist within my office over the 24 years I've employed them.

Why go to all this bother? Two rooms and a full-time assistant dedicated to hygiene? While many intangibles can be identified in favor of the system—such as the psychological advantages of establishing a supportive hygiene team to help stave off the hungry wolf of rejection—the definitive answer lies in an analysis of the numbers. **(It's about PROFIT, remember?)**

Our Office Numbers from Expanded Hygiene

I am going to illustrate my proposal using statistics from my practice where we have collectively reaped the fruits of expanded hygiene for approximately 14 of my years in private practice. Please digest the concept, then employ fee and salary figures from one's own office to personalize and enhance the meaning of my example.

Some of you may be concerned that my numbers won't be representative of your situation. True, Keokuk is the Mecca of fine dentistry, but remember, I am one of nine dentists practicing in a Midwestern community of 13,000—mostly blue-collar—souls. Insurance fees are low for our rural area, much below those paid in the Iowa City, Iowa, area (a community 95 miles due north of Keokuk), where the level of dental excellence is seemingly perceived to be significantly better by insurers and/or providing care much more expensive.

I have employed four hygienists during our 14 years of expanded hygiene and have had similar fiscal results with each. In short, it's not the practice, it's not the community, it's not the staff or dentist . . . *it's the system.*

When we began utilizing two rooms and a dedicated hygiene assistant we were instantly able to expand our hygiene schedule from eight to 12 patients a day. In the pre-expanded era, our hygienist spent roughly an hour with each patient. Today, with two staff seeing an average of 12 patients daily, each client receives 80 minutes of staff time. (Sixteen total hours of staff care divided among 12 patients = 1.33 hours per patient.) This leads to enhanced relationships and case acceptance, with more time being available to reinforce vital concepts, and the existence of a more leisurely hygiene pace.

Recall from the previous chapter's monitors (Page 1, Line 34, under December) that Melissa produced an average of $118 per hour in 1997. A single hygienist working an eight-hour day generates a daily production of (8 x $118) = $944. If patients are seen a conservative 200 days annually, total hygiene production is (200 x $944) = $188,800. (Our actual 1997 totals were 175½ eight-hour days of hygiene worked and $171,274 collected. Our numbers were somewhat reduced by Melissa's marriage and honeymoon last summer. Again, best wishes, Sunshine!)

Take a moment and focus on this number. How does it compare to your current hygiene production, or to published national averages? (According to the May 1998 *Dental Economics* practice survey article, the average hygienist produced $6,835 per month or $82,000 per year. Assuming a 40-hour week, this calculates out to $43 per hour. Melissa produces at approximately 2.75 times this level!) I hope each reader is motivated by the realization that if such production is achieved in our little country office, it is possible in his or her office also.

Sure be nice if one got to keep all that! You don't, so let's examine overhead. (My focus on net doesn't waver regardless of our topic.) Your hygienist will probably wish to be paid. Let's assume one is considering my suggestion to establish hygiene compensation as a percentage of production. The harder one's hygienist chooses to work, the greater her compensation . . . just like you, doctor. Depending on the competitiveness of one's practice area, the range of remuneration could be from 20% ($23.60 per hour at $118 production) to 33% ($39 per hour at $118 production). To enhance these figures' relevance, our wonderfully talented Melissa, with six years of experience, was paid $14.50 per hour in a nearby office from which we rescued her.

Hygiene assistant is an entry-level position in our office, requiring outstanding people skills more than dental experience and expertise. (We'll detail the hygiene assistant's duties shortly.) Let's assume the beginning salary range for this team member varies from $7 to $10 per hour.

One must factor in overhead in addition to salary—a difficult figure to define for hygiene—but in our low-overhead, highly efficient office, this averages approximately $18 per hour of hygiene care.

This $18 overhead beyond salary is my best educated guess. I arrived at this figure by noting (see Page 2, Line 11 of Chapter 3's monitors) that hygiene produced 25% of our total office revenue. I assume 25% of rent, phone, utilities and front-office salary is dedicated to hygiene's behalf. I had a staff member total typical hygiene supply expenses (gloves, prophy paste, disposable prophy heads, fluoride, toothbrushes, floss, etc.) for a six-month period and double this figure to estimate annual total dollars of hygiene supply expenses. Adding all items results in total hygiene non-salary expenses, which I divide by the number of hours hygiene saw patients during the year reviewed to reach this $18 hourly estimate.

We have now established a low range of $24 plus $7 plus $18, or $49 per hour of total overhead, to a high range of $39 plus $10 plus $18, or $67 per hour of total overhead. **At $118-per-hour production, this leaves the practice with a remaining hygiene profit of from $51 to $69 per hour.** (Recall the *Dental Economics* figure for average hygiene *production*—not net profit—was $43 per hour.) Based on 200 eight-hour days, we're discussing an **annual NET PROFIT from $81,600 to $110,400 occurring from hygiene alone!**

If this example has failed to excite, take a pulse! The next step is to use one's fees to determine the rate of production one's hygienist would achieve seeing 12 patients a day, rather than eight, thus personalizing my numbers. (To get an estimate of expanded hygiene's effect, add 50%—the increase from eight to 12 patients—to your most recent six months' average hygiene production.) Now repeat my overhead computations with figures from your practice to determine:

a) one's profit or loss from current hygiene.

b) the potential that exists with expanded hygiene.

(Consider that all hygiene overhead except a few supplies and added salary is fixed, so **the additional 50% production is almost entirely profit!**)

Hypothetical Calculations

I'm about to indulge in a pastime that, at least while writing about dental matters, I attempt strictly to avoid: **I'm going to make something up!** Please understand this to be a hypothetical example, useful only to illustrate a bare-bones comparison between conventional and expanded hygiene, the numbers included being nothing more than experienced conjecture on my part.

Let's consider a hygiene department that treats an average of seven patients a day for a prophy fee of $49, resulting in $343 per-day production—very close to *Dental Economics* $344 per-day average. (I'd hope every dentist employing a hygienist would AT LEAST KNOW THE AVERAGE DAILY PRODUCTION OF THIS DEPARTMENT. If not, find out, but please follow my thoughts using your figures.) I'm using a seven-patient average to take into consideration the failed, unfilled cancellations and just plain unscheduled open time that unavoidably appear on most hygiene schedules.

Let's **make up** a hygienist's salary of $20 per hour, for a total gross salary of $160 per eight-hour day. (This is NOT a suggested compensation—plenty of people are already mad at me—merely a modest estimate. I know of hygienists earning twice this amount.) Add to this a non-salary expense of $12 per hour (**made up**), times eight hours = $96 per day. Thus we have total non-expanded daily hygiene overhead of $160 + $96 = $256. Reducing our $343 of production by this amount leaves a net of ($343 - $256 =) $87 per day—about the fee for a two-surface restoration. (Could you place an MO composite during the time it takes to conduct seven examinations? What about two units of crown and bridge at $____?)

These rough (**made up**) calculations are in no way inclusive, as they make no attempt to consider x-rays, sealants, etc. on the revenue side; or social security, workman's compensation, and the inevitable five-patient day (when $245 production results in a negative $11 net) as overhead considerations.

When my thought processes (using **made up data**) are supplemented by accurate figures from one's office, I hope these scribbles, when compared to our previous expanded hygiene figures, allow more light to be shed on the potential of expanded hygiene.

One's calculation should clearly illustrate adding a hygiene assistant will present no financial burden. Can one justify adding a room of equipment to make this concept feasible? If one has the additional space, the practice will pay for top-of-the-line equipment from increased hygiene production alone in about six weeks. Even at our most conservative annual figure of $81,600, one can finance the building or expansion of an office easily on expanded hygiene NET alone.

One last critical hurdle: Do you have the patient load to keep expanded hygiene productive? Even if one's current hygienist is completely booked, a 50% increase in patient load (from eight to 12 daily patients) is required to make the system viable.

In addition to the many patient recruitment ideas that comprise Chapter 3, allow me to advance the following suggestions to enhance one's level of patient flow, all of which our office has implemented for years.

1. Share this information with one's hygienist

Don't be reluctant to reveal my projections of enhanced office net. Your hygienist will be more interested in his or her new salary estimates. Be certain you have completed your homework by using office fees and production to make the example personally relevant. Dentistry may be the only industry embarrassed or reluctant to create a system that improves staff compensation, enhances patient care AND increases the owner's net—an example of the free enterprise system at its finest. (No wonder third parties threaten to engulf our profession.)

Success of expanded hygiene requires the complete and enthusiastic cooperation of one's hygienist. I strongly suggest enlisting his or her zealous support for these proposed practice improvements by offering to change compensation to a percentage of production.

To reach an equitable salary percentage for one's office, take total hygiene production from the last calendar year—say $100,000—and divide that into the hygienist's total W-2 compensation for that year. If the income figure was $28,600, one's new agreement would establish his or her hygienist's salary at ($28,600/$100,000 =) 28.6% of production. If production for the following year was again $100,000, the hygienist's compensation would be unchanged. But, for every dollar above $100,000 produced, the hygienist would earn 28.6 cents. (Again, 28.6% is not a suggested compensation, merely an example to illustrate how easily and accurately percentage of hygiene production paid in salary can be calculated.)

What about paid benefits? All are included in the hygienist's W-2 information, so every existing perquisite—paid vacation, holidays, sick leave, paid staff meeting time, prophys for fellow staff, family and perhaps friends for which there will be no charge—is contained within our hypothetical 28.6%. Be very clear here. While there is no longer a need for separate accounting of benefits, these fringe-benefit dollars haven't been eliminated, but are already factored into the total compensation package.

It has been my experience that hygienists are hard-working professionals, as enthusiastic about enhancing performance and income as any dentist. The idea of two rooms, plus their own chairside dedicated to hygiene, should be attractive, if presented properly. The data we've shared should excite both dentist and hygienist with the vision of a more mutually fulfilling and financially rewarding future.

Hygienists sometimes fear expanded hygiene will leave them burned-out "scaling machines." Just the opposite is true. Freed of the drudgery—unless he or she enjoys exposing and developing x-rays, scrubbing instruments, reviewing medical histories, cleaning and setting up rooms, giving oral hygiene instructions— their work environment becomes more pleasant. Allow me to present the definitive example of this contention for any dentist to comprehend: Would you enjoy working a day without your chairside?

2. Chart audit

We discussed this topic at length in Chapter 3, but now one's office has a hygiene assistant to help with this important, never-ending duty. She too should make five calls per day and be a leader in this task. If one has been in practice a few years, there are probably hundreds of patients out of relationship with one's office available to fill hygiene time, their records accumulating dust in one's file cabinets as their oral health deteriorates.

3. Practice enhancement and marketing

A famous author once stated, "if you build it, they will come."

He referred to ghostly baseball players, but the same concept holds true for patients. An office's physical capacity will establish the absolute limits of practice growth. Expanded hygiene revenue can be used to enhance marketing, or provide the financial foundation and patient flow to allow an associate to join one's practice. (More on group practice in the chapters to follow.) Expanded hygiene may even provide the profit boost necessary to allow a new and expanded office facility to become financially viable.

Expanded hygiene allows patients to experience more individual staff time and attention, thus enhancing the overall dental experience and stimulating referrals.

Expanded hygiene will end the national shortage of licensed hygienists, as with our system each dental office is now capable of an instant 50% increase in patient care.

Rather than injuring the hygiene profession, expansion allows increased remuneration—**without decreasing owner's net**—and improved working conditions, as tedious jobs are shifted to less skilled staff.

A markedly more profitable hygiene department creates higher net for the office, plus performing 12 daily exams, rather than the previous eight, will lead to diagnosis of additional restorative needs and thus increase demand for the dentist's services, especially if hygiene uses its intraoral camera effectively.

(Our dentists request an intraoral image of every patient seen in hygiene be on display when the doctor's examination is begun. The hygienist will usually indicate the tooth or area that requires enhanced dentist and patient attention, while the hygienist assistant actually records the picture. This visual aid greatly facilitates patient education and case acceptance, while saving a lot of that most precious and limited commodity, dentist's and hygienist's time.)

Expanded hygiene is the gas pedal for office acceleration. What dentist wouldn't be supportive and committed to nurturing a profit center of this magnitude?

Our Soft Tissue Procedures and Fees

If one is serious about maximizing hygiene, it is incumbent upon the dentist to hone his or her expertise concerning soft tissue or periodontal treatment. Allow me to suggest two fine courses that can quickly and inexpensively jump-start one's hygiene department. I've attended both, and found each enjoyable and useful.

Dr. Rick Kushner, of *Lean and Mean* seminar fame, founder and editor of *The Simple Truth Newsletter*, offers an excellent and pragmatic course on hygiene. Rick is a marvelously successful dentist and wastes not a word in either lecture or office. He'll provide the real meat, the vital factual knowledge one needs to jump into expanded hygiene on the run. One may obtain information concerning all of Rick's products and activities by calling 1-303-277-0001.

ProDentec, manufacturer of the Rotadent toothbrush I've discussed, also offers courses on soft tissue management. (Dr. Joe Dunlap, one of my heroes, is among their group of lecturers.) I purchased the two piezo scalers Melissa and her patients love from these nice folks, at a significant discount, while attending their course.

I repeat, I have no relationship with ProDentec, other than believing their products to be excellent and the happy fact that my dealings with all their staff have been universally pleasant for a decade. (Bet Jo wishes she could claim the same concerning me.) They have never disappointed our office concerning service or support for any of their products.

I'm sure many other fine periodontal courses are available, but these are the two from which I've benefited the most. Both unerringly focus, not on the biology of the inflammatory reaction, the complexity of various micro-surgery procedures, or other such fascinating minutiae, but on how to establish an efficient, profitable hygiene department that offers state-of-the-art soft tissue management.

In the nature of full disclosure, allow me to share our hygiene fees, not to suggest what another office should charge, as every situation is unique and fees must reflect this, but to en-hance meaning when one compares his or her numbers to ours. We offer five levels of soft tissue management, the degree of individual care determined by the periodontal health of the patient. I won't get into insurance codes, or precise clinical de-scriptions—the class of cleaning is based on the periodontal charting Melissa and her assistant perform—but here are our five prophy levels, complete with fee and ROUGH description. (These fees were as of 1 January, 1998.)

Class A. This is a basic cleaning of stain and light super-gingival tartar, with little or no inflammation present, for which we charge $48.

Class B. This is a heavier prophy, frequently required after a patient is overdue for a routine cleaning. While stain and debris may be heavy, there should be little inflammation, bleeding or pocketing. Our fee is $81.

If one charges a standard Class A fee for a prophy that is months past the professionally recommended interval of peri-odontal maintenance, the message given to the patient is that the cleaning is unimportant, and dentist- and hygienist-suggested time intervals insignificant or contrived. Such a message is un-fair to one's office, to the hygienist who must provide care—often without being allowed sufficient time—and **not consistent with maintaining ideal oral health for one's patients.**

In a behaviorally sound fashion, one must explain how far after the suggested recall interval the patient has arrived. Mirror and/or intraoral camera must be employed to illustrate prob-lems or areas of concern, demonstrating more frequent cleanings are needed and why the fee must be increased. To do less—perhaps due to fear of rejection—is to fail in one's professional duty to obtain and maintain the patient's ideal oral health.

Class C. This is a no mans land—not frank disease, but an unsightly mess, with heavy stain and calculus accumulations, but without significant pocketing or bone loss. (Pretty sophisti-cated clinical description for me!) Any patient with suspected class C or ABOVE cleaning is scheduled for full mouth peri-odontal charting, so I don't get in trouble for incorrectly scheduling the required periodontal treatment. Our fee for a class C prophy is $107.

Class D. This is periodontal treatment—not a cleaning. Multiple pockets, many in the 5 mm range, will be present, most with bleeding. Anesthetic will be used and the entire treatment process will include three visits—two for ½-mouth scalings and a third regular prophy and healing check. The fee is $92 per quadrant plus $48 for the final prophy appointment—a total of $416.

Class F. This is a D gone sour. Lots of 7 mm or greater pockets, with heavy bleeding and often suppuration. Treatment will be completed using anesthesia and be spread over five appointments. (One quadrant per visit plus a regular prophy and healing check at the end of care.) Our fee is $154 per quadrant plus $48 for a total investment of $664.

Melissa and the treating dentist decide when to refer a patient to a periodontist based on disease level, oral hygiene, history of tobacco abuse, the state of his or her general health, pocket and bleeding information, past compliance record, the mood of the patient, etc. Basically, we try to transfer cases we fear might fail.

Due to the level of Melissa's ability, our referrals to a periodontist's office are rare. I have no recollection of any periodontal patient we've treated ever losing all his or her teeth. After initial care is completed, class C, D and F patients are customarily scheduled at three-month intervals for routine recare prophys. (I have no idea what happened to E—maybe E is considered bad luck, like having a 13th floor in hotels?) In addition to these soft tissue fees, all D and F prophy patients are required to purchase and use a Rotadent brush.

One can't perform periodontal treatment at prophy fees during the course of a one-hour appointment, any more than I can do an excellent crown preparation in the time reserved for a class one restoration. Being repeatedly asked to do so by patients and dentists is a topic over which hygienists are rightfully frustrated. To make this request compromises professional values and on this issue hygienists have my complete agreement and support. No dental team member should ever knowingly be placed in situations where time constraints interfere with one's ability to do one's best.

The dentists, hygienist and staff must become educated as to optimal periodontal treatment, including the use of Peridex, when and how to chart pocket depths, ideal frequency of recall interval, and many other topics. **If one doesn't comprehend this basic data, get thee to a course immediately before attempting to upgrade one's hygiene department.** Take your hygienist, her assistant and a front-office staff member with you. (The courses I've recommended discuss ideal hygiene scheduling and the wonderland of periodontally related insurance codes. I get in enough trouble as it is! I sure don't want to be responsible for correctly relaying insurance data to my front-desk people!)

Hygiene Procedures

Here is a partial listing of the main procedure our hygiene department routinely performs, in addition to the afore-discussed A through F periodontal treatment. These valuable services enhance the excellent level of care we provide, while increasing office revenue.

We stress in-office fluoride treatments, especially for adults, who grow increasingly prone to root caries, and for patients of every age with any active decay. In addition to in-office fluorides, we dispense or write prescriptions for Prevident 5000 for adult patients with exposed roots, active decay, extensive restorative work, or in fixed orthodontics.

For children over age 5 with active caries, we prescribe Colgate's .2 fluoride rinse to be used once per week. I strongly suggest each parent select a specific day and time to administer these powerful adjuncts, to be sure they aren't forgotten. I explain that my kids used .2 just before bed every Sunday night. (We live in the country. Until a few years ago, when our residential area was annexed by the city and supplied water from their reservoir, we didn't enjoy a fluoridated water supply.)

As previously mentioned, we also insist all patients in fixed orthodontics, or receiving D or F class periodontal therapy, purchase a Rotadent toothbrush. (ProDentec sells only to dentists, so if this is the brush one prefers, one must make it available in-office. Again, I have no relationship with the company—am no expert on electric brushes, though I've personally tested many and prefer Rotadent—I'm just relating what we do.)

We charge a separate fee for Rotadents, making no attempt to disguise the investment by lumping in the fee as part of over-all treatment costs. I want patients to appreciate this tool as an expensive and important portion of dental care. (Our fee for a Rotadent is $116. The cost varies, but if one buys in LARGE BULK ORDERS, and we do, the price per brush may dip below $60. To earn our fee, we train the patient in proper usage, and handle any problems that may develop with the brush, return-ing it to the parent company ourselves if it requires replacement or repair.)

Over the years, I've had a few periodontal patients refuse to buy an electric brush. We've proceeded with treatment, but I can't recall a single one who completed their required care. (Pur-chasing the brush may indicate patient understanding and acceptance of responsibility concerning his or her dental prob-lems . . . a critical portion of successful periodontal treatment.)

We enthusiastically support sealant use, and have since 1974. We place sealants on ALL kids' permanent molars, seldom on premolars, and almost never on primary teeth. We place them on adult teeth with pits, as I'd want sealants on such an area in my or my loved one's mouth. (Again, I'm not claiming our office policies to be ideal, merely explaining what we do.)

Most of the sealants are placed in hygiene, where having a chairside is invaluable. Our office policy prohibits any provider of care from placing a sealant without an assistant, as it is my strong feeling such a solo effort would result in a diminished quality of care. (I'm certain it would if I were the care provider, as the critical task of keeping a 6-year-old's lower molar dry during sealant placement is fairly challenging when I have help! I refuse to consider that others might possess superior skills al-lowing them to perform the job well without assistance!) If the hygiene assistant is occupied, a dentist's chairside or front-office staff member is borrowed to facilitate this procedure.

Nitrous oxide is available in all five of our operatories, and is a big help during periodontal care and sealant placement. As we've discussed, nitrous oxide eliminates gag reflexes and slows down the peripatetic movements of kids' tongues, greatly aiding efforts to keep teeth dry while sealants are being placed. Nitrous is ideal for procedures that might prove slightly uncomfortable, but don't require local anesthetic for most patients.

I mentioned earlier the extreme value of health-care providers' time, and how, in our office, every possible piece of equipment that can enhance efficiency is provided. Each hygiene operatory has nitrous oxide, an x-ray head, intraoral camera, virtual reality glasses, high-speed fiber optic handpiece (restorative care can be provided in hygiene, but the handpiece is most often used to smooth a chipped tooth or filling, adjust a partial, etc.), piezo and ultra-sonic scaler, and I'll gladly add anything else Melissa might desire.

We're also enthusiastic supporters of tooth lightening procedures. (I had my teeth lightened in the early days of the procedure, when drippy, unpleasant-tasting solutions had to be worn 18 hours a day. I was desperate for ANYTHING THAT MIGHT IMPROVE MY APPEARANCE. So are most of your adult patients!)

The hygiene assistant asks every patient if he or she is interested in whiter teeth. If the patient responds positively, the assistant takes a shade reading and records this data along with a note on our doctor communication pad asking the dentist to discuss tooth lightening with this patient.

Certainly we ask patients multiple times about their desire for whiter teeth, but people's interest and situations evolve. Three consecutive "no" answers might be followed by a "yes" if a relationship change has occurred, or the individual noticed a few more wrinkles.

Our hygiene assistant takes study models, and prepares the whitening tray. Our hygienist inserts the lightening appliance and evaluates the patient every week until we achieve our desired results. **Consult state laws to see what auxiliary functions concerning tooth lightening are legal in your state.**

Our hygiene assistant also exposes the majority of FMX we require for all periodontal patients. (We use a Panorex routinely, but demand an FMX for perio patients.) She also takes routine bitewings, Panorex and PAX as indicated by the dentists.

Let me confuse you in the name of clarity. (Who said I've been doing that for hundreds of pages?) Our office includes examinations as a portion of hygiene production. We do this as, when we first converted to hygiene compensation based on percentage of production (not collection for hygiene), our past records included examinations as part of hygiene production. These figures had no influence on compensation—we then paid our hygienist an hourly salary—but were compiled only for internal use. To establish a compensation percentage we had to either go back and remove all examinations done during the years (this was B.C.—before computers), or leave examinations in our production total.

This seems to perplex folks, but when determining the percentage of production to be paid as hygiene compensation, it makes no difference if examinations are left in or removed. Calculated either way, the forthcoming percentage assures identical production will result in identical future compensation. (The percent figure will change based on excluding or including exams, but the final dollar compensation paid for identical treatment won't be altered.)

Of course, hygienists aren't allowed to perform examinations by law, and if one can easily remove exam fees from hygiene production figures, this would be ideal, but hardly worth forcing someone to re-figure a year of data to accomplish.

Expanded Hygiene Assistant Duties

Besides polishing, flossing, administering fluoride treatments, taking x-rays, performing chart audit calls and the routine tasks we've already discussed, I'd like to mention additional ways in which our hygiene assistant's efforts add value to our office.

We frequently ask her to take orthodontic records and routine study models. There exists a block of time each morning and afternoon, when Melissa begins treatment on her first case, when we have a chair and 20 to 30 minutes of hygiene assistant time available. Also, Melissa is happy to occasionally finish treatment on her last patient of the morning or afternoon, freeing up another segment of hygiene assistant time. (You may have correctly guessed, I'm not one who likes to see anyone I'm paying have nothing to do. Idle hands are the devil's tools . . . at least according to my grandmother.)

Having a chairside's assistance during treatment of advanced periodontal disease and placement of sealants, to ensure a clean field by rinsing, suctioning and retracting tissue, is essential to optimal hygienist efficiency and performance.

Likewise, periodontal charting can be done in half the time, with enhanced accuracy, if an assistant records these numbers into our computer as they are called out by the hygienist.

In Iowa an assistant can perform a toothbrush and prophy-cup fluoride. (Of course, no one but a licensed hygienist or dentist can remove calculus, and any child with tartar buildup is scheduled for a prophylaxis with Melissa.) For child fluorides, we disclose kids' teeth, have them brush away all discernible debris, then polish only any remaining stained areas before administering fluoride. Pumice removes a portion of the super-hard outer layer of enamel, so we avoid polishing kids' teeth unless visible stain is present. Hygiene and chairsides both perform these preventive fluoride treatments in our office, based on who's available and what is most convenient.

Our hygiene assistant also duplicates x-rays for insurance company use, referrals to specialists or for patients leaving our practice. (We never send original films!!) She also makes trays for fixed and removable prosthodontic cases, and tooth lightening stints.

Don't let this wonderful array of skills disguise the fact that the hygiene assistant's main reason to exist is **to optimize patient relationships, answer questions, and be certain each patient feels special attention was given to him or her during recare** visits. Hygiene assistant is primarily a people-skill, communica-tion-intensive position. However, if they can create extra income for the practice at the same time, so much the better.

Hygiene Monitors

In addition to the office monitors we've previously discussed, our hygiene assistant generates internal monitors for hygiene staff and my edification.

February Hygiene Monitors

1	Date	Canc	Filled	Fail	Filled	Open	Filled	Total
2	2	0	0	0	0	0	0	0
3	3	0	0	40	0	0	0	40
4	4	40	40	30	30	30	30	0
5	5	30	0	0	0	0	0	30
6	6	0	0	0	0	0	0	0
7	9	30	30	90	60	0	0	30
8	10	0	0	0	0	0	0	0
9	11	0	0	40	0	0	0	40
10	13	30	0	0	0	0	0	30
11	16	40	40	50	30	30	40	10
12	17	20	20	0	0	0	0	0
13	18	0	0	0	0	0	0	0
14	19	30	0	90	0	0	0	120
15	23	30	30	50	0	0	0	50
16	24	0	0	70	0	0	0	70
17	25	0	0	70	0	0	0	70
18	26	70	0	0	0	0	0	70
19	28	0	0	70	0	0	0	70
20	18 days	160		480		over 10 min		630
21	8.9 min			26.7 min		630 %18 days =		
	canc per day			failed per day		35 min		

35 min lost per day

Consider the February 1998 monitor for unfilled hygiene time. Begin by examining Line 3 which illustrates that on Feb-

276

ruary third, there was 0 cancelled (canc) hygiene minutes (of which 0 were filled). There was 40 minutes of failed (fail) time, all of which remained unfilled, and 0 minutes of open (or unscheduled) time (of which 0 was filled). Thus for the entire day (under total), 40 minutes of hygiene time was unproductive.

Line 4, February fourth, illustrates 40 minutes of canceled time was filled, 30 minutes of failed time was filled and 30 unscheduled minutes were also filled, so no open time existed in our hygiene department that day.

This is a propitious moment to reflect on the likely scenario within your office if 100 minutes of hygiene time was unscheduled for a variety of reasons during any given day. How much would you estimate was likely to be filled, and if you don't have monitors, how would you know? Before hygiene was paid based on production, I can almost guarantee none of this 100 minutes of open time would have been scheduled in my office, posing a severe threat of a potential hygienist caffeine overdose.

Skip to Line 7, February ninth, where 90 minutes of failure occurred, 60 of which was filled, leaving 30 minutes of the day open. See how this works?

Line 21 is the month's summary. An average of 8.9 minutes of cancelled time, 26.7 minutes of failed time and virtually zero minutes of unfilled time existed each day of this month for a composite 35 minutes of open time per hygiene work day in February of 1998. (Often a 40-minute scaling appointment will be scheduled for a patient requiring only 30 minutes of hygienist time, so 10 minutes will remain unfilled—a problem with which Melissa and I can survive.)

We keep monitors concerning open time successfully scheduled to assess our aptitude at the difficult task of filling open time on a hygiene schedule that day. To help fill open time, we offer a 10% discount on all hygiene fees for someone willing to be treated on the day we have open time available. We have nurtured a small community of stay-home folks—basically comprising the retired and moms with all children in school—who expect to be called on short notice and appreciate this price break. We, in turn, are delighted to fill this open time with 90%

of normal production, as even with my rudimentary math skills I understand 90% is more than 0!

Unscheduled hygiene appointments for the next several days are posted on a piece of paper hung next to each provider's day sheet. Thus the entire staff is aware of time available and can help fill these openings from among the patients they treat. Often an additional visit to our practice is saved by our awareness, as a patient already in the office for other care needs a prophy and we can provide it that day. The patient is as grateful for the consideration as we are for the additional opportunity to provide care.

Now let's review the hygiene annual summary monitors.

December Year-To-Date Hygiene Monitor

	Days Worked	Cancel	Fail	Open	Total Loss
January	19	23.3	23.6	0	46.3 min
February	18	7.2	28.8	0	36 min
March	18	12.7	38.8	0	51.6 min
April	22	9.5	16.4	6.4	32.3 min
May	23	17.4	23	7.8	48.2 min
June	17	5.3	18.2	1.8	25.2 min
July	17	8.8	35.9	9.4	54.1 min
August	21	5.7	22.9	21.0	49.6 min
September	21	13.3	21	35.71	70.0 min
October	22	11.46	5.9	18.6	36.8 min
November	18	4.4	22.8	3.3	30.5 min
December	17	6.5	20.6	0	26.7 min
Yr to Date Total	233 days	125.5	277.9	103.37	507.3 min
Average Month	19.4 days	6.5 min cancel	14.3 min fail	5.3 min open	26.1 min lost

Allow me to explain a discrepancy in total days worked between hygiene's and our whole-office monitors. The entire-office monitors break numbers down based on eight-hour days.

I work a five-hour day, Dr. Long around seven, and Dr. White's days vary in length, based on patient demand. We need a common denominator—the eight-hour period—to be certain our comparisons of provider achievements are fair and accurate.

Hygiene monitors consider every day they see any patients as a day worked. Thus their year-end total shows 233 days in the office—an average of 19.4 days per month—compared to our whole-office monitor total of 175½ eight-hour days. Hygiene monitors compare only current hygiene performance with their past performance—apples to apples—so eight-hour segments or not makes little difference, as long as records are consistently kept. If one chooses to implement similar monitors, he or she might be wise to base everything on eight-hour units, just to avoid having to someday provide such a silly explanation!

Our year-to-date hygiene monitor shows an average of 6.5 minutes of cancelled time, 14.3 minutes of failed appointments and 5.3 minutes of open or unscheduled time, for a total annual average of 26.1 minutes of open time per day.

When one begins to monitor, an average below 40 open minutes a day is excellent. One might review his or her office's preceding past few months of hygiene records and calculate how much open time existed, on a daily average basis, in one's own situation, to establish a foundation for comparison. I predict most dentists paying a hygienist a fixed salary—whether hourly, weekly or monthly—are going to receive an unpleasant surprise when faced with accurate totals of non-productive time.

Hygiene production is basically determined by the fullness of their schedule. Although D and F periodontal treatment, sealants and tooth lightening are more lucrative, the large, high-revenue cases possible for dentists don't exist in hygiene. This is why, to be optimally productive, one must carefully control unfilled hygiene time and why we monitor to 1/10 of a minute!

If cancelled time were a problem, it might indicate we'd grown negligent about reminding patients of our long-standing two failures or two same-day cancellation policy, after which events he or she will be dismissed from the practice.

If failed time was increasing, we might concentrate on con-firming all appointments directly with the patient, being sure not to just leave messages.

If unscheduled time was a concern, chart audit or new pa-tient recruitment might require one's attention.

Hygiene also keeps another sheet of monitors for their own information.

Hygiene Monitor Three

	White & Bright	Rotadent	Pt has Rotadent
February 2	1	1	1
3	1	2	1
4	1	1	0
5	1	2	1
6	1	3	1
9	2	2	1
10	2	3	0
11	1	2	0
13	1	1	0
16	2	3	1
17	0	3	2
18	0	3	0
19	0	3	0
23	0	2	0
24	0	2	0
26	2	2	2
28	0	1	0
Total	17	42	11

For February, 1998, we see 17 white and bright treatments were suggested, 42 Rotadents recommended and 11 patients seen are already using a Rotadent. The topics measured on this monitor are determined by Melissa and her assistant and are based on our old friend, the premise that **measured behavior improves.** The hygiene department monitors whatever facet of hygiene they most wish to see grow, and their targets vary as time passes.

For several months they monitored how many warm face towels were handed out, to develop the habit of using this value-added service when the machine was new to our office. Monitoring how many patients had images displayed on hygiene's intraoral camera, or number of tooth lightening cases suggested and accepted, might be worth considering.

Hygiene Recruitment

There exists no advantage to believing in and being committed to an outstanding, profitable hygiene department if a dentist can't employ an excellent hygienist to share one's dream. I believe every dentist can identify and hire this key staff person if he or she is properly motivated by understanding my philosophy and accepting how critical hygiene is to success. If a doctor is thus aware, he or she will pursue a hygienist with a zeal similar to which the drowning seek air!

As a personal credo, I don't accept "can't." I do accept "It isn't worth my trouble," or, "I'm too lazy." My kids are sick of my rejection of their explanations of why something wasn't done with a dismissive wave of my hand and the affirmation that, "People do what they truly desire to do."

I've never been without a hygienist for more than a few weeks, and that single opening was many years ago—probably the event that led to the creation of my hygiene recruiting system. As you'll soon witness, I leave no opportunity unexamined in my hygienist quest. Let's consider doing what everyone else does when they need a hygienist first—only performing it better—before examining a few more original efforts. What follows is the ad we place in dental journals and area newspapers:

DENTAL HYGIENIST

Are you kind, compassionate, people-oriented and motivated to succeed? We are seeking an exceptional person for our progressive office. We focus on warmth, caring and expert communication with our clients. We emphasize personal development through continuing education, full participation with other team members and high involvement with clients. Applicants should be career-minded,

personally stable and health-centered in their lifestyles. If
you are searching for a real opportunity to grow and fulfill
your potential, please call us at 319-524-8811. John A. Wilde,
D.D.S., P.C., and Staff, 1610 Morgan Street, Keokuk, Iowa,
52632.

Every aspect of staff recruitment is covered in great detail
in Chapter 9 of *Focus*. All the forms: applications, phone interviews, patterned personal interviews, and critical **reference
checks** we employ when filling any staff opening are reproduced
there in full, and won't be repeated here. But the first vital step
in any hiring is identifying qualified people and motivating them
to contact one's office. (With 30 Iowa-schooled graduates a year
shared among 1,400 dentists, this is especially true for hygienists.)

Notice our ad avoids all the usual topics and assertions—
good pay, benefits, hours, boss doesn't have too much B.O.—and
focuses entirely on value and character. I don't desire to hire
just a body with a hygiene certificate! I want the special person
described in the advertisement for my exceptional office. I hope
this ad will intrigue hygienists who aren't actively seeking a job,
but also aren't completely happy and satisfied in their current
office. (Reading *RDH* leaves one with the inescapable conclusion that their numbers are legion!)

This ad is placed in all the customary places like *RDH*, 918-
831-9742, *JADA*, 800-621-8099, and every nearby state dental
journal. It often takes two to three months for these advertisements to be published, and I rarely have the luxury of such time,
but I'd rather waste a few hundred dollars on these advertisements and have a hygienist in place when they are run, than risk
still not having a hygienist two months later, and place the ad
then. The profit potential of our hygiene department makes
running the ad an easy decision.

I've also placed these notices in the want-ad section of every major city paper within 250 miles of our office (including
Chicago, St. Louis, Kansas City and Des Moines). This is expensive! In the two times I've run these advertisements, I've yet to

receive a single response; however, I'll try this approach again if I'm ever desperate.

Our hygienist before Melissa gave us one week's notice, which makes one a little tense, when patients are booked solid for the entire year! Melissa was working part-time for us and, to our delight, she left her other office and was working full-time in ours within two weeks. If one lived in or near a urban area (where one hunts what? Pigeons?), a city newspaper want ad might prove successful. Local dental or hygiene societies might also be of assistance in metropolitan settings.

So much for what everyone else does. Now let's deal with the methods whereby almost every hygienist I've ever employed has been recruited.

Most state hygienist associations will provide one with a list, complete with addresses and phone numbers, of every member of their organization. In my experience, it's hard to track these groups down. Usually one has to reach the society's president at home after work, but the lists cost little, as I assume the associations are motivated to help identify employment opportunities for their members.

The ADA (phone number same as JADA, listed above) also provides an inexpensive book listing every hygiene school in America along with the name of the hygiene department head, plus address, phone, fax and e-mail information. We send the following letter to every hygienist listed by state societies and every student in each school within our 250-mile radius of interest:

Dear ,
We are in need of a Dental Hygienist to join our strongly team-oriented dental practice. Our staff is dedicated to helping each other grow as individuals and fulfilling not just the dental needs, but the human needs of our patients. We are seeking a people-oriented individual who desires to develop personally and professionally.

Ours is a general dentistry practice in which care from all dental specialties are included. We are strongly preventive and periodontally oriented, treating advanced periodontal cases. We encourage use of sealants, recommend fluoride aggressively and stress optimum oral health.

Our office is fully computerized (nine (9) terminals), features five (5) fully equipped operatories, all with their own x-rays, N20, intraoral cameras and virtual reality glasses. Two of these completely equipped rooms are reserved for the use of our hygienist and her assistant exclusively. Our staff of three (3) dentists, three (3) chairsides (including expanded hygiene assistant) and three (3) front-office staff are committed to providing the highest quality of care for our over 5,000 patients of record.

We are located in Keokuk, Iowa, a town of 13,000, located on the banks of the Mississippi on the extreme southeast tip of Iowa. We are 95 miles south of Iowa City and midway between Burlington, Iowa, and Quincy, Illinois. Keokuk is a typical friendly Iowa community with an excellent YMCA and downtown mall. The area is sports- and family-oriented, with a mixture of businesses (there exists no one large employer whose labor problems could threaten office prosperity) and a rural flavor.

We appreciate your assistance in our quest for a qualified and motivated individual. This is an outstanding opportunity for the right person and we look forward to hearing from you soon.

Sincerely,

John A. Wilde, D.D.S., P.C., and Staff

As stated, this letter is mailed to every member of the state hygiene association. I personally contact the head of each hygiene school in our tri-state area of Iowa, Illinois and Missouri about a week after the letters are mailed. (I believe speaking directly to a person in authority creates a much stronger impression than merely sending a letter.) Often the school's dean is aware of a graduate looking for work, or has an idea of a possible suitable candidate. The dean will usually agree to place a copy of our letter in each student's mailbox. We also send photos of our office, especially of our two fully equipped and beautiful hygiene rooms, to each educational facility to place in their job-opening files, along with a copy of our letter.

After two weeks, if we've not had several calls expressing interest, either I personally, or a key, experienced member of my staff will contact by phone each member of the state hygiene association to whom we've sent a letter, greet them warmly, inquire if they have any interest in our opportunity and answer any questions. Sometimes the person we call isn't interested, but can direct us to another hygienist who he or she has heard might be a candidate. (Not all hygienists are members of their societies.)

I've never failed to identify a qualified applicant by the combination of these methods. Yes, it's a lot of work and somewhat expensive. If that concerns you, flip back to review the figures of our net profit from hygiene.

As I stated, application forms, patterned interview, etc. are provided in *Focus*. I would caution every dentist to **always perform reference checks on any staff member one is considering employing—including associate dentists and hygienists.** I've heard many horror stories concerning staff embezzlement, alcohol, drug, and other personal problems of a severe nature—all clearly identified in the previous place of employment—if only the new employer had taken a moment to investigate.

Our staff is carefully coached to provide nothing but dates of employment and beginning and ending salary concerning inquiries about any of our previous team members. To volunteer more puts one at legal risk!!! Fortunately, most dental offices aren't aware of this, and especially if one calls staff at home, he or she—including dentists—will often be candid in their comments.

Summary

I reiterate, no modern office can achieve maximum potential without a sophisticated, profitable hygiene department. One now possesses the understanding, resources and motivation needed to begin making this a reality in his or her office. The systems we've discussed throughout this book are integral to optimizing success, wealth and joy. Establishing profitable expanded hygiene is foundational to employing successful associate dentists—who will multiply the impact and advantages of all the previously described practice segments—and who comprise the topic of the following chapter.

REFOCUS FIVE:
THE FRUITS OF OPTIMISM

"But, Ms. Parsimonious, we picked the shade out together, remember? We even went outside to use natural light. You told me they looked great yesterday, before we permanently cemented them in place."

"I remember quite well, Dr. Impecunious, but these teeth are too white and so big and shiny, I look like a horse! And I lispp-p-p when I speak. When my husband walked in the door last night, he took one look at me and laughed! I've been a wreck ever since I got home from your office yesterday. These teeth of yours will ruin me!"

You half-listen to the continuing litany of bitter complaints. Despite an over-all sense of shock-like numbness, your pulse is racing and sharp pains radiate from your stomach. This is a big case for you—replacing an unsightly, discolored, badly worn partial with a six-unit anterior bridge. You planned the case meticulously and worked hard to do your best, plus you need the money to pay this month's bills. The latter thought only adds to your distress.

"Will I have to redo the bridge? The margins and occlusion are excellent. With the resin cement I used, I'm sure I'd have to section—destroy the whole thing—to get it off. Will the lab charge me a second fee? How will I meet payroll if Ms. P. refuses to pay?" These thoughts further cloud your mind as the diatribe continues.

Your entire body slumps as your mental distress intensifies. "I guess I'm a lousy dentist. I'll never be able to make people happy. Who am I trying to fool? Dad was right . . . all that schooling was a waste. I just can't cut it."

Your pulse is now roaring so loudly, you can barely hear your patient's complaints. You feel sweat trickle down the side of your flushed face, adding to your embarrassment and distress. You risk a glance at your assistant. She looks as horrified as you feel. "I wish I could die."

Sorry to put you through that. I'm afraid this, or a similar scenario, is familiar to many—if not all—within the dental profession. Take a moment and calm down. I bring good news. You may never satisfy Ms. Parsimonious, but I'm going to demonstrate some simple techniques to relieve your pain, make your personal and professional life happier, more satisfying and successful, while enhancing your health.

There are **three legs to achievement's stool**. Used together, they will allow one to escape Dr. Impecunious' unpleasant fate. The first two are common knowledge, and we'll touch on them but briefly.

1. *Talent*. None can go far without this essential ingredient, especially in our demanding profession. Dr. I., and the rest of us, can and must labor diligently to enhance skill levels, but increasing talent is slow, difficult work and there is a limit to the talent level each can achieve. (Again, this cruel fact explains my failure to make the NBA.)

2. *Desire*. Few are capable of great achievement without possessing the vital component of desire. This is a trait much more quickly and easily influenced than talent. It is the topic on which many eminent dental leaders focus. A great book, moving speech—or unpaid and overdue bills—are among the many forces that can virtually instantly increase one's desire to excel.

But there is an ebb to desire's flow. An unhappy patient, personal problems, fatigue, illness . . . can deflate desires as quickly as they escalated. How many dentists have returned from an inspiring meeting, arriving at the office ready to slay dragons, only to be carried home on their shields that very night?

There is a third vital component to achievement, unknown to the masses. The psychiatric discipline of cognitive therapy is working to make all more aware of this integral factor. I would recommend the superb text, *Learned Optimism,* by Martin E. Seligman, Ph.D., to anyone interested in further discoveries concerning the fascinating and valuable subject we are about to broach.

3. *Level of Optimism.* There exist two basic ways in which one can view the world. When faced with **adversity,** one will exhibit the mental **beliefs** that distinguish his or her predominant mind-set. In Dr. I. one witnessed the beliefs of a *PESSIMIST.* Faced with conflict, his self-doubt emerges.

The pessimist sees problems as **permanent**—I will NEVER be a success; **pervasive**—I will fail in ALL I attempt; and **personal**—failure is entirely MY FAULT.

The **consequence** of such a belief system is deep melancholy and loss of energy. An overpowering wish to somehow—anyhow—escape a situation that seemingly can't be improved. The pessimistic view of life leads to depression and hopelessness. To heartache and shattered dreams.

Everyone must deal with adversity. But the *OPTIMIST* differs in his or her basic beliefs and reactions. He or she sees adversities of every ilk as **temporary**—Ms. P. too, will pass; **specific**—the problem I face is confined to this individual and time; and **non-personal**—neither he or she, nor one's efforts are to blame for the patient's displeasure.

All are familiar with the "power of positive thinking." Think positively and life will improve. "Every day, in every way, I'm getting better and better." Nothing wrong with programming one's mind in this upbeat manner, but often these carefully nurtured optimistic feelings don't survive one's first confrontation with conflict. (Or next experience with ethyl alcohol.) Any healthy person can feel good when things go his or her way. **It is** the manner in which one handles adversity that most significantly influences success levels in life.

Let the good news begin! There are simple, easily understood and specific ways to transform painfully crippling negative beliefs and, through this process, grow to be an optimist. The first step is to become **aware** in times of adversity and start to listen to one's internal beliefs. (In case you've failed to note this trend, awareness is the vital first step to all growth.) One doesn't need to wait for hard times to begin this growth.

Find a quiet, comfortable place, and reflect on a recent unpleasant event. It might involve a patient, staff or family member. Be courageous, and relive—not just remember—the exchange, allowing yourself to feel the emotions. Listen carefully to your internal dialogue. Do you recognize the agonizing symptoms of self-doubt? What do you tell yourself, and how does this message make you feel?

Here is the crux of my message. It is within the power of everyone to **dispute**—to argue with—their internal beliefs. On reflection later that night, Dr. I. may realize he honestly did everything within his power to make the case a success. Here is one form such an internal dialogue might assume:

"I worked hard with the patient and the lab on this bridge. Maybe if the incisal edges were slightly shortened, the patient would be happier? Anyway, Ms. P.'s displeasure doesn't mean I'm a failure. I was in the top portion of my dental class. It's been tough getting an office started, but most of my patients are pleased with the care I provide, and our office is growing. I doubt many people have ever pleased Ms. P. about anything. No matter what happens in this situation, I'll be fine."

Where pessimistic doubts led to fear, pain and paralysis, the disputing beliefs **energize**. Dr. I. is alive with ideas on how to deal with the situation, and this is to both his benefit and that of the patients he treats.

I must issue a warning. There exists value in pessimism. While optimism leads to vision and energy, it often causes one to overestimate his or her true position. **Studies have shown pessimism**

to be a mind-set that most accurately reflects one's situation. An optimistic mind-set leads one to over-emphasize positive aspects. This affirmative bias distorts reality and can prove dangerous. When one is in an unfamiliar, or critically important juncture—such as about to make a large investment, or decide on a location for a new office—the reality of pessimism will serve one well. But in the great majority of cases, optimism will tremendously enhance quality of life.

Let's return to the office and see how newly optimistic Dr. I. manipulates this fabulous tool.

It's a month later. The newly aware Dr. I. has been carefully examining his internal dialogues and disputing his pessimistic beliefs. Mr. Frugal is in the office for his new-patient examination.

"Doc, the lower left back teeth have chipped some, and once in a while I get a sharp pain when I bite there."

A visual examination reveals teeth 18 and 19 have four-surface, badly worn amalgams. Dr. I. shows his patient in a hand mirror, or with his intraoral camera, what is causing the problem.

"See the chips and roughness along the edges of these two fillings?" Dr. I. explains. "That's caused by the metal aging, and such defects, called ditching, are where decay starts. This dark vertical line is a crack in the tooth. Our x-ray shows no abscess and the roots and bone are strong. These teeth can last a lifetime, but they need to be covered and protected with crowns."

There is an uncomfortable moment of silence before Mr. F. looks Dr. I. straight in the eye and delivers his pronouncement. "Just fill them, would you, Doc? I'm not made of money, and if you need a new car or would like a trip to Hawaii, don't expect me to pay for it."

Thus, adversity knocks, and the doctor's beliefs answer. The senior resident begins the internal dialogue. "I can't believe this. The lecturers I hear and read about get all their patients to commit to these cases routinely. The teeth are symptomatic and this care is desperately needed. What's wrong with me? Maybe I should get my old college job back, flipping burgers."

This is as much of the old garbage as Dr. I.'s strengthening new-found beliefs will tolerate. They dispute these pessimistic ideas vigorously. "Mr. F. may have financial problems, or maybe, for whatever reason, just doesn't value his oral health. He's not been a patient here, so I haven't had a fair chance to gain his trust. I've recommended the right care—exactly what I'd choose for myself or a loved one. I explained and demonstrated as well as possible. It's a compromise I don't like, but maybe with pins and bonded amalgam, the teeth will be comfortable and stable for a while. I'll get a chance to demonstrate my skill, and at a later date, Mr. F. may accept ideal care."

Dr. I. is now energized and motivated. "If you insist, we'll try the fillings, and I'll do my best. We have some newer materials that improve the chances of this treatment's success, but I want to be sure you understand the fillings are a temporary measure. The ultimate need is to cover and protect these teeth with crowns."

Mr. F. nods his understanding, tension melting from his brow. "I want to keep my teeth, Doc. I'm just not sure about these crowns, and money is tight now. I'd appreciate whatever you can do to hold them for a while at least."

Here, in capsule form, is a prescription for joy and success.

1. When faced with adversity (and dentists won't have to be too patient to get there), discipline oneself to listen to one's internal dialogue—a reflection of one's most deeply held convictions.

2. Where beliefs are negative and rob one of energy and joy, **DISPUTE THEM.** Observe the situation from every angle, and study the facts as if it is a problem one needs to solve. (It is!) As one comes to a calmer, more reasoned, less reflex plan of action, note the freedom from distress and the energy to act that is now enjoyed.

Pessimism has its place, when one must accurately and carefully make a major decision, but the fruits of optimism—energy and joy—are addictive. It's one obsession that's good for everyone!

Chapter Six

Multiple-Dentist Offices

We've accomplished much to this point, but all has been merely setting the stage—constructing a solid foundation capable of bearing the weight of a concept that will allow a dental practitioner to **leverage himself or herself and his or her career investment to enjoy net PROFITS that can provide MULTIPLES of solo practice returns.**

I'm going to share my professional history—the bald-faced, unblinking numbers—in even greater detail, as in all candor, we are going to be discussing NET profit possibilities within a group practice venue that achieve a level most solo practitioners don't believe possible. (As support of this assertion, I submit that if they did, they would be doing everything possible to become involved in a group practice.) Such an astounding premise demands the support of concise documentation. Let me open this factual barrage with a mere tidbit . . . an hors d'oeuvre to pique one's appetite as to what follows:

During July and August of 1997, I saw patients a total of 3½ eight-hour days. (Page 1, Line 3 of monitors.) For this two-month period, two weeks of which my family played in the hot sun of Cozumel, Mexico, I had a **personal NET, from my office alone of**

295

$52,000! That's a NET of ($52,000 / 28 hours =) $1,856 per hour, or ($52,000 / 3.5 days =) **$14,857 per day**.

I freely confess to taking a relatively short time period and presenting it to maximize—to sensationalize—the profit possibilities of group practice. However, the figures are the gospel truth, and for a more lengthy and comprehensive evaluation, we'll study my annual net profit totals for all of 1995, 1996, and 1997 later in this chapter.

For now, spend a moment considering how one's vacation plans might be adjusted if faced with a similar financial situation. Then, tropical breezes still stirring one's hair, the smell of coconut perfuming the air, with a smile still on your lips, let's focus on how such a level of income, with so few days devoted to patient care, can be achieved.

Before launching our odyssey, let's be certain all are clear as to our standard unit of measurement. Every reader should be aware of his or her **net per hour**—the most important of all practice statistics, at least in my mind. All one need do to obtain this critical statistic is divide net profit (collected dollars retained after all expenses are paid) by total hours worked per month.

One can adjust net and lower total profit, perhaps for tax purposes (as by deducting various forms of insurance, an automobile, costs of dental meetings and social events related to one's practice, etc., as business expenses). One can also define hours worked in a variety of ways—hours one is physically present in the office, hours actually treating patients (not counting unfilled time, as failed appointments, time on the phone or taking a break) or total hours invested in all aspects of dentistry, including staff meetings and planning sessions. There exists no absolutely ideal definition. Pick a method that has maximum meaning for you, and compute this fundamental hourly net figure.

For the reader's information, we choose to use actual hours spent providing patient care—not time scheduled in office—as our time factor for dentist and hygiene monitors. If a provider has an unfilled hour, that time is not considered. If one works an hour later than scheduled, that time period is added to one's total.

This is not the "correct" way to compute this data—merely the method we feel gives the data maximum relevance. The main consideration is choosing a clearly defined system, then always following the pattern faithfully, so one is perpetually comparing identical situations.

The Average American Dentist

What do we know of the work habits and average hourly net of the typical American dentist? The most definitive study of which I'm aware comes to us from the ADA and consists of 1994 data. (More current information is available, but not as complete. We'll touch on some 1997 numbers, but as I'll be reviewing back to around this period in my personal history, I believe this 1994 information will suffice as a basis of comparison.)

This ADA study found the average U.S. dentist spent 1601 hours at the chair performing dental care and 205 hours a year dealing with tasks they lumped together as "administrative." Thus the average dentist worked 1806 hours (1601 chairside + 205 administrative) or the equivalent of 225¾ eight-hour days. (Author comment . . . My goodness! The mere thought of such hours makes my knees shake!)

In 1994 the average American dentist grossed $317,960 and had a net of $107,780. Overhead averaged 62.7% and collections 95.6%. Now it gets interesting. Annual net computes to ($107,780 / 1806 hours) = **$59.67 NET per hour.** (For the math-adverse, that is substantially LESS than my summer hourly average of $1,856.)

(Allow me to update this information using the May 1998 issue of *Dental Economics* practice survey, which stated that in 1997 the average American general dentist produced $360,000, collecting 96% ($345,600). They had overhead of 68%, resulting in a net income of $110,592. Comparing this to the 1994 ADA numbers above, one sees an approximate 1% increase in net annually. This doesn't compensate for inflation and decidedly will not feed the bulldog. Noting the overhead increase from 62.7% to 68% in three years should give every dentist cold chills! **To suggest how to reverse this rapidly increasing overhead/slowly increasing net dilemma is why this book was written.**)

One may quibble with this 1994 ADA data. Perhaps administrative hours shouldn't count, as who can help but enjoy figuring payroll, working up cases, preparing for and attending staff meetings, performing periodic team member evaluations, composing stirring insurance narrative reports, meeting with unhappy hygienists or patients, etc.? How could such rapture be included as work!?!? So if one removes administrative hours (205), one is left with $107,780 / 1601 = $67.37 per hour average. Let's add 10% to compensate for the pernicious effects of inflation on the purchasing power of the dollar since 1994 to increase our total to $74.11. Take your choice of which figure you believe most accurate. This fact remains:

It is possible to produce $1,856 per hour, rather than $59.67, $67.37 or $74.11. I've done it—am doing it. In Keokuk, Iowa. The guys and gals I believe comprise my audience are, at this point, not incredulous, not jealous, but chomping at the bit (Iowa horse talk) thinking, "Quit babbling and get to telling us **HOW?**"

Of course, the answer lies in group practice. (I don't care what fees are charged, or how clinically skilled the dentist, it's hard to net $52,000 in 3½ days working by oneself!) Dental offices remain mostly solo practices, although the percentage of groups increases, slowly but steadily each year. Probably because of our profession's relatively modest size, dentistry has become the last bastion of the cottage industry. There is great joy inherent in this freedom, and none savor this independence more than I.

But a solo dentist today is as vulnerable as a single, isolated tooth . . . in hyper-occlusion! Perhaps the main message of this book is to allow my readers to come to grips with the unhappy fact that **the days of the small, independent businessperson are GONE** . . . for dentistry as well as every other segment of modern industry. If dentists don't proactively address the realities of the ever-changing world, but continue to insist on fighting insurance giants (whose advertising budgets are greater than total dental care dollars produced per year) and other third-party be-hemoths one-on-one, dentistry as we know and love it is doomed! We are in danger of becoming nothing more than one additional proof of Darwin's theory of survival of the fittest. The independent practice of dentistry will follow in the path of the dodo bird!

Allow me to refresh your memory. Think of the small fam-ily-owned businesses some of you are old enough to recall. Virtually all have passed from existence. Consider the Wal-Marts, super-markets and such that replaced them, or, closer to home, the changes of the last decade as regards optometry, pharmacy and medical professions. (Each possesses unique skills and li-censing protection that amounts to a professional monopoly, now controlled by various and sundry bean-counters!)

I believe dentistry still retains a modicum of control con-cerning our fate, but only if we develop what is demanded to independently evolve into more efficient and competitive group practice alignments. Let's thoughtfully examine this alternative that may still allow dentists to retain personal freedom and profit opportunities unknown to those who toil for a paycheck. (I be-lieve there will always be a niche available for the "super-dentist," those gifted in clinical and behavior skills who can attract pa-tients willing to pay any price for their care. These blessed few need no help. My message is addressed to the remaining 98% of dentists.)

All are aware of how difficult successful associate relation-ships and group practices are to develop and maintain. They are fragile as the most delicate orchid, and their high failure rate is common knowledge. (I like to describe group practice as being similar to marriage—without sex!) What isn't so well under-stood is why these affiliations frequently flounder (dental groups . . . not sexless marriages; most of us can understand the latter's problems), and I believe the numerous demises of dental groups should be the first topic addressed.

Why Group Practice Relationships Fail

Dental groups are subject to the normal pressure that makes any long-term relationship difficult, compounded by the bloated egos inherent within too many doctors. But, in addition to the common, ubiquitous reasons any affiliation might fail, dental groups face these unique challenges:

If each care provider within an office doesn't possess excellent clinical abilities,

If an office isn't a team, dedicated to common goals, proficient at communication and people skills,

If an office isn't highly sophisticated regarding patient attraction (marketing) and patient retainment techniques,

If an office doesn't employ excellent business systems on a perpetual basis to facilitate self-understanding and growth,

If an office doesn't already have a highly profitable expanded hygiene department in place (I really hope these indispensable topics ring a bell???),

Then adding another dentist will likely result in chaos and dismal failure!

One must have all his or her ducks in order—have maximized one's ability within a solo dental setting—before considering group practice. Bringing another provider into a disorganized office, whatever the motivation for the decision, is akin to having a child to "save" a troubled marriage, or attempting to extinguish a spark with gasoline. Like every other "shortcut to success," it's **not going to work!**

In 1985—the last year I had brown hair, and my final year as a solo dentist—my office featured five fully equipped operatories, enjoyed successful expanded hygiene, had effective systems in place allowing us to produce $40,000 per month working four days a week . . . In short, I'd done everything possible to maximize my productivity. (I was also working and drinking way too much!)

Let's segue to 1986, my first year with an associate dentist on board. I'll be the first to admit this was a learning experience, in which I committed many mistakes (recall the cardinal sin of my paying an associate dentist based on production?), but let's compare my 1985 office statistics to 1986 and see if we can begin to sense the nascent power visible within the group concept even during this early trial-and-error period.

Analysis of My Final Solo and First Group Year of Practice

Because our office had done everything possible to optimize productivity, we needed to make almost no changes in our physical plant to add an associate. (No outlay of capital was required, other than modest recruitment expenses—covered in the following chapter—and the procuring of a few "special instruments" without which no dentist can seem to adequately function.) We expanded office hours to include evening and Saturday appointments, so two dentists were able to share five rooms comfortably.

The fixed costs of utilities, rent (paid by my professional corporation to me personally, as I own our space), business insurance (not malpractice, of course), depreciation, etc. remained about the same with two dentists as they had been with one. In 1986 our office overhead, with two dentists and two additional staff working in the office, dropped from a 1985 total of 65%, to 58% (excluding all dentists' compensation), while our average production steadily rose from approximately $40,000 to around $60,000 per month by year's end.

Let's analyze these statistics. In 1985, with myself and seven staff working, we produced $40,000 per month, or $5,714 per staff member. In 1986, with two dentists and nine staff, we produced $60,000 per month, or $6,667 per team member. **Adding almost 17% of productivity per staff member employed** is one easily illustrated economy of scale we enjoyed.

There are many advantages—as well as disadvantages—to group practice, and we'll discuss both pro and con, but make no mistake as to what I consider constitutes the critical benefit: **Total dollars brought into the office increases, while the percentage of overhead decreases, providing a DOUBLE BOOST**

to the dear friend of any business hoping to survive and/or thrive
... NET PROFIT.

In 1985 we produced $40,000 a month with a 65% over-head (35% net) for an average profit of **$14,000**. In 1986, after a number of months of a steady growth trend, two dentists produced $60,000 with a 58% overhead (42% net) for an average monthly profit of **$25,200**.

Granted, this additional net must be shared among two dentists, and the level of compensation for an associate varies greatly by geographic area and supply of dentists. (I've spoken with dentists paying associate compensations ranging from 14% to 42%, but the consensus seems to remain near the 30% of collections mark.)

Our first associate's skills developed to enable him to produce around the $20,000-per-month level. Our agreement was to pay him 30% of production. This awarded him a take-home pay of ($20,000 x 30% =) $6,000 per month. (This was a propitious income for a first year in practice by 1986 Midwestern standards. This young man is an excellent clinician with a strong work ethic and wonderful personality who opened his own office and has gone on to great achievements.) Deduct this compensation from the practice net of $25,200 and the practice owner retains ($25,200 - $6,000 =) $19,200 per month net!

This is ($19,200 - $14,000 =) $5,200 more per month than I was previously making, and my work schedule had not changed, except for an increase in my hourly and total production as a result of short operative appointments and half of the hygiene checks being handled by my associate, freeing me to provide more complex and lucrative care.

I didn't add an associate to increase income and had prepared myself to accept a drop in net. (We'll discuss motivations for associate relationships in a moment.) I was stunned when I realized the level of increased profitability that had occurred. (This enhanced profit developed over a number of months as our recent graduate's clinical efficiency steadily increased, and as collections took their customary six months after adding a provider to return to our office norm of near 100%. After the first six months with an associate paid on production, my net was $15,000 LESS than the previous year, and I was concerned.)

My first reaction to awareness of the enhanced profitability our office had achieved (well, I guess it followed a very full, Cheshire-cat smile) was to be concerned that I'd stolen money from this fine young man. Remember, this was my first experience with multiple dentists, and I was making up rules as we went along. Let's continue to analyze this data.

I had reduced office overhead, as is the duty of any skilled manager, by 7%. Seven percent of $60,000 is $4,200. So all but ($5,200 - $4,200 =) $1,000 of my enhanced income came not from the associate's pocket, but from my managerial ability to decrease the average percentile expense of dental care provided.

For this $1,000 per month net not resulting from better management, I provided my associate with patients, trained staff, excellent office systems, dealt with the great majority of problems concerning staff or patients and created a vision for his future within the profession. Would any of you running your own practice be unhappy to invest $1,000 a month for such benefits? I personally believe this to be an unparalleled bargain!

One last point: this additional profit accrues month after month, unless the office finds methods in which to grow and improve. Then it increases!

Why Consider Group Practice?

We've already touched on what I consider as the most compelling argument for multiple-dentist practice configurations by reviewing the first year's enhanced profitability in my office. I'd leaped from a very respectable $168,000 annual net as a solo dentist in 1985 to an amazing (to me, at least) $230,400 net per year with no change in my treatment hours. (I'm too lazy to adjust these figures precisely for inflation, but if stated in terms of today's dollars, assuming a 4% inflation average, the equivalent of my 1986 total stated in 1998 dollars would be approximately $391,400.)

This data was all discovered in retrospect, about a year after my first associate joined my office. As I've mentioned, increased profit was not my motivation (or even dream) for seeking an associate. My purpose was entirely to reduce the pressure of patient care from which I had to have relief. (I entered treatment for alcoholism near the end of my first associate's year in our practice, and suspect my addicted behavior played a role in his eventually leaving our office.)

Before adding an associate, our office had not accepted new patients for four years, but we still had approximately 5,000 active patients and I frequently treated **10 emergency patients a day**. I recount in *Focus* how I returned from a week of skiing/ drinking (guess the drinking part of the story is new) in Colorado to a completely booked week's schedule and a list of 45 emergency patients plastered to my laboratory wall, each waiting none too patiently to be seen. During the course of that week approximately 40 additional patients with acute problems had to be cared for.

I was exhausted from driving 18 straight hours to Colorado, then 18 hours back, attending continuing education meetings early mornings and evenings, and skiing all day, every day. (This was at the peak of my addiction, and I don't even want to consider the level of my alcohol consumption. I do remember drinking 18 beers during the drive out—carefully pacing myself to one an hour. Just the idea today makes my liver swell!) By the time the week of my return mercifully ended, I was exhausted and, perhaps for the first time in my life, scared and desperate for assistance. I knew I had to have help!

So much for my story. Before we proceed in our discussion of the benefits of a group, be aware that not every practice is blessed with the option of being able to employ an associate immediately. If the office isn't running smoothly, then system problems exist that must be addressed before adding a dentist. If one has open time on his or her schedule, no matter how compelling the following arguments appear, one is not ready to have another dentist join his or her office. This doesn't mean one can never form a group, but indicates additional effort is required first. We of the Heartland clearly understand that one must prepare the soil properly before planting a seed, if one wishes a bountiful harvest.

Common signs that it might be time to add an additional dentist include:

1. One's practice is overly busy

The solo dentist is working nights, through lunch, on scheduled days off, to fulfill treatment demands. Patients are forced to wait weeks for necessary care. Under such circumstances the most desirable patients—the ones most serious about their dental health—will be abandoning this too-busy office.

2. One's office has reached a financial plateau

No matter how or what is attempted—what courses are taken, consultants employed, concepts incorporated, new equipment purchased—revenue has remained basically flat for several years. In an already ultra-efficient office—maximized as regards physical plant and staffing, proficient in the areas and systems we've been considering—this means one has attained the peak of practice capacity and no further growth is possible without adding additional dentist help.

3. One's energy and/or interests are flagging

Your body is strongly suggesting it is time for you to cut back, to reduce the pressure. This is one message I'd earnestly suggest each doctor honor—based on personal history—for the sake of his or her physical and emotional health, in addition to the well-being of one's office and patients.

In light of these three factors, should the timing seem propitious, let's consider common reasons why an established practitioner might be motivated to add an associate dentist to his or her staff:

1. Reduce the pressure of providing treatment in an overly busy office, or provide help for a clinician wishing to slow the pace at which he or she practices.

2. Diminish the strain of steadily escalating overhead, (increasing 1% a year on average for over a decade!) and, when this is combined with increased productivity, dramatically increase profits.

These two topics have been previously, I trust adequately, discussed.

3. Expand hours and available treatment.

As mentioned, with the addition of an associate our practice began to schedule evening and Saturday office hours. We also opened the doors earlier in the morning, as while two dentists and a hygienist can co-exist in five operatories, it's a whole lot roomier if they work contiguously only a few hours per day. One dentist is optimally scheduled for predominantly morning care each day, the other for afternoon and evening hours, with no more than a two-hour overlap occurring at midday. (Each provider works some morning, some evening hours, so patients with every possible time requirement, except Sundays, can be treated by the dentist of their choice.)

It's quite possible the new dentist will also provide treatment the senior dentist had referred, be it oral surgery, endodontics, advanced periodontal care, veneers, implants, etc. Undoubtedly due to my limited ability/interest, almost every associate we've employed (there have been seven dentists share my office over 11 years, including Lowell and Joe, who currently work with me) has expanded available services.

It was after I added an associate that I found time to pursue orthodontic training and personally enhance the breadth of care our office could offer. I was also allowed to focus additional study and clinical time on TMJ—an area of treatment both challenging and (for me, at least) fascinating. (But I'd sure hate to try feeding my family—hell, feeding my pets—on the income that accrues from my TMJ treatment in Keokuk, Iowa!)

4. Bring in a potential partner or future office owner

Much has been written on this topic. With some of the ideas I am in agreement, with some I disagree. I don't want this issue to become a focal point of our discussion, as the subject is complex, and I fear only appeals to the relatively few in my audience nearing retirement. However, let's briefly contemplate the associate as an office purchaser.

A typical practice transition scenario involves a very senior dentist (read "old") selling a badly declining office, for a fraction of what it was worth a decade ago, to a recent graduate. The practice owner is usually forced to finance the purchase himself or herself, as few banks or financial institutions want to touch an unknown and unproven commodity (a new graduate) with $100,000 in debt and a 10-year-old car, a cat and battered suitcase as his or her only collateral.

The worst possible outcome might be for the practice purchase to be consummated, then the new dentist to capitulate after two years of near-starvation and quit making payments, returning ownership to Dr. Senior. The senior dentist, now living blissfully in a no-children-allowed, walled community, somewhere near an ocean, mountain or desert, is forced to come back to re-open and re-sell the practice, or forfeit this source of income.

In contrast, let's consider a buy-out where an established associate purchases Dr. Senior's practice. From the young dentist's perspective, after working in the office for several years, having created warm relationships with staff and patients of record, while establishing a predictable stream of income, his or her chances of success as the office's new owner are greatly enhanced. A financial institution would probably be willing to invest in what is now a stable and predictable (two things banks appreciate more than I love hunting!) business venture, removing the risk of the transaction from the slumping shoulders of Dr. Senior (with whom I empathize!).

Of course, the senior dentist is also greatly benefited by this stability, and by bringing in an associate at an earlier date, (this infusion of youthful energy, abetted by wise counsel, allowing the practice to expand, despite flagging interest by the founding dentist), it's possible the office might be more valuable . . . or at least not have diminished in worth when eventually sold.

This is one broad, over-simplified example of a complex subject with virtually unlimited variables. Despite the short-comings of this illustration, I believe it is apparent how both associate-buyer and owner-seller chances for success and joy can be enhanced if the practice purchaser is already a successful employee of the office.

5. *Leverage one's investment*

How many businesses of any description can afford to invest hundreds of thousands of dollars in equipment and facilities, and be open 32 hours a week, 48 weeks a year? Answer: none but dear old dentistry.

As a Midwestern analogy, the fact that family farms that only grow crops (not raise livestock too) are workable for approximately seven months of the year has proven an almost certain death sentence to this capital-intensive industry. (The cost of one major piece of modern farm equipment would fully equip a dental office, and they aren't giving the land away either.)

It saddens me to witness the many abandoned farm homes in Iowa, Illinois and Missouri as I traverse the beautiful countryside while hunting. We are forfeiting not just a small industry—nothing new there—but what I consider a wonderful and badly needed way of life, that fostered good health and close families with strong personal values and rock-solid work ethics, at a time when our culture desperately needs such attributes.

Small farmers who have survived have second, primarily winter jobs and wives with employment providing additional incomes to allow them the luxury of continuing this inefficient but often beloved business. Dentists who insist on the 32-hour/48-week use of assets better consider a similar second-job strategy. (Marrying wealth is a viable option I dearly regret not considering. Dad always told me it is just as easy to love a rich woman. Would I had listened!)

Being open more hours and days significantly enhances the return—both average and total—on the tremendous fixed cost of a modern dental office. (A solo dentist typically cares for patients 48 weeks x 4 days = 192 days. With an associate the same facility may see patients 52 weeks x 6 days = 312; a **120-day addition**, not including daily expanded hours that probably **double the total time one's capital investment is in use.)**

Extra or non-essential equipment—the computers, intraoral cameras, etc.—are more affordable when using longer hours to greater effect, and purchases of such high-tech, high-price assets represent a much smaller percentage of group practice revenue. Multiple dentists also leverage the return of marketing efforts. (The cost to advertise a five-dentist clinic is the same per ad unit as for a solo office, but the expense is split five ways.)

6. Create passive income

Passive income is money made NOT as a direct result of one's labors. (Investment income is a common example.) Here is an apparently difficult paradigm shift the dentist/entrepreneur must make: **It is acceptable to make money by employing one's brains, not just one's fingers**. (This is the crux of the famous admonition to work smarter, not harder.) My time spent visualizing, planning and enhancing practice systems is of more value than my efforts in treatment. (Of course, that might not be so strongly the case had I any proclivity toward the treatment end. One does what one can! And in any service industry, if the office leader is focusing on systems and vision, and isn't providing care, someone else MUST BE.)

I believe I've spent sufficient time astride the soapbox concerning this central financial topic, near and dear to my old ticker. I also believe the analysis of my office in 1985 / 1986, as well as three years of additional figures that will be considered later in this chapter, demonstrate my contention more effective than further words might—so I'll shut up!

7. Reduce out-of-office referrals, thus enhancing office productivity within the same space and office population

We've touched on this topic before. It's probably impossible for any dentist to remain current as regards every facet of care available today. (My good friend, Dr. Craig Callen, is the exception that proves the rule, as his understanding of technical dentistry is simply astounding!)

The more each dentist in an office is able to specialize, the more skilled, efficient and profitable he or she becomes in that concise area of expertise. Focusing on clinical techniques one enjoys enables one to decrease treatment that proves not of interest or reward, thus enhancing both profitability and joy.

As one small example, adding Dr. Joe White to our office as a third dentist greatly decreased our referral of oral surgery, as this is a procedure Joe enjoys, while I detest pulling teeth, and Dr. Long doesn't enjoy this task. I'd conservatively estimate our office referred 10 extraction cases a week, and over the course of years, performing this treatment in-house adds significant income to our practice, and enhances patient appreciation, as few enjoy referral to an unfamiliar office. (Better the devil one knows? Also, it's always a comfort knowing where the bathroom is located!)

The ability to offer a diverse menu of services attracts patients, as most prefer all their dental care be completed in a single office setting. Little extra expense or overhead is required to perform these additional services, so office profit is sharply enhanced.

8. Built-in disability coverage

Not only is some income guaranteed the owner dentists who employ associates in case of disability (recall, our profit from hygiene is ongoing, even when I'm not in-office, as long as dentist supervision is possible), but one's staff is assured employment—thus not forced to seek another job—even if all must endure slightly reduced hours.

Also, one's patients will be cared for while the disabled dentist is out of the office and not be required to go elsewhere for needed treatment when their dentist of choice is unavailable due to health problems. Often new patients are attracted when their solo dentist (whom they often haven't seen for five years!) is unavailable and our office is open to provide emergency care.

Vacations, holidays and weekends are also much easier to cover in multiple-provider offices.

Buy-out agreements and even cross life insurance policies, taken out by each partner on the other to fund office purchase in case of death, are valuable, attractive and relatively inexpensive built-in options possible for all parties—be they senior or junior—involved in dental group practices. (We have never used life insurance in this manner. Due to my fortunate financial situation, even in 1985, I felt no need of additional income protection, and no associate has ever suggested such an arrangement. If the practice owner has minor children and debts, such insurance arrangements should be given serious consideration.)

9. *Flexibility to phase out active patient care slowly*

This has proven a significant, totally unplanned benefit to me. **During their entire existence, the time in which men are most likely to die occurs during the first six months after one retires.** Being allowed to make this critical transition, from worker to retiree, slowly—a difficult accomplishment for a solo dentist who must bear the full burden of office overhead, plus commitments to staff and patients—can literally be a lifesaver!

I am aware of no similar data for women, but assume their longer life-span would make this grim prediction unlikely to be true for them. My guess is, as is the case with cancer and smoking-related deaths among women increasing steadily, females in the work force are "gaining ground" on men in this morbid category too.

In over a decade of working with associates, I have gradually reduced my annual time commitment to patient care from 200 days to the current 30-something (while watching my net income remain comfortably above the dental average, as will be detailed in a moment). I've allowed myself to naturally and slowly grow into other areas of interest and passion such as writing and speaking, as well as hobbies such as hunting, reading, gardening, tennis, racquetball, investing, fishing, etc.

I'm often asked what I do, since I work so little. My totally candid reply of "whatever I wish to" doesn't seem to be completely comprehended or appreciated by most as the wonderful blessing such freedom assuredly is. What a gift to be unfettered to pursue whatever (not whomever!) in life creates passion! To be allowed to live precisely as one chooses. After 25 years chained to a 10-minute-unit appointment book, few can savor freedom more than I!

But perhaps the transition of greatest significance has been in enjoying the luxury of slowly redefining myself. I am no longer limited to being what I do to make a living. (The standard response to the query of, "What do you do?" with "I'm a dentist" now seems pathetically confining. This constricted awareness is nothing more than a quirk of the time and culture we inhabit. Aren't we all a great deal more than how we make a living?)

I no longer judge myself based primarily on how hard I labor or how much money I make. As are many who come from relative poverty, for most of my life I was rigid in this regard, and at first felt guilty as I tentatively reduced my office hours. I can empathize with the fatal shock so many experience when they realize their long-desired retirement has robbed them of their identity and reason to exist.

Some of you may have attained sufficient rings around your personal tree of life to understand that a portion of the aging process means one gets tired more easily, more quickly. (I was born December 14, 1946. I've had to give up basketball, and three sets of singles tennis is becoming a rarity.) Shorter days, with more breaks and relief from all financial pressures, are true blessings as the weight of years evermore stridently calls for one to slow down! This segues nicely to our next topic:

10. The office is elevated by the youthful energy and enthusiasm of a new associate. (Especially the Preternatural Vitality of Youth Inspired by Being Buried Under a Mountain of Debt)

There is much to be said for youthful enthusiasm—as well as much to be concerned about—but we'll consider the cons of associate relationships later. Eager, hungry (literally as well as metaphorically today) young dentists can provide a lift to staff

312

and senior dentist, challenging them to abandon possible complacency and "hardening of the attitudes," and continue to grow.

These young dentists, with time and energy available, can engage in personal marketing, calling on other dentists (and begging for referrals, as I once did), meeting pharmacists, realtors, hospital emergency room staff and others in the community who might be in a position to refer business to one's office, thus fueling the primary source of vitality—more patients—of any practice.

I believe it incumbent upon the senior dentist to provide precise guidelines as to what practice-enhancing activities he or she feels appropriate for the new associate, but also to be sure timidity doesn't prevent these important tasks from being accomplished.

Our office still bears my name, and I don't wish any member of my team to engage in behavior—no matter how well intended—I would find embarrassing. On the other hand, while I've never asked an associate to undertake anything I have not done, many young dentists "feel uncomfortable" performing these basic practice-enhancing activities. (Such discomfort results from facing one's fears of rejection, and invariably accompanies growth.)

I was completely booked from the day my office first opened, yet did all of the above mentioned practice-enhancing actions, as I had a wife, two kids and a smattering of cats who kept getting hungry. Reality was an incentive vastly superior to the hindrance created by my fear of rejection. I'd have a great deal of concern about the future of an associate unwilling to do his or her part to help one's practice grow.

11. Enhanced revenue makes adding equipment more feasible

Dentists are in a competitive market situation. (To grant some perspective, 20 years ago I paid money to attend courses on how to properly dismiss patients!) As in any industry so challenged, a dentist must discover ways to differentiate his or her office from the masses. Certainly the behavior skills we've discussed are essential, but computers, air abrasion, intraoral cameras, digital radiography, electric anesthetic and a plethora of other new techniques and devices create interesting reading in the local papers and present one's office in a progressive and positive light.

(I recall my horror upon seeing a local newspaper article, clipped from a wire service, concerning a dental office offering patients virtual reality glasses, as we'd had these glasses available for some time in our office! Today, with the time I have available, and a single staff member in charge of our office public relations, I hope such a lost opportunity for our office to be impossible. Has your local paper ever run an article concerning dentistry that didn't come from your office? How did you react to this situation? If you've made no deliberate effort to become acquainted with people of influence on the local newspaper staff, you've forfeited a great opportunity for free practice promotion. **WHY?!**)

These practice adjuncts are expensive, and while many enhance productivity potential, some are hard to justify on a return of revenue basis, especially for a 32-hour / 48-week solo office. Splitting the bill among two or three providers whose office is open twice the hours (or purchasing them in mass quantities, at deep discounts, as can an insurance- or other third-party-owned large group practice) seems essential for one to remain "cutting edge" competitive, and still profitable today.

12. Attracting additional new patients

Within a few months of our first associate joining our office, we'd experienced a **50% increase in new patients.** Enhanced capacity for treatment, expanded hours, some external marketing (in 1986, this consisted mainly of a photo and article in the local paper welcoming the associate to our office), and the energy and presence of this young man and additional staff within our community are among the forces that resulted in this increase.

I can't speak to new-patient flow as regards solo to multiple-provider practices from a statistical basis after my first year in a group, as we've virtually always had at least one other dentist, making further comparisons to solo days impossible. Our office performed 356 new-patient examinations in 1996, and 298 in 1997 (Page 3, Lines 8,9 monitors). Perhaps one can judge the effectiveness of our group at attracting clients by comparing our office new-patient flow to one's own.

13. *Internal and continuous peer review*

These are dangerously litigious times in which dentists exist. Legal pressure, plus one's own moral compass, should provide sufficient motivation and guidance to offer the best care of which one is capable. But, knowing a colleague and friend will be observing one's work enhances one's incentive to always perform at his or her best. One can also benefit from gently constructive criticism given by another dentist, totally familiar with one's practice situation, thus replete with almost perfect empathy.

The other dentists in one's office may be forced to treat the same difficult patient, and understand how a procedure might lack the perfection one desired. Nobody—not wife, lover, child, staff member or dog—can possess the complete and honest understanding to which another dentist is privy who faces the same trials and tribulations attempting to provide the best care of which one is capable.

All dentists within the same office are rewarded by successful care provided by any member of the team, as this production adds to total office revenue, so they have strong motivations to keep the best interests of each staff member in their heart and do whatever is possible to assist them in achieving optimal success. A fellow member of one's group who doesn't do his or her all to support team members is exhibiting immaturity and foolishly diminishing his or her, as well as the group's, prospects for prosperity.

These lucky 13 advantages create a powerful motivation for practice owners to investigate multiple-dentist offices.

Why a Dentist Might Seek to Join an Established Group

Let's consider motivations a dentist might find compelling enough to encourage him or her to join an established practice, rather than opening a solo office. As mentioned, I've had seven associates; four have been veteran dentists—I believe two slightly older than I—and three have been recent graduates. (I've never been fortunate enough to recruit a new graduate of a residency or military dental program. It would seem such experience would be ideal, as the dentist would have gained enhanced clinical ability, confidence and finesse, yet not be totally set in his or her ways, or have developed a powerful office vision that might conflict with the practice culture he or she will be joining.)

The following comments represent nothing more than personal reflections based on the sum of my years working with associate dentists. I make no claim to understand what may define the ideal associate candidate for any given office. I have no idea how valid the following thoughts and experiences might prove outside my little country office (and my smaller country brain). That caveat issued, the only dentists with which I've had long-term success have been recent graduates. I suspect the following two reasons explain my failure to establish enduring relationships with more seasoned, clinically skilled practitioners:

1. It's very hard to have experienced the autonomy of running one's own practice, then be forced to suffer any other boss. Yet commonly accepted values and consistent systems are essential for all within a group to uphold. Any deviation from these instigated by a new doctor disrupts office harmony and efficiency.

Being compelled to conform to a system whose beliefs one doesn't share seems an unavoidable source of friction. I don't think there's any way I could work as another's employee . . . at least for more than a day! (Obviously, the experienced dentists weren't too successful in running their previous offices, or they wouldn't be seeking new employment. But freedom—even when diluted by minimal accomplishments—is still a heady brew!) Recent graduates have no prior practice experience with which one's office systems and values might conflict.

2. When a dentist is 40 or so, and beginning one's career all over again, no matter how plausible the story explaining the circumstances, something is wrong.

Allow me to further quantify my experience and bias. (All have bias—the enlightened are more aware of theirs, and thus able to temper judgement in light of this realization.) I have never joined another group, or—other than as a student extern—ever been employed by another dentist. While the reasons for adding an associate to an existing practice are tried and true segments of my experience (earned with sweat, tears and years), the information that follows concerning motivations for a dentist to join a successful office are of an intellectual—not experiential—nature. A world of difference exists between these two sources of potential wisdom. My lack of bona fide credentials and background in this perspective of group practice stated, let's examine possible reasons for dentists to consider joining an existing practice.

1. Lack of funds to open an office

File this under cold, cruel reality. The customary financial plight of today's graduates (unless parents paid their educational expenses) is horrific! I've bored you with my story of working eight years, married three of those years, and Jo and I having a child without benefit of insurance; and, while paying 100% of my living and education expenses, graduating a mere $5,000 in debt. (Five thousand dollars didn't seem "mere" at the time!) I damn near killed myself, but *DEBT WAS NOT, IS NOT, ACCEPT-ABLE TO ME.*

The far too typical $100,000 debt of today's dental graduates places him or her another **decade** in arrears as regards financial achievement. (He or she is already at least eight years behind the high school buddies who entered the work force directly.) Our nation, our society and our baby dentists must somehow learn that, despite its deceptive allure, debt is NOT a portion of the pathway to success, wealth and joy.

Fiscal sophisticates successfully borrow money to use as a tool, but debt in our current culture is more commonly employed to purchase toys designed to disguise the emptiness of one's existence. Debt as an instrument of wealth enhancement is a nuance beyond the grasp of almost all dental students, and most dentists. The concept of using other people's money to advance financially is far too potentially destructive to be dabbled with by the great majority . . . including me!

Borrowing money is a **decision—a choice one makes—that MORTGAGES THE BORROWER'S FUTURE.** If such a choice must be made—and to achieve an education, open an office, purchase a home, it usually must—it is imperative the debtor fully realize the significance of the obligation he or she has incurred. That they understand the total effect of compounding interest payments on personal wealth. (As we study finances in Chapter 8, my diatribe concerning debt will continue, and we'll consider how the **behavior** of most proves them lacking in this central awareness.)

In addition to existing student debt pressure, the investment required to open a modern practice is staggering! We're not talking one chair in a 200-square-foot space over the bank any more. (This description recalls my family dentist's practice when I was a child. Those 20-some steps that ascended the shadowy stairwell to Dr. Wilson's office seemed steep and foreboding to me, even in my youth.)

To open an office enabling one to successfully compete with established practices could add another $100,000 in debt, if it's possible for a new graduate with no collateral and NO PATIENTS to find a lending institution willing to commit to such a risk. (My third book, *How to Create the Dental Practice of Your Dreams*, deals with several possible ways in which this office financing might occur; none of them simple or without peril.)

The encroachment of insurance, government, and other third-party forces, the continued oversupply of dentists, diminished rate of decay, the frequency with which inexperienced

318

dentists feel compelled to join plans offering remuneration that makes profitability impossible for all but the most efficient, are all major factors adding to the fiscal pressures of a modern dental practice. The influence of these debilitating forces is even greater upon beginning practitioners.

In the early days of my practice no such third-party forces significantly impacted dentistry, and the supply of dentists was inadequate to meet patient demand. Many established practices routinely referred patients they were unable to find time to treat to our office. Annual insurance limits of $1,000 were GENEROUS in those days of $200 crowns. My goodness, how times have changed!

2. Lack of business skills

I am aware of no period during which a dentist completed his or her eight years of education being even slightly prepared to make a living in the world. Despite my perpetual whining (of which this is but another example), there is no discernible trend to rectify this glaring deficiency by any dental educational institute of which I am aware.

If it helps any, my M.D. brother, lawyer son and even my master's-in-finance, business-school daughter were no better prepared than dentists by their educational experience for the realities of earning their daily bread. Possibly college educators honestly don't know how to provide for themselves, let alone guide another, except by cashing their salary check. Teachers who have never been forced to "make a payroll" represent a level of blissful unawareness of reality akin to Marie Antoinette who, when informed the starving masses of Paris had no bread, suggested they eat cake!

A generation ago, one could survive this lack of fiscal preparation. Today the debt burden graduates carry and the much more competitive nature of our profession have reduced the margin of error for many beginning a dental business to practically nil. The subsequent stress and strain under which recent graduates suffer is many times greater than the significant level of tension I endured. Residency, military, and other training pro-

319

grams enhance clinical skills, but consume energy or add debt, while only prolonging the ultimate facing of fiscal reality that is private practice.

Under these circumstances, it seems logical to begin one's career within the sheltering confines of an established practice to guarantee an immediate patient load and cash flow, as well as being afforded an opportunity to enhance clinical skills while learning the business end of the dental industry. Often this is seen as a method by which recent graduates may gather themselves prior to launching a solo practice.

However, again speaking only from personal experience, no associate in our practice has ever demonstrated more than a slight interest in the business end of our office, seemingly completely at ease with allowing existing staff to be solely concerned with such matters. If financial education was augmented in any of our associates, said learning must have occurred through osmosis.

3. Additional guidance required in some facets of clinical care

When I taught senior students at the University of Iowa College of Dentistry during the 1974-1975 school year, I was amazed by the markedly varied levels of skill these almost-graduates exhibited. Some were capable of performing almost any dental procedure at an acceptable level; others struggled mightily to place even the most simple restoration. As a student, I had no perception of how great the talent differences were among my classmates. (This could well have been a form of self-protective ignorance. If such was the case, I'm grateful. My self-esteem needed no further damage!)

Certainly the military or resident route will result in augmented technical ability, and for those needing a great deal more guidance in ALL FACETS of clinical care, the supervision available under such programs probably makes them the ideal selection, despite added debt and more time sacrificed from an already late-starting career. (No private practice owner will—or can afford to—tolerate an associate taking four hours to place a simple restoration, as is typical of many dental students, if for no other reason than that the chairside's salary is greater than the income generated.)

But many recent graduates are competent in some clinical areas, adequate in others, and clueless in a few. (I fabricated one complete denture—an upper—during my dental school years. I doubt my removable prosthodontics skills were adequate for solo practice, had it not been for the excellent and generous advanced removable prosthetics training I received in the military.)

If this typical recent graduate, of mixed abilities, can find an office in which he or she will be properly supported—left alone when he or she feels competent, aided when certain procedures require help—one's learning will not only be vastly accelerated, but prove considerably less painful for neophyte dentist and patient alike.

4. Lack of interest or ability in the "business part"

It is one thing to have not received training in the business of managing a dental office. (All dentists start even, at least in this regard.) It is another to have no interest in this aspect of private practice. (The first deficiency is correctable, the second, almost by definition, is not.) As I've (over-) stated, the days of being able to ignore the "business part," and avoid bankruptcy, are over! The stakes, the pressure, the competition, have simply grown too intense.

I'm old enough to recall times when any dentist could simply open his or her office doors, muddle about, and still enjoy a successful career. One-chair offices, with one staff member, were the norm, and bankruptcy was unheard of among professionals (as was staggering debt). The demand for dental care then (exploding when insurance first entered the dental universe) far exceeded the profession's ability to supply, and patients waited months to have dental work completed, as virtually every office was booked far in advance.

The economic reality of our times precludes any solo-practicing professional from success unless he or she is willing to make the effort required to become proficient as a business manager. No dental graduate lacks the ability to learn such skills. (If one can perform endodontics on an upper second molar, one can learn to read a profit and loss sheet and understand office monitors—I promise!) The question is more one of attitude. Can one achieve the goals of success, wealth and joy if forced to concentrate on an area of the profession, no matter how essential, that he or she dislikes? A personal answer must be forthcoming (through value clarification) before a decision to open one's own office is reached.

Also, possible levels of dental achievement seem to me, in great part, to depend on acceptable levels of self-esteem. Without getting all touchy-feely, or psychoanalyzing the point to death, I believe some individuals lack the self-confidence required to deal with elevated degrees of success and consequently sabotage their progress in ways apparent to everyone but the self-saboteur, thus remaining on a plane of attainment consistent with their view of personal worth.

Such a deficiency in self-confidence is limiting and seems tragic in one who has survived the rigors (horrors?) of long years of professional education. Even the unavoidable bottom student by class ranking in every dental school graduating class has attained a position within the top 1% of educated Americans.

My advice is succinct: If one has invested the required lonely thought needed to clarify values and honestly determined he or she dislikes dealing with management of staff, patients and other essential business portions of the dental profession, identify a good opportunity working for another who excels in these areas and seek one's future there. If one's self-perception has been accurate—not fear-induced—such reduced pressure will enhance one's chances of achieving joy.

5. A wish to be productive and earning money at once

I might be old-fashioned, but I believe offices that employ other dentists should be busy, successful and well organized to a level where they can create an immediate patient flow that will keep the newest member of the team reasonably active providing patient care from his or her first day in the office. Thus the newest team member is learning, producing income and, most likely, happy. Certainly, the newest dentist will be required to put forth the effort needed to establish his or her own patient flow. But I believe the office should be able to schedule something near a 60% full appointment book indefinitely, or the joint venture will fail.

One might review Dr. White's 1997 monitors to gain a clearer understanding of my contention. Our office has been able to schedule sufficient patients to enable Joe to produce and remain above the $15,000 level from his second full month in our office. (An office with sufficient patient volume to completely fill another dentist's schedule indefinitely would probably be one so overburdened as to be near chaos. It's unlikely that such an over-stressed office—and I've been there—could have excellent systems in place that are mandatory to establish before adding another dentist, although having too many patients seems a burden many would gladly shoulder.)

I believe Joe's skill level makes him capable of producing $25,000 per month, if fully scheduled. Growth above his current "60% of capacity level" will come when patients begin to call the office requesting appointments with "that nice new dentist."

A typical recent graduate, in mid- to late twenties, probably with a wife, perhaps a child, and our ubiquitous and crushing debt (and I've spoken to new graduates in their thirties with four kids and even more substantial financial obligation), can't afford to wait a year or more to begin earning a living wage, while watching debt mount ever higher, as is often the case when one begins an office on his or her own.

I can't imagine the agony of a new dentist, neck-deep in financial obligations, office overhead running, praying for the shiny new office phone to ring. An additional year of struggle to achieve a profit presents a challenge to one's pineal gland and self-esteem. I would venture such a first year of practice to prove tough on gastric lining, brain cells and relationships down to and including the essential affinity with one's dog. My advice to one who chooses such a daunting challenge—hunt, fish and pray all one can! Better to physically and spiritually work off tension than to inflict distress upon those closest to you. There is no need to add divorce or an alienated family to the suffocating pressure one is forced to endure.

As a personal aside, I've guaranteed a minimum salary to some of my associates. **I dislike** accepting this responsibility for his or her success—such behavior is inconsistent with my beliefs—but the honest need of some graduates makes it almost impossible for them to make a commitment to any office without some minimal degree of financial assurance.

The arrangements I've reached have varied by the individual's need. I've chosen never to charge interest, feeling these poor kids are suffering enough pressure, but **always** had a signed agreement concerning how this debt is to be handled as an addendum to our employment contract. To date, these salary guarantees have caused no problems, but do place additional stress on the already fragile owner-employee relationship.

6. A wish to enjoy a badly needed supportive environment

We've discussed clinical support, and it is critical. But psychological reinforcement—being part of a team with a common goal, surrounded by people who wish one to succeed—is also vital to a dentist starting a new venture, especially if he or she is facing the frightening prospect of private practice, while still suffering from the combat fatigue and shell-shock of the denigrating dental school experience.

I started practice on my own, after two valuable years of military experience. There were many times when a veteran hand and brain could have saved both patient and me a great deal of grief. I often reflect, during the thousands of times I've attempted to solve associate dentists' problems—both great and small, behavioral and clinical—how wonderful it would have been in my early years to have a source of support and hoary wisdom available to lean on, to count on, that I knew invariably had my best interests at heart. Simply being reassured I was on the correct path would have been of inestimable value.

7. Creating an opportunity to buy into an existing, profitable practice where one is already established, and success almost guaranteed

We've touched on this topic. Purchasing an office in which one is currently employed, where the staff and patients already know and accept the new dentist, affords a much greater likelihood of success than buying an office from a complete stranger, the purchase based on only an analysis of the practice numbers (by a recent graduate, totally unschooled in such a venture), then hoping to be accepted by existing staff, who view anything performed other than how "old doc Smith" did things as wrong, and struggling to win the trust of patients who would greatly prefer being treated by their lifetime friend, good old Doc.

(Too often the new practice owner discovers ole Doc's retention was based on a complex pattern of OVERHANGS! How to explain this type of clinical problem—or why, after 30 years of regular checkups, a patient now has periodontal disease—is a slippery slope that must be traversed if one is to succeed.)

Of course, having an existing and predictable cash flow from which one may accurately estimate one's financial future elevates buying an office from the realm of hopefully gazing into a murky crystal ball to a matter of making a fact-based decision in the lucent light of day. Making this critical business judgment based on existing office history, rather than conjecture and extrapolation, greatly enhances one's probability of success.

Also, an established associate enjoys the advantage of knowing he or she feels at home in the community, as well as with patients and staff—a factor not to be underestimated. Purchasing an office, then feuding with existing staff, can prove a death knell, as patients relate to known staff more than the unknown dentist. I've also lost associates who were doing well, happy within the office and town, but whose spouse couldn't adjust to life in Keokuk, away from her loved ones. (This female reference is not sexist, merely a reflection of the experience within our office. I've never had a single female dentist seriously consider our practice opportunity.) In our office, an unhappy dentist's spouse has meant the family will usually soon be moving closer to the wife's relations.

The Problems Inherent Within Group Practice

I've candidly admitted my bias in favor of group practice, and attempted to describe and begun to document the personal experiences and practice results that have created said enthusiasm. But the problems and inherent disadvantages that lead to the dissolution of so many groups are compelling. Significant obstacles exist that should not be ignored by any wise man or woman who is intrigued by the promise of a dental group.

As previously mentioned, I think many senior dentists attempt to form a group practice before placing their house in order. This is perceived as a short cut to success, but in reality is as certain a recipe for disaster as exists. Let's reflect upon additional concerns accompanying the group concept.

1. Loss of shared vision

This is by far the most troubling problem of group practice for me, as it threatens my personal value structure. After years of struggle, it is a conundrum I feel can't be totally avoided, but must to some degree be endured. When I had a one-dentist practice, the office vision was an extension of my personal conception of the ideal dental clinic. I strived to clarify that insight and discussed it endlessly with staff, attempting to communicate and inspire my team toward the same lofty goals that established meaning and excitement in my professional life. There is great joy and energy inherent within a group of people working toward a clearly defined and shared destination—be it a basketball championship or forming the best possible dental office.

None of the seven associates employed in our office has shared my vision in the manner virtually all non-dentist staff who continue as members of our team do. (I seldom have to dismiss employees who disagree with our values. Mainly because

326

of our staff meetings and communication exercises, staff often sense their beliefs are in conflict with our culture and values, feel uncomfortable, and move on.)

After years of concern and frustration over dentists who join our office, motivated to accept this position at least partially by our documented success, then almost immediately begin to rebel against many of the central concepts that allow us to achieve these results (staff meetings and monitors are two common examples), I'm almost as puzzled by the phenomenon as I was the first time it occurred, and have had limited success in changing this behavior. (This is the most significant, embarrassing and painful admission of a book seemingly comprised of a list of my failings.)

I believe the ego of dentists (by ego I refer to a sense of self—not a bad thing—if appropriate and controlled) forces them to rebel against a powerful culture, such as exists among our team, in an effort to create their unique identity. Psychologists refer to this fear of losing one's individuality as "engulfment issues." I can tell one more than he or she wishes to hear concerning this thorny subject that has so plagued me, but won't, as none of this conceptual understanding has allowed me to positively impact the problem one iota.

I am more aware that associates need a manner in which to establish their unique identity that is more constructive than bucking the prevailing system. I attempt to identify areas within our office where new dentists can exercise leadership in a positive way. It might be as head of our annual OSHA review, taking over management of our lab work, investigating a new material or technique—anything in which the associate has an interest and that affords him an opportunity to express his unique self.

The problem is that, as long as the tasks are appointed by me—not the associate's idea—the threatening feelings of lost identity can still exist. The more the owner-dentist is present within the office, the better able he or she is to enforce office values, but efficient use of equipment and space limitations reduce the practicality of such possible joint occupancy, even for dentists still seeing patients full time. All I can do is sound a warning concerning this troublesome, seemingly unavoidable reality. Maintaining any form of relationship in which diverse central values exist is a challenging feat.

2. Decreased control of office owner

It is difficult to see patients you've treated for years being cared for by the new dentist . . . even though that is precisely what one desired to happen! When this first occurred in my office, I recall thinking, "How can Ms. Smith trust anyone but me with her care?" Of course, it was precisely her faith in me, and the trust of many faithful patients in me, transferred to the dentist **I had selected to join our office**, that allowed a successful group practice to develop.

For an associate relationship to have any chance of survival, the senior dentist must be prepared to undergo the gut-wrenching task of allowing the new dentist the freedom to express himself or herself as the unique individual he or she is. The associate will perform technically and (especially) behaviorally in a manner differing from the owner's approach, and the senior dentist must allow this variation, **assuring only that quality of care isn't diminished**, and attempting to wait until requested to assist before offering advice and suggestions.

(With kids, significant learning occurs only when the parent is asked for help. Part of being an effective leader is having the fortitude to hold advice until the proper moment, when it is desired and won't be resisted and rejected. However, patience is not numbered among my natural strengths, even during the critical times I'm sitting in a deer stand.)

If one hasn't employed an associate, allowing another dentist freedom within one's office might not sound difficult. After all, one desired a decreased workload and this is how that goal must be achieved. Let me assure all that relinquishing control over an office one has slaved and sacrificed to build is anything but pleasant or easy. Who but you can give painless injections, establish abiding relationships, and create undetectable margins? Now that your associate is here, how can you trust him or her to treat YOUR PATIENTS?

The key is developing the awareness that they are no longer your patients, but rather OUR PATIENTS! Remember the heart-wrenching feeling you experienced the first day you sent your child off to school? The pain of observing another dentist care for your flock is similar, only longer-lasting. Controlling one's ego and sharing ownership—a frightening act of faith—is a barrier one must surmount to have any hope of achieving a successful and joyful group practice. It may help to consider this discomfort as merely another step in one's growth.

3. *Accelerated staff conflict*

What we've all heard is true—staff friction increases geometrically as more people are employed within the same space. The sheer weight of numbers—of unique personalities—guarantees more interpersonal problems developing. The resulting conflicts usually, ultimately, end up being the responsibility of the practice owner to resolve. This added friction can mean more disruptive turnover within a profession already severely decimated by short staff tenure, if not anticipated and pro-actively handled.

Cliques tend to form around each dentist. Our office purpose (the year-long creation of our office purpose—our Magna Carta—is documented in *Focus*) begins by stating that our office exists to serve the patient—not ourselves. It is essential for every office to develop a written mission statement, but, no matter how committed one is to a purpose, all humans have affection and loyalties that vary in strength from person to person. (One who denies this assertion in the name of fairness is likely to lie about other things as well!)

It is perhaps normal and appropriate that people who spend a great deal of time working closely together forge powerful personal bonds. It is unfortunate when such positive relationships result in the choosing of sides and expanded office conflict. It is the duty of the leader of any organization to continue to focus all members on achieving a common goal greater than themselves. Focusing all visions beyond personal needs is essential to forming a cohesive unit. In our case, this effort takes the form of working together to realize the fruition of our office purpose.

I can offer some help concerning the painful problem of team conflict. Staff meetings that encourage excellent, honest communication become even more essential in a group practice. (Again, Chapter 8 of *Focus* deals with the mechanism of our **VITAL STAFF MEETINGS** in minute detail.) Staff meetings are where group values form, and where individuals are forged into a cohesive unit with shared goals and purpose. Excellent staff meetings are important for any office, but are indispensable to the development of a dental group, where additional staff and split work-shifts compound communication difficulties. We've increased staff meeting to half-days every two weeks (instead of our standard one half-day per month) after new team members are added.

4. Increased legal liability

The more procedures an office performs, the greater the likelihood of being sued. All make mistakes, or at least witness outcomes that are frankly short of what was desired. Often personal relationships—affection and trust between dentist and patient—prevent legal action, even in these diminished-results situations. (This phrase—"diminished-results situations"—sounds like my lawyer-son talking! I felt I needed a phrase more substantive and forgiving than "screw-ups"!)

Our office makes every effort to schedule the same patients with the same dentist, but scheduling errors, especially for hygiene recare appointments, do occur. Also, in a group practice, patients are often treated by a different dentist, either due to certain specific clinical needs, or the logistics of patient and dentist schedules. (The patient insists on after 5 p.m. appointments on Friday. Only Dr. Smith works that late on Friday. Or molar endo is required. Only Dr. Jones performs that procedure in our office.) I believe the resultant loss of personal loyalty and friendship that occurs when a strong personal dentist-patient bond isn't fashioned enhances the chances of a lawsuit being filed.

Our office (knock, knock) has never had a suit or complaint filed against any employee . . . although I have probably deserved a few. I talk tirelessly (or at least endlessly) about proper documentation and procedure. I consider it my personal responsibility to be certain our office complies with OSHA guidelines, although we have an excellent team member of 20-plus years on staff who acts quite capably as our OSHA coordinator . . . Thanks, Carol! (I can delegate authority, but not responsibility . . . Right?)

Our employment contract requires associates to carry a preset amount of malpractice insurance that fits snugly against the $2 million umbrella policy the corporation holds. (Personal malpractice coverage is to the $300,000 level, while the umbrella policy begins at $300,000 and extends on to $2 million.)

Despite our fortuitous history of no malpractice problems, I believe one can't be too careful concerning legal risks. The fruits of years of effort can be erased by one careless action, and the doctor involved suffer great emotional distress throughout the process. There is no question in my mind that adding dentists enhances the likelihood of my facing litigation, as the practice owner will almost certainly be named a defendant in any action against an employee dentist. (The owner is vulnerable if for no other reason than having more money—the "deep pockets" lawyers covet with the zeal of a bear seeking honey!)

Awareness, preaching perpetual caution, insisting on proper procedures and documentation, and adequate malpractice insurance allow one to moderate these risks. But the surest way to avoid court is for every team member to treat each patient as a valued friend, going out of one's way to do whatever is required—not just what's fair—to create long-term relationships by absolutely assuring each patient's satisfaction. A short-term focus on immediate income—understandable, but not forgivable in one deep in debt—is the arch-enemy of efforts to avoid litigation.

5. *Additional office mistakes*

As with interpersonal conflict, errors increase geometrically as more staff are added and lines of communication grow

331

muddled. Expanded hours means the same person who began a task might not finish it.

For example, office and patient convenience might dictate study models being taken by someone other than the prescribing dentist's chairside. In such cases, lab work may be left uncompleted—such as a custom tray not being fabricated in time for the following impression appointment—each of the staff thinking another will do it.

Perhaps post-op calls aren't placed, or the same patient is called twice by two different staff . . . disturbing and irritating the patient and making our office appear inept. These are but two among many errors that can be made, even among dedicated, hard-working and experienced staff, in a group situation.

The solution to this confusion and resulting errors lies with excellent staff meetings, where the entire team is present as concerns and misunderstandings are discussed, and clear, mutually agreed-upon solutions reached. It is also vital for the office to create a system for every task—including monitors—that is easily implemented and concise.

In our above-mentioned error examples, a sheet posted in the lab area can list every lab case in progress, the date of the next appointment and which staff member is in charge of its completion, each task initialed by the one who completes it. A master list of post-op calls can be fabricated and each patient checked or lined off when contacted. (But brace yourself, as you'll almost certainly suffer some increased errors, no matter how excellent one's systems.)

6. Equipment breakdown and supply system failures

More people working more hours, performing more dentistry means more vital pieces of equipment breaking down. (The quality of maintenance grows suspect as extra people are involved, and again, more concise systems are required. We have a monitor sheet hanging next to every major piece of equipment in our office which is dated and initialed by the staff member performing assigned periodic maintenance.) The expense of repairs and replacement is a concern, but the frustration of not having a needed piece of equipment available is a much more disturbing problem.

The chance of running out of key supplies also increases as more hands are involved in usage. Again, a concisely monitored, team-developed system (we use a card inventory system), with one employee totally in charge of ordering and checking in all supplies, is vital to efficient group practice. Staff should accept the fact that running out of any supply is an avoidable error, as is ordering in too large a volume, thus cluttering the office, and risking expensive materials passing the recommended usage date and having to be discarded.

Extra equipment and supplies will be needed in a dental group practice, and to a point that is acceptable, but one must carefully monitor these expenses. Constructing a fully equipped, nine-operatory office with a 400-square-foot central supply fortress would solve equipment and supply problems, and be flattering to the owner's ego. (I'd build it on a hill, facing a shallow reflecting pool.) Such an office would also destroy a great deal of the economy of scale that creates the enhanced profit I feel to be the major advantage of a group.

7. *Reaction to the failure of an associate relationship*

When the associate informs the owner he or she will be leaving, or when the owner advises the associate their relationship has failed, it hurts. Many hours, intense planning and precious energy from the entire team has been devoted to helping the associate succeed . . . and these resources are now virtually wasted. There have also been the expenses of recruitment and the purchase of those aforementioned vital "special instruments," required, it seems, by every dentist. (Forgive my pettiness, but one might as well make a going-away gift of these instruments, as I can almost promise they will never be touched by human hands again! Giving them away makes the owner look good, while freeing valuable storage space.)

A sense of loss, of personal failure, has accompanied every dissolved associate relationship in my office, no matter what the reason for its demise. It's a feeling to which I've never grown accustomed.

A dentist leaving also means a staff member, perhaps two, will be thrown out of work. It is not a pleasant task for the office leader to dismiss these people, especially when they are forced to leave through no fault of their own. However, I've come to consider this situation as an opportunity to "prune the staff." To employ "addition by subtraction," as employees I perceive as least valuable are the ones let go. (The last one hired is not necessarily the first one fired. My decision as to who remains on our team is based ENTIRELY ON SKILL, ATTITUDE, MERIT AND VALUE TO THE OFFICE. At least the loss of an associate allows us to condense our team into the strongest possible unit.)

An associate's leaving also means office, dentist and hygiene hours must be readjusted. Perhaps the most telling blow is that **patients resent change**. Unless totally discouraged, the owner is also faced with beginning the time-intense task of finding a replacement associate and then introducing him or her to the office culture and now more skeptical patients. (I was done with associates forever after our first one left—until I'd worked alone for two weeks—long enough to remember why I'd desired help in the first place—and had completed a detailed analysis of my profit and loss figures at year's end.)

No one should enter an associate relationship without considering the statistically most likely outcome—that of the associate eventually leaving. (I guess the same can be said of modern marriages!)

Dr. Rick Kushner, whom I deeply and sincerely admire, and who has enjoyed success that dwarfs the modest levels I've accomplished, attempts to eliminate failed associate relationships by selling portions of his multiple offices as partnerships, thus binding the associates in an equity situation. Financial obligations make it more difficult and complex to leave an office, similar to the difference between breaking up with a girl friend, and ending a marriage. The buy-in arrangements also enhance initial income for the part-owner.

I've never wanted a partner. I feel I've worked too hard and sacrificed too much to turn part of my accomplishment over to another. Perhaps I'm too mean, insecure, greedy, stuck in my ways or lacking in vision. Also, I'm concerned about the attitude of a dentist who wishes to leave one's practice, but is unable to do so, due to financial obligations. Whatever my fatal flaw, one can't argue with Rick's level of achievement, merely admire it. His philosophy is certainly worth examining before one begins any associate relationship. (Rick can be reached by calling 1-303-277-0001, the office of his Table Mountain Seminars.)

Perhaps the critical question one should ask himself or herself before considering a group practice concerns the owner's personality and interpersonal abilities. Can you live with a submerged ego, giving up some control of the office (which, at least partially, defines you) to another? Do you understand and are you motivated enough to perform the supplementary work required to reap the potential rewards of a dental group? In your mind, are the benefits I'm documenting sufficient to justify suffering the additional problems and enhanced effort? Are your management and behavioral skills adequate to handle the more daunting challenge of a group? What changes, what growth are required in you and your office before a group practice is feasible?

Examine my motivations. I find clinical dentistry to be difficult, demanding, exhausting work. To have any chance of enjoying my work—my life—I must be well compensated for my efforts. My management and behavioral abilities—deficient as they may be—still prove more valuable than my limited technical abilities, so managing others in practice seems a viable option in my situation.

Make no mistake, for me the primary reason to consider a group is **the singular opportunity to make more money while providing fewer hours of patient care**. It is this flow of cash that bequeaths the freedom I find so valuable and exciting. Allow me to end this chapter by precisely illustrating and documenting the cash flow that purchases my treasured freedom.

The following information describes eight-hour treatment days and W-2, IRS reported income from my practice of dentistry alone. (No investment, book, newsletter or other revenue included.)

YEAR	ANNUAL TREATMENT DAYS	W-2 INCOME	DAILY AVERAGE
1997	38⅔	$229,000	$5,900
1996	52	$347,000	$6,673
1995	72	$251,000	$3,500
Totals	162⅔	$827,000	$5,074

Average Annual Income, 1995-1997 = $275,670.

This is roughly **2.5 times the national average** of $110,592 as listed in the May 1998 *Dental Economics*.

Average Net Income Per Eight-Hour Day, 1995-1997 = $5,074.

I don't believe I have to apologize for a three-year average daily net of $5,074, but allow me to explain the fluctuation in numbers. (From $3,500 to $6,673 per day, and $229,000 to $347,000 per year.) My office is incorporated. (Although the advantages of incorporation are much less compelling today than when I incorporated, 20 years ago.) This corporate status allows me some freedom to shift income between years. As mentioned, I own my office space personally and rent to my corporation, thus I can raise or lower rent to alter my personal income. We also use corporate retained earnings (detailed in Chapter 20 of *Focus*) of up to $150,000 to hold profits within the corporation, tax-free, if we so choose, rather than paying the money out as taxable personal income.

My point is not to examine these somewhat complex features of business, but to demonstrate my ability to increase or decrease net income during any given year based on tax and other business considerations. Without the need and opportunity to adjust net for tax reasons, each yearly and daily average would be similar.

Were I seeking to sensationalize, rather than inform, I could extrapolate data from my best day or week to arrive at an eye-popping annual figure. (Remember discussing July and August, 1997, at the beginning of this chapter, with the $14,857 per-day net I hope captured your interest?)

Or I could have used precise and accurate figures from only 1996—$347,000 per year net, or $6,673 per day—to represent my situation. Averaging three years provides more comprehensive and accurate data. I'm detailing a philosophy that has the power to change lives! I want you to have complete facts available—not just highlighted numbers containing my most recent and impressive results.

With this personal data, you witness precisely how I define working smarter, not harder. (Note the trend in days worked, declining from 72 to 52 to 38 .) I believe such NET INCOME (the only numbers worthy of one's focus) created in a **modest number of clinical days** can only be achieved in an extremely well-run group office where multiple doctors significantly reduce overhead percentage while boosting total dollars collected and thus increase my beloved net income. I also believe this to be *Dentistry's Future*.

Conclusion

Allow me to state it one more time, as the message sounds sweet to my ears: Group practice allows decreased overhead percentage combined with increased production to give a double boost to net profit for ALL INVOLVED. These advantages can be employed, as I choose, to create freedom from one's office that allows me to live a life of choice and maximum meaning. For some this ideal life might well consist of 200 days per year invested in providing dental care in precisely the manner one chooses, freed from the pressures and worries of finance.

Others might make the choice of expanding income within a group situation—or have no other realistic fiscal option at this time. My son once asked me how much money I could make if I chose to work a normal 220-day year of patient treatment. The answer is A LOT, as all fixed overhead expense is already paid, and **I'd guesstimate 85% of my additional production would be profit**. That's not my path or calling, but the potential for revenue well beyond the numbers I've shared exists for those to whom maximizing income appears attractive.

Make no mistake ... A lot of time, energy, vision and painstaking attention to detail is required to create a revenue stream that affords complete financial freedom. The systems we've discussed in previous chapters are of significant value in their own right, each empowering an office that employs them to grow, but when all are efficiently combined within a group practice, one has created a rocket!

The economic realities of our times will force many into groups, either as owners or employees. I believe only a few charismatic and gifted individuals—the promised remnant—can successfully buck these great exterior forces to thrive in a solo setting. But I feel the goal of obtaining the freedom and joy inherent within success is worthy of the effort and sacrifice required to achieve an optimal practice, even if such were not dictated by external circumstance. The benefits of a group free one from more mundane concerns and allow one to achieve what Abraham Maslow described as man's highest calling ... self-actualization.

I trust the above information has, at the least, interested every reader. If one has decided to pursue dentistry's future in the form of a group practice, let's consider how one goes about attracting and hiring associate dentists.

REFOCUS SIX:
SERVING A HEARTLESS MASTER

Virtually every member of the human race (and this defini-tion—at least marginally—encompasses dentists) suffers throughout his or her existence due to the never-ending pres-sure of a merciless and undeniable master. The cause of this omnipresent pain? One's own instincts.

Instincts that pass the "survival-of-the-fittest cut," and thus are bequeathed to succeeding generations, are those that im-prove one's odds of remaining extant and enhance reproductive opportunities. To live and reproduce are the two primary drives of all life, the factors that determine which species thrive, which enroll on the "endangered list."

Examples of life-affirming, reproduction-enhancing traits among humans (tree frogs and such have their own list) include any characteristics or behaviors that lead to health, strength, wealth or status. (Their vital nature explains why losing any of the above-named attributes causes intense pain and sadness.) These genetically favored traits are chosen by "the great unseen hand," based entirely on efficiency. Failures or triumphs of the life force are unrelated to the attainment of either pleasure or peace—just not part of the job description that requires one to survive and recreate.

Nothing sinful here, we are merely describing evolutionary reality, basically the same for humans as it was for dinosaurs. (A somewhat unsettling thought!) During humankind's meager hunter-gatherer past it was impossible to obtain too much and the specter of death hovered closely around those unable to acquire enough.

Although times and circumstances have dramatically changed (today, in first-world nations, the burning aspiration is to find a way to consume more—without gaining weight), the veteran engineer on one's train of life has retained a single unrelenting characteristic that causes tremendous anguish in our relatively safe and prosperous modern world. This fact must be understood if one desires to maximize opportunities to achieve personal happiness. **Man's genetic drive has NO BRAKE!** No achievement is ever enough. The throttle is perpetually locked all the way forward, stuck, quivering above the phrase ACHIEVE-EVER-MORE.

Humankind's inherent propensity for continual questing and contesting—admittedly essential in our species' past—today leads to a life of perpetual restlessness, bereft of peace. Life's motto is, "Never stop, brothers and sisters, as someone might be gaining on you." The great majority have no awareness—let alone understanding—of this hard-wired genetic imperative that unceasingly motivates and torments, and thus are unable to temper its influence with reason and wisdom.

What's a poor dentist to do? How can one attain his or her goal of bliss—under the hardened hand of this ever-demanding master? Guided by a wonderful book, *How to Want What You Have*, by Timothy Miller, Ph.D.—which is written for a lay audience and that I'd strongly recommend reading—I'd like to share a four-part prescription for happiness that has **significantly enhanced my peace and joy, while simultaneously increasing my personal power and competence.**

Step One: Awareness of the Human Condition

Ancient Eastern wisdom advised that within desire lie the seeds of all unhappiness. Yearning subjects one to the pain of disappointment and failure. See, feel, taste and smell the pain caused by never-ending ambition in one's life. I have so often set goals, reached them, and still lacking joy, set new, greater goals and willingly lived in torment as I continued to pursue the attainment of some self-contrived achievement that I believed would finally grant me contentment. No such golden fleece exists! (As a clue for the enlightened, the Gospel of Thomas states the kingdom of heaven lies upon the earth, but men see it not.)

How many dentists believe they're prosperous enough, wealthy enough, have sufficient patients, and thus are satisfied— even among the ultra-successful elite within our profession? How many billionaires breathe their last, scheming to discover a way to make a few more dollars? Being aware of this inherent tendency to ceaselessly acquire is essential, if one hopes to moderate this portion of the life-force, and thus achieve the peace of mind each desires. (Recall, this drive is labeled "greed" by society in its attempts to control individuals' power and thus allow humans to co-exist within society.)

Step Two: Attention

French philosopher Albert Camus told us, "If there is a sin against life, it consists perhaps not so much in despairing of life as in hoping for another life and in eluding the implacable grandeur of this life." A more contemporary way to state the same premise: "Wake up and smell the coffee!" or "Seize the day!" Does the message not have a familiar ring? It implores one to live in neither the shadowy past nor impenetrable future, but within the **precious moment of NOW.** To exist within that brief interval between stimulus and response, where choice resides.

Guilt rules the past, worry is the god of the future, joy is possible only in the present moment. Many invest a great deal of time judging both themselves and others, and this focus distracts from the present and thus dilutes the richness of life.

An example: Many days the care of 20-some patients goes flawlessly, yet I come home saddened and beset by thoughts of the one patient whose treatment results didn't satisfy my goals. The patient with the deep filling who needs endodontics, a crown I seated 10 years ago that has failed, or the patient on whom I had difficulty achieving complete anesthesia. I engage in lengthy mental dialogues with people who aren't there, explaining, justifying. (To reassure my audience, I **know** he or she isn't there.)

341

I've awakened at 4 a.m., unable to sleep, focusing my consciousness not on the current, malleable moment when action and change are possible, but on some unpleasant past or dreaded future event over which no human possesses influence.

What to do when one finds half-a-worm of guilt (past) or dread (future) in one's apple? Center all one's attention on the unpleasant emotion. Experience the feelings—perhaps a cold, physical knot in one's stomach, or tightness in one's chest—fully. Insist the fear, anger or regret give one everything it has and allow these amplified feelings to run their course. Exaggerate the emotions and they'll weaken, then disappear. Repressing, denying or attempting to ignore feelings only enhances their power. (The blessed oblivion of alcohol served as a fuel upon which my demons grew in influence and might.)

Make a determined, conscious effort to live in the present—the only time over which one has control. The following final two steps will help one achieve this difficult goal.

Step Three: Compassion

Compassion grants the ability to SEE ONENESS—that you are no better, no worse, than all of humankind. Compassion includes an awareness that others justify their means of getting what they desire in a fashion similar to one's own. All humankind has a "hungry heart" that demands continually more from creation. Every life has in common the suffering of pain and death.

There is a legend of a distraught mother who had lost her only child and was unable to contain her grief. Fearing for her sanity, she came to the Buddha seeking solace. He gently advised her to tour her village until she found someone who had not suffered such a loss of love, and bring that person back with her that evening.

In the purple of sunset the woman returned. She had spent the day searching for one who had not suffered . . . and found no-one. She had come to the self-realization that life is pain, and all are born into death.

Or consider Arthur Schopenhauer's suggestion that in moments of supreme crisis, a level of one's mind beyond consciousness is able to pierce the illusion of our separateness to see the essential oneness of humankind. This, he claims, explains the many instances where one risks his or her life to save a stranger. (I've been in such situations, and have no better way to explain the tendency, past thought, to endanger one's survival—in defiance of our strongest instincts, and seemingly common sense—to rescue one unknown to us.)

Let's consider an everyday example of how compassion can increase joy and simultaneously result in more efficacious behavior. The next time a patient fails an appointment, reflect with empathy. Perhaps he or she had no money, was deeply frightened, or simply forgot. Aren't these circumstances to which all can relate, and thus accept, free of anger or fear? (Recall Buddha's caution that you are not punished for your anger, but by your anger.)

Does this mean one must cheerfully welcome failed appointments? Not in the least. But, that the patient has failed is an unalterable fact. One can make an effort to embrace sympathetic understanding, or be angry. Which approach promises to be more helpful? Which mind-set, the waves of which permeate one's office and influence all within, will free one's mind to plan and thus make further failures less likely? Which mental basis will allow one calm, healthful, joyful interaction with staff and future patients?

Lack of empathy leads to isolation and anger. If one suffers from these painful emotions, exercising empathy is the way to end them. Those able to express compassion are viewed as likable, friendly, non-judgmental . . . not a bad description for a beloved health-care provider.

Step Four: Gratitude

One forfeits gratitude for life's many blessings if he or she allows one's never-slaked instinctive desires to control life's journey. To re-achieve the benefits gratitude bestows, challenge the premise that one must achieve certain things to be happy. One will obtain fulfillment, peace and joy when he or she realizes *one's desires are not important.* Attaining one's every wish won't bring happiness and the effort to accomplish this impossible genetic demand could cause pain.

As proof of the above bold assertion, reflect on the major achievements of one's life. Did graduation from school, at any level, requite a legacy of unending joy? Did opening a practice, developing it to the point of living comfortably and beyond bequeath peace? Has any achievement of your goal-driven life ever redounded to a deep and permanent sense of contentment? Despite one's genetically determined instinct's insistence that it should be so, achievement never creates lasting peace or joy.

Listen to these so-true words of Susan Ertz, "Millions long for immortality who do not know what to do with themselves on a rainy Sunday afternoon." I'd find this thought amusing, if it weren't so tragically true. But perpetual restlessness doesn't have to be one's fate.

But, if one practices awareness, attention, compassion and gratitude, will one become a non-competitive, non-productive, mindlessly happy, impecunious idiot-savant of dentistry? Despite one's effort to control one's nature, virtually all will continue to strive. Humans' inherent nature can be modified, but not denied. However, with enlightenment one can choose to live within the **precious moment**, deciding to attain that which has true meaning—not jousting with every windmill—while maximizing joy and thoughtfully choosing one's challenges.

Life becomes not only more joy-filled, but healthier—as stress is reduced—and more successful. In the serenity of now, aware of one's innate drives and thus able to monitor their effect, one is free to choose goals that will lead to lasting bliss, and not frantically pursue the perpetual chimera of happiness hiding behind a few more possessions and/or dollars.

Family, staff and patients will note and appreciate the changes forthcoming from this maturity. Wisdom and peace thus attained are forms of success by themselves, but also act as platforms upon which one may advance to even greater achievements in worldly pursuits, while creating and enjoying the great gift of a life in balance. (Recall our discussion concerning how patients will be drawn to an office brimming with peace and happiness?)

Wealth, health, reputation and regard of peers—all enhance survival and reproductive opportunities and thus give one a sense of pleasure. It is possible to achieve our genetic demands joyfully, if their attainment is approached with understanding and wisdom: to possess the objects our instincts demand, as well as peace of mind.

Chapter Seven

Associate Recruitment

Let's assume one has maximized every office system, carefully pondered his or her personal situation and motivation, and studied the documentation of my group practice results. (This data is no guarantee of another's experience, but merely a report of my personal history.)

During the course of this reflection, if one has discovered his or her office is overly busy, one's energy or interests are drifting elsewhere and thus other creative outlets appear desirable, yet one wishes to maximize return on the tremendous investment of time, energy and money that is the dental office, and is not ready or able to retire, adding an associate might be an appropriate response to personal needs, as well as a timely reaction to the external pressures impacting the dental profession. (Such as growing third-party influence and steadily increasing overhead.)

But, how does one identify attractive associate candidates? How does one determine if an individual will successfully complement and enhance one's office? And once an associate is on board, how can his or her opportunities within one's office be maximized? Let us sally forth to consider all these important queries.

347

It behooves one to be brutally candid about the challenges he or she is about to face. As we've discussed, there may be no more demanding undertaking in dentistry than the establishment and successful continuation of a multi-doctor practice. (Our sexless marriage!) Many complex factors are involved, but none more critical than the initial choice, by both the owner of the established practice and the doctor seeking an office to join, as to with WHOM they wish to develop a professional relationship.

To some degree behavior can be modified, but basic beliefs and values can't be changed by any external force. No matter how attractive a candidate appears, if the beliefs that define him or her differ sharply from those of the practice, both parties will soon discover the office isn't big enough to hold them.

Let's first consider how one goes about the essential task of identifying a large number of associate candidates, from whose numbers you may then select someone possessing an ideal complement of valuable skills and compatible values.

After making the initial decision to bring other dentists into our office, I began to search for the proper individuals or organizations to help me identify appropriate candidates. I still remember my surprise and distress when I realized that, in my estimation, no viable, trustworthy entity existed to aid me in this critical task.

Because of the dearth of neutral parties available to lend unbiased assistance to either the dentists seeking an associate or the doctor in search of the proper opportunity in which to practice, and the critical nature of associate recruitment to my perception of dentistry's future, I've recorded my thoughts and experiences on the "recruiting trial."

Again, I'm no expert here, but have learned a bit, enrolled as I've been for over a dozen years in this particular school of hard knocks. While most of my history comes as the dentist seeking an associate (with the sole exception my original search for a practice in 1973 and 1974), I believe the following information will also assist associate candidates by revealing where and how established dentists conduct their recruitment efforts.

348

Preparation for The Recruitment Process

Recruitment of an associate is a lengthy, difficult, and somewhat expensive task. Before one begins, I'd urge you to be as certain as possible as to the nature of your commitment to have someone join your practice. Time spent in careful study, reflection and planning (value clarification) before recruitment begins can save a lot of wasted effort and distress later.

One must develop a mental image of the perfect associate for his or her unique office; must visualize the preferred final outcome. What would be the exact combination of clinical skills that would complement the services the office currently offers? (It seems everyone likes cosmetics, but, in rural Iowa at least, it's hard for one dentist to make a living with bonding and veneers, let alone two or more. Consider what procedures are now referred out of the office, or those you don't enjoy performing, and would be delighted if an associate took over. Attempt to find a dentist with skill and interest in these complementary areas.)

One also needs to define ideal associate behavioral characteristics. Our office is outgoing, tends to be a little loud, and we laugh a lot. A quiet, introspective soul—no matter his or her other gifts—would most likely find this environment uncomfortable. An essential portion of any staff hiring is identifying individuals who will fit smoothly within the existing team the doctor has carefully established.

I know successful offices where business suits are the dress of the day, and others where jeans comprise the official office uniform. Both can become dominant practices, but the owner's vision and direction must assure every detail—including hiring people with compatible personalities—is consistent with the office's identity. In a similar manner, an associate dentist must determine if he or she meshes with the new practice environment. (I think such seamless integration is a rule of nature, and explains why one seldom sees a blue or orange deer!)

Precise skills exist to help one identify associate candidates, values and accurately assess compatibility (as detailed in *Focus*),

349

but before they can be of assistance, the practice owner must be clear in his or her own mind as to the practice's vision.

Physical Plant Preparation

One's mind and beliefs clear, one's purpose resolute, I'd strongly suggest a dentist seeking an associate fully equip his or her office—redecorating and augmenting one's physical plant in any way possible, to make it as attractive and functional as feasible—BEFORE beginning to identify candidates.

I realize physical changes to offices represent expensive and time-consuming tasks. The temptation is to wait until the associate is hired before updating and enhancing one's office. However, after an associate is in place, the motivation to make these changes may not be as compelling.

Most of the work undertaken to allow one's office to achieve maximum beauty and efficiency is helpful whether another dentist joins the team, or not. The equipment one adds will improve function and enhance productivity, as well as elevating the image of one's practice in patients' eyes. (Remember how we've repeatedly stressed the need to maximize one's office and refine systems BEFORE searching for an associate?)

Also, one will be able to put an associate to work the day he or she is able to join the office, and not be delayed at this critical emotional and financial juncture by incomplete office preparations.

MOST IMPORTANTLY, enhancing the decor and equipment of one's office in preparation for an additional doctor demonstrates to potential associates that the practice owner's commitment is sincere. To the best qualified candidates—those you'll have to compete with other practices to hire—a fully equipped and beautiful office is more compelling than explaining what one plans to someday accomplish. If one's systems are maximized, expanded hygiene profit alone should allow renovation, expansion or even moving into a new office facility.

Before beginning the recruitment process, one must also clarify his or her preferred future relationship with an associate. Do you wish a long-term commitment? Is a partnership, or even practice purchase, on the horizon? If you seek only temporary assistance, you must plainly tell each candidate. If you aren't candid at this early juncture, there will be pain and justified anger when the truth is revealed.

Buy-in Agreement

If you desire a long-term commitment—and I'm unable to detect any advantage to an office arising from bringing in a different associate each year—I believe the practice should be valued by a professional dental practice broker and a tentative buy-in contract implemented before one's search process begins.

We had our office appraised in early 1998, by a professional broker in the business since 1964, for a flat fee of $1,000, but received quotes as high as $3,000 for this service. One should definitely interview candidates and solicit bids for this job. Brokers are listed in the JADA want ads.

The tentative buy-in agreement establishes that on a mutually selected date in the future—usually one year from the date the agreement is signed, with annual renewal dates—should both parties be willing to proceed, a permanent buy-in or practice purchase can be executed. One will require an attorney to draft an associate employment contract, and the buy-in agreement can be created at the same time. This agreement will define what **FORMULA** will be used to value the practice at some appropriate future date.

I see no fair way in which an exact value can be established for any practice to be sold at some as yet undetermined future date. It IS POSSIBLE for owner and associate to agree on a formula that, when the proper and agreed-upon practice numbers are inserted in predetermined slots, will yield a practice value accepted by both parties as equitable on the date of their choosing.

Sadly, potential associations often fail, even when both doctors have been happily working together for some time, when it is realized owner and associate disagree on the specific arrangements for buying into the practice. I am aware of two incidents where the perception of office value differed by 100% between the owner doctor and the established and successful associate seeking to purchase a share of the practice. Instead of a sale that would continue an excellent working relationship and viable business for both, each felt the other party to be grossly unfair and the relationship ended in bitterness and a courtroom, instead of mutual benefit.

These unhappy events occurred after years of successfully working together, because no attempt to provisionally agree on a buy-in was made at the onset of their relationship. Owner and associate felt an agreement could be "reached later, when both were sure things were going to work out." Now both parties must start over in their respective searching, hopefully wiser, if sadder, from the experience. It is tempting to ignore the creation of a buy-in agreement when beginning a relationship, especially when one is unfamiliar and uncomfortable with how to proceed, but this pre-agreement represents a critical portion of a future group's foundation.

The ADA has a simple booklet, *Successful Valuation of a Dental Practice, Volume Two* (one may reach the ADA by calling 1-800-621-8099), that is extremely helpful in establishing a method or formula to determine a practice's worth. I've read several books on the subject of practice valuation that were longer, more complex and harder to comprehend than the ADA's slender text (51 pages in length), but to me, none was as valuable and easy to implement.

You'll need professional help from accountants and lawyers, but the basics of a buy-in arrangement that will assure mutually fair treatment are clearly detailed in the ADA publication. **Do the necessary homework yourself!** Bringing an associate into an office is too critical a decision to be left entirely to the discretion of a third party (said lawyer or accountant) with no vested interest in the eventual outcome.

I realize practice evaluations and buy-ins seem foreign and imposing to the majority of dentists. It is normal to fear and avoid the unfamiliar, but this lack of understanding is not a valid excuse for failing to acquire this essential learning. Consider the academic courses one was "forced" to take in order to achieve one's goal of a dental degree. None of us loved each and every discipline. We were required to study subjects we didn't necessarily enjoy or naturally have an interest in, because they were essential to the attainment of our ultimate goal.

In today's world this accurately describes one's need to be aware and concerned about the business of dentistry. Too many powerful forces outside one's control—be they IRS, OSHA, or the initials of one's choice—affect dentistry's future to be ignored. I may have previously mentioned this point (no more than 10 times!), but the game of dentistry has changed, and whether one agrees with or approves of the contemporary situation, one had better get used to playing by the new rules.

I understand examples of my employment contract and buy-in agreements would be helpful, but sharing such exposes me to more liability than I desire. (I guess I'm getting old and scared.)

For years my associates were employed as **independent contractors.** Today the prevailing wisdom strongly suggests they must be considered employees—as are both Lowell and Joe—or one risks incurring severe IRS penalties. I'd recommend contacting the ADA for help crafting employment agreements and buy-in documents, but one must still work with his or her personal attorney and accountant so one's unique legal and tax situation can be carefully addressed. These areas are too critical, too complex, to be handled without adequate professional assistance. (Again, delegate authority, but educate yourself to the level required so acceptance of personal responsibility for the outcome can be assumed.)

At this juncture, the established doctor is certain she wants to bring in another dentist and has proven this to herself and to a potential associate by fully equipping and enhancing the office, while diligently refining and maximizing office systems and procedures.

The nature of her commitment to a future associate—as long-term or short-term, buy-in or office sale—has been clarified. No option is good or bad, but it is essential that both parties be precise and candid as to what they seek. Some recent graduates desire only a year or so of employment in another office to gain experience, and perhaps save some money, before launching their own dental venture.

A definitive image of the desired character, clinical skills and behavioral characteristics of an ideal associate has been placed **in writing** by the practice owner.

An employment contract has been prepared by the owner's attorney, and a valuation formula within a tentative buy-in agreement has been crafted. (Allow me to reiterate that these documents can't be finalized at this early date, but can be mutually understood and accepted. They will serve as the framework for a final agreement when both parties are prepared to make this step. Neither owner or associate—at least assuming they are in their right minds—would consider agreeing to a permanent arrangement before working together. That would be akin to marrying someone on a blind date!)

Our remaining task . . . how to locate this clearly defined, ideal associate.

Associate Recruitment

I started my first recruitment process by placing an ad in the *ADA Journal*. This became a major instrument in our office's efforts to locate recruits, especially those no longer in dental school. Here is an undated version of the most recent ad our office ran. It's no masterpiece, but we consistently receive excellent responses.

American Dental Association
Classified Advertising Department
Box #B271
211 E. Chicago Avenue
Chicago, Illinois 60611

We have an outstanding opportunity for a full-time associate with buy-in available. Our staff of nine, five fully equipped and modern operatories, complete with nine computer terminals and five intraoral cameras, and over 5,000 active patients are eagerly awaiting. Our very successful office enjoyed 1997 collected revenues of $665,720 and 48%

overhead. We are located in Keokuk, Iowa, on the banks of the Mississippi, an outdoor- and family-oriented community of 13,000. Immediate patient load and income is available.

Please call Dr. John Wilde at (I placed both my home and office phone numbers).

In this advertisement, I attempted to stress the positive aspects of our office (what a unique concept! I should have gone into marketing), such as the size and sophistication of our physical plant, past financial performance, and our immediate patient load. (I believe using precise figures, as our $665,720 collection total, adds verisimilitude, when compared to such generalizations as "excellent collections.") This information is intended to draw a response from as many candidates as possible.

The brief description of the community will eliminate those interested in an urban setting, while encouraging those seeking a more pastoral location. The size of the practice—over 5,000 patients—will discourage those seeking a quiet, lower-pressure situation. Mentioning "buy-in available" should encourage those desiring a long-term relationship, while discouraging those with a short-term frame of reference. The goal of this ad is to maximize responses from candidates with a genuine interest, while eliminating those searching for either a quiet office, temporary position, or a big-city location, so neither the applicant nor I will waste time.

I place the identical ad in the state dental journal that tends to reach publication sooner, has fewer ads with which to compete (in Iowa, at least), and is less expensive than the *JADA*. I have not advertised in any other journals, although we'll shortly discuss a publication related to the Student ADA I believe to have promise.

The *JADA* ad is critical to recruitment, but it takes over 90 days from the time our ad is mailed until it is published in the journal. This length of time seems totally unreasonable and certainly not the way I'd run a business, if one may take the questionable liberty of considering the ADA as such.

I've been an ADA member and loyal supporter for over 20 years. Of all my frustrations with the ADA (and they are too numerous to discuss here), the delay in ad placement is one of the most annoying and least understandable to me, especially when our small-town, local paper can have a want ad in print in 24 hours. I assume the explanation is similar to why it takes months to be notified as to the results of board examinations. (And neither explanation has a chance of being acceptable to me!)

I have had dealings with a number of brokers and professional placement agencies. Mostly I filled out forms and had long phone conversations with them. When I discovered how expensive it would be to employ them, I decided to avail myself of their service only if no other efforts to identify viable candidates proved successful.

Some of these entities demand a percentage of the associate's first year's collected dollars as a portion of their fee. I freely admit I'm CHEAP, and wish my wife and kids were too, but it seems to me one who signs such an agreement is confessing, not to mere extravagance, but that he or she is insane! I hate to think how I'd feel if an associate told me she was leaving after I'd spent thousands of dollars employing some organization to recruit and hire her.

So far, I've been able to locate excellent people using the other methods we are discussing, and haven't been forced to resort to availing myself of the costly assistance of brokers or agencies. This has saved me paying them a substantial fee, but more importantly, **I've learned by my personal involvement in the recruiting process**. I have no bias against these businesses, no cautionary tale of misfortune or mistreatment from them to impart, but if one chooses to let others perform a job he or she may not find appealing, **one will eventually pay dearly for the cardinal sin of delegating responsibility**.

By far the most meaningful sources of candidates, after the *JADA* ads, are the dental schools. Our staff developed a photo album of our attractive office and sent it, along with a two-page cover letter describing our practice, to every dental college within a 250-mile radius. This mailing was followed a week later by a phone call from me to the appropriate party at each institution.

Names and addresses of dental school officials are acquired from The American Association of Dental Schools publication, *Directory of Institutions and Members.* (Call 202-667-9433.) The cost of this book is $50, but this is the most up-to-date information of which I'm aware and gives the names, numbers, e-mail and snail-mail addresses of the individuals in charge of student placement at every American and Canadian dental college.

Often the person the dental college has put in charge of handling this information is a secretary or librarian whose job description includes "putting these things out." It's sad and frustrating that after four years of involvement with students, many colleges' commitment to their graduates' futures involves nothing more than having someone "put something out" for someone to peruse. However, some dental schools are more helpful, frequently updating potential job information, and a few even publish available opportunities in newsletter form. It won't take long to discover the commitment and support level of every institution with which one has congress.

Here is a copy of the letter I sent to every University of Iowa dental senior that resulted in Dr. White's joining our office. The dental school was kind enough to place our message in each senior student's mailbox. This communication was sent in early fall, and after getting to know Joe, I was so impressed that we reached an agreement by January of the following year and I had no need to involve myself with any other recruitment.

But recall, I've recruited associates seven times over more than a decade, so have a precise concept of the individuals for whom I'm searching. If one is engaged in this exercise for the first time, I'd strongly suggest he or she complete each of the recruiting methods we'll discuss. This will identify a maximum number of candidates, thus enhancing one's chance of success, while affording valuable experience with every facet of the entire potential associate identification process.

Dear University of Iowa, College of Dentistry Senior:

Congratulations! The day you've long awaited is rapidly approaching: GRADUATION! You will finally begin to reap the rewards earned by your years of strenuous labor.

I'm writing to inform you of a rare and exciting opportunity. Our office in Keokuk, Iowa, wishes to establish a long-term relationship with one of you. We offer an active patient population in excess of 5,000 and last year saw an average of 29 new patients a month, so you'll be busy with patient care (and making money) at once. Five completely equipped operatories, each featuring fiber-optic handpieces, nitrous oxide, x-ray unit, one of our nine computer terminals, and one of our five intraoral cameras connected to cable television and virtual reality glasses means you can enjoy state-of-the-art facilities in a warm, friendly environment immediately after graduation.

We are a values based-office that stresses teamwork, communication skills, personal growth and the creation of joy. I believe that is best illustrated by:

OUR OFFICE PURPOSE

Our office exists to serve the people we have dedicated ourselves to—our patients. We will create an environment of honesty and professionalism where each patient will feel comfortable and welcome. All patients will be aware of the quality of treatment they receive and of the sincere commitment of the staff to their best interests.

We pledge to be positive, supportive team members and to create an environment where we are able to have fun while encouraging and supporting personal and professional growth.

I opened our office on August 17, 1974. Dr. Lowell Long, also a University of Iowa graduate, joined us 10 years ago. Our practice's long history of growth has created an opportunity for an additional dentist to join our "dream team."

Keokuk, Iowa, is a town of 13,000 located on the southeastern tip of Iowa, on the banks of the Mississippi River, 95 miles due south of Iowa City on highway 218. The economy is diverse and thriving. Keokuk is a family-oriented community where life is safe and the citizens unfailingly Midwestern-friendly.

I enjoy speaking to dental audiences and am the author of three books on dental management as well as over 50 magazine and newsletter articles. If you wish an insight into my beliefs, you may find a copy of my most recent book, *How to Build the Dental Practice of Your Dreams,* in the Iowa dental library. The book deals with the art of establishing a successful, profitable and joyous dental office.

If this position sounds appealing, and you desire more information, you may reach me any evening or weekend at 217-847-2816. It will be in your best interests to give this unique offer your most serious consideration. Please act promptly, as opportunities this attractive are rare and will be quickly filled!

Again, congratulations and
best wishes for your future,

John A. Wilde, D.D.S.

The following letter is somewhat redundant, but was prepared for a different audience—every dentist already engaged in practice within a 100-mile radius of our office. (I planned to NOT mail to any dentist in our community, wishing to cause no ill will among neighbors.) Since Dr. White joined our office, there was no need to send this letter, but I offer the information for your edification and possible use. (In both letters I've updated practice statistics to 1997 figures to avoid possible reader confusion resulting from having different years' figures appearing in similar documents.)

To identify the people one will be mailing this letter to, lists or labels of dentists of any possible description—one-eyed, left-handed, with B.O.—can be obtained from any number of companies dedicated to providing such information. I'd suggest calling the ADA, which sells the master list, to obtain the names and phone numbers of such businesses if one is considering a direct mailing effort of any type to fellow dentists.

GREETINGS!

If you are currently enjoying the dental practice of your dreams, congratulations!! You need read no further and I offer my apologies for having bothered you.

However, if you desire to achieve more in your personal and professional life, I have an offer of interest. Our office is currently seeking to establish a long-term relationship with a fellow dentist committed to excellence. Our office cares for over 5,000 active patients, and last year averaged 29 new patients per month. We are very efficient and profitable, collecting $665,720 with a 48% overhead in 1997.

Our practice focuses on teamwork, personal growth and providing the best dental care we can offer. Our beliefs may best be illustrated by our office purpose, which we read before each staff meeting, and which has hung on the wall of every room in our office for many years:

OUR OFFICE PURPOSE

Our office exists to serve the people we have dedicated ourselves to—our patients. We will create an environment of honesty and professionalism where each patient will feel comfortable and welcome. All patients will be aware of the quality of the treatment they receive and of the sincere commitment of the staff to their best interests.

We pledge to be positive, supportive team members and to create an environment where we are able to have fun while encouraging and supporting personal and professional growth.

Our practice has been located in a professional building in Keokuk, Iowa, since 1974. This Midwestern community of 13,000 souls sits on the banks of the Mississippi River in the south-eastern corner of the state. It remains a bastion of family values in a changing world.

Our current staff consists of myself, Dr. Lowell Long—with the practice 10 years—our hygienist and seven wonderful and talented staff members. (We have several inept and mean staff members, but have no plans to discuss them!)

We are proud of our modern, attractive office that boasts the finest in equipment. Each of our five operatories features nitrous oxide units, fiber-optic handpieces, an intraoral camera system connected to cable television and virtual reality glasses, and one of our nine computer terminals.

I've published three books and over 50 articles in dental magazines and newsletters on the subject of practice management. Lecturing to dental groups on how to create an efficient, enjoyable and profitable dental practice is something I enjoy. I firmly believe in mutually beneficial mentor relationships within the profession.

If you are searching for more in your existence and career, are tempted by the lifestyle of a wholesome community and are willing to work hard to achieve your desires, give me a call any evening or weekend at 217-847-2816.

I'm looking forward to meeting you.

John A. Wilde, D.D.S.

Despite the limited assistance of some colleges, we've always been contacted by a good number of students as a result of our letters. The synergism of our photo album, letters, and personal call to each school not only garners a greater number of responses, but attracts the interest of the most aggressive and highly qualified persons.

It seems today's students, at least in the Midwest, are making their post-graduation commitments very early, often a year before receiving their degrees. I applaud this preparation, and I suspect it may be due in large part to their accurate perception that it is difficult to find good opportunities "out there."

It is a little frustrating to me, when I desire immediate help, to find the senior class completely committed before January of their final year. However, my advice to both those offering and those seeking associate positions is to plan well in advance. Never allow something as critical as the search for an associate or for the office position that will define one's future to be rushed. (Remember the admonition that those who decide in haste may repent in leisure!)

Once contact is established with a student, after you've met with them and they've visited your office (a process we'll detail shortly), assuming both parties remain interested, I'd recommend the practice owner schedule a trip to the applicant's dental school. Obtain the student's permission to review his or her grades and transcripts (one can't see school records without the individual's authorization), but the primary advantage of visiting the school is to gain insight concerning one's candidate by discussing the student with some of his or her instructors. Both clinical and behavioral attributes can thus be revealed.

I'd only make this effort with candidates I'm seriously considering, because a whole day is usually involved. However, the depth of commitment you and your associate must make to each other, if a permanent relationship is to result, means this is time well invested.

One may choose to combine this trip with a continuing education opportunity. If there exists an instructor at the potential associate's school you admire, you may be able to arrange some time spent talking with this paragon of academic achievement or perhaps watch him or her treat patients, thus enhancing the benefit of your journey. Be certain to schedule time with specific individuals one feels will prove helpful in advance.

At Iowa, each clinical instructor is required to spend time each week treating patients. This is a wonderful concept, as I doubt some of my dental school instructors had treated a patient in years . . . and it showed! During my visits to the university, I've called and been granted permission to observe Dr. Gerald E. Denehy, noted author, speaker and clinician, personally perform his cosmetic miracles. Jerry's a great guy and a superb clinician! The one-on-one experience has been inspirational and educational.

In our rural area, contact with local or area dental societies has not proven beneficial in identifying recruits. In a metropolitan area, I'd assume such organizations could be extremely helpful, and I'd suggest one explore this possibility if he or she lives in or near a densely populated area. Little time, money or effort would be required to investigate such regional opportunities, and one might be wise to BEGIN a search with these resources, where applicable.

Another possible source of assistance in one's quest for an associate is to contact state dental association headquarters. (ADA head-quarters can provide one with their phone numbers and addresses.) As with schools, I think one will find the effort expended to assist interested dentists in finding each other to vary significantly from state to state, but this is another quick, easy and inexpensive avenue to pursue.

I've always contacted area dental-supply dealers when searching for an associate. They are usually enthusiastic and immediately fill out a form describing the details of the situation one has available. I've never had a candidate referred by the supply companies, but contacting and providing them with information is a simple process for which no fee is required. (One can't beat free!)

Jo and I dedicated a year to the search for our practice location, and spent an exhausting four weeks driving through Iowa, carefully evaluating possible opportunities. A supply representative guided us to our first and only practice location. Their motivation is self-serving . . . and I like that! If a supply-company representative can provide assistance in establishing an associate relationship, he or she will create goodwill with that office that should result in years of business directed to them.

Nearby dental laboratories can also assist in one's recruitment efforts. Sometimes technicians or lab representatives are aware of an unhappy dentist considering a change in his or her location. Laboratory representatives who call on area dental offices might be privy to information concerning a dissatisfied dentist, even before the dentist begins to actively explore career changes. Again, it's quick, easy and without cost to contact laboratories and garner their assistance.

To my amazement, over the last 10 or so years, I've been approached by four area dentists, who suggested I purchase their office and they continue to practice as my employee. I've looked into, but not acted on, these offers, partly out of concern the dentists would leave, and I'd have another office to run. But these unsolicited occurrences illustrate how frequently local dentist might be willing to consider a major change in their professional employment status. (I think this fact also testifies to how many dentists hate and/or are inept at the vital business aspects we've been discussing, and are willing to allow anyone else to manage their professional future. I fear this distaste for business will be the door through which third parties achieve control of dentistry.)

Besides state and *JADA* ads, one might consider the Student ADA journal as a potential source of locating associate candidates. I've written several articles for this magazine, and read it regularly in an attempt to remain informed as to the issues about which students and recent graduates are concerned. I'm impressed with the work this organization does, and have a strong belief that experienced dentists need to assist recent graduates, rather than leave them adrift, then complain about the choices—like joining low-fee plans—they make.

The SADA may be reached by calling 312-440-2795. Their offices are located within the ADA headquarters building in Chicago.

The last information source I'll mention is one of which I only recently became aware and with which I've had no dealings. It is called dentistTREE, and is a "national dental employment source" that has "teamed up" with the SADA. DentistTREE publishes a monthly newsletter listing over 1,000 job opportunities, said to include dentists, hygienists, and other staff. They may be reached at 1-800-624-2904, or www.dentistree.com.

Again, if this is one's initial associate recruitment experience, all the above sources should be fully explored in an effort to identify as many candidates as possible. I'd strongly suggest the practice owner personally handle recruiting. The time and expense required to exhaust all these resources is trivial compared to the potential benefits of successful multi-dentist offices that have been documented.

Let's assume the necessary labor has been completed and one is ready to harvest the fruits of these recruitment efforts. A number of candidates have been identified, and preliminary phone discussions and an exchange of letters have eliminated some, while thrusting a few others to the fore. The time has come for you to meet the potential associates face to face.

The Office Visit

I believe it mandatory the visiting dentist bring his or her spouse (or significant other, if involved in a serious relationship) to examine the office and community they are considering joining. To make the task of writing a little less cumbersome (and by now you realize I need ALL THE HELP I CAN GET!), I'll not mention another visitor in the course of our discussion, but recall that I previously warned how an unhappy spouse can doom the most solid of associate relationships? I would NEVER CONSIDER hiring an associate without his or her partner's having seen and approved of our practice and town.

When I meet with a candidate I try to be completely frank, telling him or her exactly the type of practice we have and candidly sharing our philosophy. I illuminate our strengths and open all financial records to them, including profit and loss statements, our much-discussed monitors and even corporate and personal tax records, if he or she is interested in such things.

Most students have no idea how to analyze practice financial figures, and spending much time on more than the most cursory of business monitors confuses them and wastes time. I sometimes sense that sharing information I consider vital to reaching an informed decision about joining a practice is perceived as bragging or excessive concern with money by students with no conception of the reality of private practice. It's possible that practice statistics intimidate (as well as bore) dental students, so be wary of such a possible negative reaction, and don't overload the candidate with data.

Conversely, an experienced dentist who has managed a practice may ask some very candid and incisive questions based on his or her review of one's financial records. Under such circumstances, it would behoove the practice owner to have pertinent fiscal information readily available for this veteran practitioner's perusal. I'm always willing to allow the dentist privacy to study such financial information, and when requested, happy to provide copies of any data.

I make a deliberate effort to reveal our office's blemishes, imperfections and idiosyncrasies. (Although not in too harsh a light.) My interest has always been for the development of a long-term relationship, and after investing many hours and dollars selecting a candidate, having an associate leave is disheartening. I never want an associate's departure to be the result of a lack of candor on my part. The relationship between the senior doctor and associate dentist must be win-win, established on a bedrock of complete honesty. If such openness seems hard to believe, one might recall how our office monitors are shared with all staff, every month, so any practice secrets I might be foolish enough to withhold will soon be revealed to any dentist joining our office.

It also does the associate no good to mislead the employer doctor concerning his/her qualifications and desires, thus being awarded the position under false pretenses, only to lose the job when unrevealed facts become apparent. (For example, if one claims clinical skills he or she doesn't possess, the truth will soon be obvious, and any chance of mutual trust destroyed.)

I would recommend a credit check be performed on a serious candidate. It is not unusual for a dentist—rookie or veteran—who is looking for a new opportunity, to be shouldering significant financial burdens. I would like to be certain he or she has been honest in sharing this pecuniary information with me, just as I have openly and candidly shared my documented financial situation with him or her. Factual awareness of financial pressures is also helpful in salary negotiations, as we'll consider later. One must obtain the applicant's permission to run this check, but a refusal would afford one a great deal of insight.

Personally checking the references of ANY potential employee—dentist or staff—is essential!! A few years ago, a physician whose office was contiguous to mine hired a very attractive young lady to be his office manager. She had extensive previous experience in medical office work (as well as an hourglass figure and Farrah Fawcett hair—not that I suggest these attributes may have influenced the 50-year-old M.D. concerning her hiring. If one is

366

suffering a mid-life crisis, I believe a sports car is a vastly superior alternative to a curvaceous staff member, for any number of reasons).

By the time the doctor realized a problem existed, his best estimate was that she had embezzled approximately $10,000. The frosting on the cake was when he discovered she had been dismissed from two previous jobs for theft. No legal charges were ever filed in any of the three incidents. I guess this or other such unpleasantness couldn't happen in your office? It won't if one diligently and personally checks references.

(Let me remind all that the demanding steps we take in our hiring process are detailed in Chapter 9 of *Focus*, and include patterned personal interviews, hiring summary and reference check forms.)

I prefer the potential associate visit our office while we are actively treating patients. The **office atmosphere** during these times, more than any other factor, should help job candidates decide if our practice represents the right opportunity for them. I advise associate candidates that new patients know if they are in the right place within two minutes of first entering a dental office, or any other service-related business (be it hotel, restaurant, clothing store, etc.). The associate candidates should be able to arrive at a similar quick, intuitive perception.

I suggest he or she attempt to suspend left-hemisphere function for a few moments—not a simple request after eight years of logic and fact-dominated schooling—and imbibe an emotional sense of the office. Does the office smell, sound, taste and look like a place in which he or she would be comfortable? In a similar manner, I place greater weight on my feelings or sense about a candidate than on factual information.

When a candidate does visit, after being welcomed briefly by me, he or she is turned over to a senior staff member for a tour of our office and an introduction to each team member, then is offered tea, coffee, soft drink or juice, and enjoys a quiet visit with our designated office guide in my private office.

We encourage the associates to wander about the office, observing whatever they choose and asking questions. Recall the

367

compatibility of staff to dentist and dentist to staff is essential, and must be determined during this visit. I also gain insight by witnessing what interests he or she has.

My staff is observing the candidate during this time. The visitor is usually unaware of this subtle evaluation, and thus more relaxed and candid with staff than he or she may be with me. In ALL staff hiring—and a dentist is no exception—I rely on feedback from, and the collective judgement of, my staff. Many times information shared with staff—often shocking in its candor—has strongly influenced my employment decision.

My guest and I get our first chance for meaningful communication over lunch (for which I schedule 90 minutes on days when visitors will be in the office). During this time we have an opportunity to get to know each other, and I can address any questions or concerns that may have arisen over the course of the morning. The type of questions asked is perhaps the most revealing factor in helping me begin to understand this individual.

Some ask repeatedly about job security. Others are fixated on patient load and seek reassurance they will make money. I have no way of predicting how any individual will perform financially, and I tell the candidate so. I don't know enough about this person as a dentist—as regards the level of skill, speed and behavioral excellence attained to date—to hazard a guess concerning future performance. We do have written documentation of how other doctors who joined our practice have performed financially during the course of their first year.

I prefer to provide written documents in answer to questions whenever possible, because my memory isn't that great, and I fear inadvertently misinforming my guest. Also, if in the future a question arises about what was said, we have a common document to which both parties may refer.

I'm most impressed with associates whose questions dwell on quality of care and service, but I'm also aware that the level of one's needs (mainly depending on degree of family obligations and debt) often dictates pragmatic concerns. However, while finance and income are essential topics that must be addressed, they should not remain the primary focus of discussion.

As I do with new-patient interviews, during this lunch/interview, I try to only ask questions, confining my declarative sentences to answering direct queries. All my senses must remain open to allow the most accurate assessment of this individual.

After lunch, one of my staff gives the potential associate a guided tour of our community. (This is invariably one of Jo's many tasks, and she's excellent at exhibiting the predominant features of Keokuk, while inquiring as to the associate's special interests—schools, YMCA, churches, shopping, tennis courts, etc.—then touring the appropriate facilities.) Again, Jo is attentive to the dentist's interests. In the relaxed, casual atmosphere of the car, after an intense 90-minute meeting with "The Doctor," often an even more candid and revealing conversation occurs.

After this tour, the associate candidate returns to our office and continues to observe (and be observed) for the few minutes remaining in my treatment day. At the end of patient care we relax in my office, enjoy a beverage, and have the opportunity for a long, uninterrupted talk. By now both parties usually sense if this relationship has a chance for long-term success.

During this quiet interlude, I answer any questions, ask a few, and try to develop a vision concerning our future together. I'll spend whatever time is needed to pose and answer queries, including an evening meal together, but after an hour or so of one-on-one, the associate and I usually feel we have sufficient information.

How we proceed from this point depends on my sense of our future together. I will reflect on this visit carefully before I reach a final decision, but having worked with associates for over a decade, I usually have definite feelings concerning our collective future before the visit terminates. If things seem positive, I give the candidate a copy of our employment contract and tentative buy-in agreement to study, and make arrangements to visit over the phone in a few days.

If I am doubtful we have a future together, I'll ask the dentist to think our day through and get back to me with his or her thoughts. Almost always when I feel things won't work, the candidates do too, and I seldom hear from them again.

Both parties must evaluate the situation objectively and be completely frank with each other regarding lingering questions or concerns. With both dentists' futures at stake, it's no time to be bashful! When each step we've discussed has been carefully completed—**especially reference checks**—and some candidates have withdrawn or been deemed unacceptable, my advice is to choose from among those remaining the individual ONE ENJOYS and with whom one feels comfortable. Trust this emotional content to outweigh the logic, research, and the reasoning. Certainly, do your homework, but after thorough consideration of the facts, I suggest hiring someone you sense will become a friend.

The decision reached, all that remains is to call, offer the job, and, if it is accepted, settle final details (such as the day and time the associate will begin offering care). The contract should have been exchanged and thoroughly discussed before this juncture.

Don't be upset if the job offer is refused, but consider this to be what should have occurred and trust it is for the best. If the offer is rejected, I wish the dentist well, offer to help in any way I can with future decisions, and continue the associate search. Those who desire success, wealth and joy must not be deterred by any disappointment, let alone one as unsubstantial as a rejected job offer.

How to Accelerate an Associate's Success

The decision has been made, the ink on the contract is dry. Finally the day for the associate to begin work in your office has arrived! Let me assure you, it's a bit scary for staff, owner, new dentist and patients, at first. How does one begin to get patients who trust only (wonderful!) Doc Senior to elect to receive care from the unknown, and often unlined, hands of this new provider?

We begin the process by having the local newspaper take a photo of all the practice's dentists shaking hands, welcoming Dr. New to the office. **We prepare an article for the paper—not trust to God as to how an interview might come out—stressing the expertise, charm, interests and any and all possible attributes of our newest team member.** (When preparing press releases, take care to write clearly and position every fact in the best possible light.) Of course, we can't control the final story, but one can make a lot of money betting on over worked and underpaid reporters allowing someone else—in this case, us—to complete their work for them, and your article may appear verbatim.

When Dr. Long joined our office we had an open house to celebrate, partly because both he and his lovely wife, Becky, are Keokuk natives. It was a lot of work and a fairly expensive undertaking. It was also deemed not worth the trouble, and we've never had an open house again. (But feel free to try this. The open house did create a reason for us to do a fair amount of advertising that might have borne fruit later. Don't feel you have to learn from my mistakes!)

Once in the office, our associate begins meeting patients by performing hygiene recare exams, unless the patient objects. (And patients must be asked! One can't force any patient to accept care, so developing skill to enhance and accelerate the new dentist's acceptance is essential. PAY ATTENTION TO THE FOLLOWING INFORMATION!) I impress on the associate—who is paid to do the exam—that each hygiene check is an opportunity to meet a new patient. Every examination should be a WOW! experience, or the neophyte has no chance of the patient's scheduling diagnosed care with Dr. New.

We also allow Dr. New to treat almost every emergency, offering the patient the advantage of being seen almost at once. (Patients will schedule with a new dentist—or accept any other office policy—only when it is perceived to be to **their advantage** to do so. Allowing them to be seen more quickly, offering

371

more convenient evening and Saturday hours, providing services otherwise referred, or treatment at a reduced fee—an act we have never believed in for associates, as it indicates reduced quality—are examples of potential patient advantages.)

We make every effort to schedule routine care with Dr. New also, explaining to patients, "These procedures are now done by Dr. New in our office." If the staff accepts such scheduling as the normal office routine, and presents it as such, the patients will generally follow along. WARNING: if the senior dentist makes exceptions to this policy, it will confuse staff and anger patients if they discover others received treatment they were refused.

Precisely what these "routine" procedures will be depends on the associate's interest and experience. Most commonly these consist of simple fillings—that no experienced dentist regrets not performing—and sealants. It is hoped one has identified an associate with talents no other staff member possesses, or chooses to use. Dr. White began doing all our extractions at once, quickly increasing his and our office's revenue.

We are seldom forced to resort to prophys to keep new associates busy—which is just as well, as almost all the dentists with whom I've worked do a substandard job with cleanings. But prophys are an alternative that allows new dentists to produce some income, keep busy, and get to know patients who may then trust the nice, gentle, young dentist to fabricate the crown they need.

During the open time the first few weeks in the office invariably includes, we have the associate observe senior dentists at work, to demonstrate the specific materials and techniques we employ, and give Dr. New the priceless opportunity to meet more patients. All staff—especially dentists and hygienists—must make a point of introducing the associate to as many patients as possible. We bunch the cases he or she is treating, to free blocks of time during the day for our newest teammate to meet every area dentist, pharmacist, emergency room staffer, etc., as we've discussed previously.

We also attempt to identify areas of unique non-technical skills the associate can employ to develop his or her identity within the office, thus avoiding the engulfment issues we've mentioned. As I've related, the enthusiasm for such tasks has varied a great deal from person to person, so I suggest one monitor the situation carefully, making the associate's projects part of each staff meeting agenda, and not have the unpleasant experience of discovering important tasks performed poorly, or not done at all, months later. (Yet another example of delegating authority, but not responsibility.)

Here is a critical, but seemingly minor or even foolish point. We instruct all staff to repeatedly point out that **"Dr. New has been PERSONALLY SELECTED by Dr. Wilde to join our office."** The foolish part is that of course I selected him or her. Who else could? The amazing part is how this precisely worded statement seems to transfer our trust to the patient, and make scheduling with Dr. New much easier. (And anything one can do to help the front office fill Dr. New's book will be appreciated.) I know it seems silly, but this precise wording works like magic!

The most critical issue, and one that must candidly and repeatedly be shared with Dr. New, is **the absolute necessity of the associate's winning the trust of the entire staff.** This is one objective I can't order accomplished. It must be earned by consistently performing careful, painless, high-quality care and perpetually demonstrating respect and concern for staff and patients.

It's not unusual for a recent graduate or veteran dentist to feel superior to staff and patients. (Routinely keeping others waiting is a clarion call of self-considered superiority.) It has always been my firm belief that our office succeeds or fails as a team. That every assignment is important—including that of the cleaning lady—and no person, including myself, is superior to another. It's heady stuff, being a new doctor. But hubris is not a trait linked to achievement or joy. Heed the ancient warning that those the gods would destroy, they first make proud!

Such a mind-set of equality eliminates any tendency for dentists to belittle or criticize staff in front of patients. (A sin beyond forgiveness in my office. I have apologized just for having annoyed thoughts about a team member.)

If an associate wishes to discover a technique to guarantee failure in an office, I recommend adopting a superior attitude. My excellent staff—who often understand some aspects of dentistry well beyond the level of recent graduates—have no mercy for such arrogance. AND IF THE STAFF DOESN'T BELIEVE AND SUPPORT THE NEW DENTIST, PATIENTS WILL SENSE THIS TRUTH, AND NOTHING I OR ANYONE ELSE CAN DO WILL ALLOW THAT DENTIST TO SUCCEED. It's that simple. It's that critical.

I trust each practice owner now understands that bringing in an associate is a daunting challenge, but also that the documented rewards which accrue when this endeavor has been successfully accomplished make the effort worth undertaking. Assume a year has passed, and the associate has blossomed beyond the owner's expectations. Office production has increased 50%; and overhead declined 10%! Despite everything going well, the owner-dentist has developed a new and pressing problem: what to do with all the extra money?

The quick answer in my family (remember my wife and three daughters?) is to insist more shopping be done! (I guess I could find a few hunting and fishing trips to blow some loot on, if pressed.) But let's move on to Chapter 8 and consider some alternative ways to utilize this burgeoning wealth. (Burgeoning wealth . . . what a felicitous phrase!)

REFOCUS SEVEN: DO YOU WANT TO BE HAPPY FOR THE REST OF YOUR LIFE?

The answer to the above query is simple: YES!!! The "how to" is a little tougher. As always, the devil is in the details.

But modern dentistry is not renowned as a repository of unadulterated joy, so perhaps those within the profession should be willing to labor to define "how to." The litany of travails—suicide, alcohol and drug problems, divorce, etc.—that plague dentists requires no expounding within our profession. Yet this tale of woe exists **in spite** of what would seem compelling factual arguments that dentists should be joyous:

1. Financially, dentists rank in the top percentile of income-earners in America, the wealthiest nation in Earth's history!

2. The personal freedom our profession affords is the envy of many. (Despite notable recent interference by third parties and various governmental regulatory bodies, one would be hard pressed to find a physician not envious of dentists' independence.)

3. Dentists enjoy the trust and admiration of society. In a recent poll, our profession was proclaimed the second most respected occupation. (Compare this to the near-bottom ranking of government officials.)

4. Every dentist has received an excellent education and ranks well above average in intellectual gifts and attainments.

Yet—despite all our blessings—many (most?) of our relatively wealthy, liberated, respected and educated colleagues exist in conditions far removed from perpetual bliss, and polls indicate, if choosing a profession today, the majority would not become dentists. Considering the above enumerated advantages, why is this sad fact so?

We'll eschew all the typical explanations—ungrateful patients, indolent staff, OSHA, HMO, PPO, increasing overhead, stress inherent within the field, post-potty training stress syndrome. All these are external forces over which one has, at best, but slight influence. Our discussion will deal with matters over which one does maintain control—the internal, if uncharted, ways. (I've advised my children for 25 years that they can confront any problem of significance that will ever occur in their lives by **looking in the mirror!**)

Despite evidence that seems to suggest otherwise, the passage to joy isn't controlled by outside events, but lies within ourselves. (Hence the famous expression, "What happens to a man is less significant than what happens within him.") Since one is responsible for internal events, it's possible for those who are intelligent, determined and courageous enough to make the diligent effort necessary to achieve joy. That each has, no matter what the circumstances, within his or her power, the ability to attain bliss is the good news. The bad news, in our society so unwilling to accept personal responsibility: Failure to be joyful is an individual shortcoming.

(Precise methods do exist that, when understood and implemented, allow for life to be filled with joy. This is the common life example and message of every spiritual master to have trod terra firma. I am forced by space constraints to focus this discussion on our professional milieu. To the discerning, our dialogue is replete with clues as to how this information can lead to joy in every facet of existence.)

Let's preface our journey to contentment with a concise review of the three familiar external forces that affect every facet of human decision making. I hope this brief reassessment will provide a slightly diverse examination, to enable some who have trouble with this basic concept to achieve the needed insight, and deepen the understanding of those already sensing the power and truth of these concepts.

As we've discussed, barriers to joy consist of *three layers of illusion,* so ubiquitous as to escape detection by all but the most perceptive, yet so powerful as to dominate the majority of one's decisions, without our conscious knowledge of their existence. To live a life of self-awareness that allows one to **deliberately choose joy** requires identification of these elusive forces. With understanding, one has the option of following these subconscious directives or selecting a path unique to one's needs and desires.

The first of these forces is one's **genetic code**. We are all animals, despite pretensions to being "higher life forms." Humankind's delusion of greatness merely obscures one's deepest and truest nature.

As animals, one's primary drive is to take every action that enhances one's odds to survive and reproduce, thus assuring continuation of one's genes. This genetic imperative is lodged in each particle of one's DNA. There is no "political correctness" mandate involved in genetic directives. Every creature is compelled by these unseen forces of instinctive self, but only the wise are consciously aware of, and thus able to intelligently modify, the demands of one's nature.

Over eons, the forces of natural selection have favored a human mind that is **constantly questing**. A mind left undisturbed for a moment returns to this thought: **I WANT!** As animals, this perpetual desire for more enhances one's odds of survival, as each achievement increases power and thus one's chances for continued existence.

This same drive also creates, within our very souls, a continual **restlessness and anxiety that is an intrinsic portion of humanness**. One's nature, left unexplored and uncontrolled, robs one of peace. There is no natural end to this innate desire for more—even in the most accomplished and wealthy of people. Only awareness of this force, and conscious efforts to limit its influence, will afford one peace.

The second force of subconscious directions comes from **culture** . . . a group acting in concert to achieve a common will. (For examples of culturally dictated behavior, consider paying taxes, or obeying laws and social customs.) A consequence of culture is a belief that one's ideals, language and customs are the best. GOD BLESS AMERICA! Or fill in the name of the nation of one's allegiance, as *every patriot is schooled to feel the same way.* (Such learned bias is essential to create the will necessary to have really good wars.)

The gifts of every culture are significant—language, customs, traditions, values, history—and surely not to be ignored. The reward for devotion to one's kind is an enhanced ability for that culture to thrive, thus enabling individuals within society to increase personal power and maximize one's genetic desire for perpetuity. (And I am grateful that my birth occurred in the most powerful nation ever to exist, where my potential to achieve has been maximized by the might and freedom inherent within the society that, due to a happy quirk of fate, I was blessed to join.)

Dentistry has its unique culture: the "proper way" to do things. These values are enforced not merely by the peer pressure of patients and colleagues, and the weight of historical precedent, but by the profound sanctions of professional organizations and governmental bodies. Those who don't comply with these cultural values are punished. (Do you really believe it's inherently logical to suspend the license of an office that promotes itself as an "unauthorized specialist"—in this land of First Amendment liberty? This is merely an example of cultural control.)

The third force that veils reality is one's **ego**. One's brain functions to convince others, as well as himself or herself, that HE OR SHE IS RIGHT! (Hasn't the sheer mystery of how you are always accurate, among the debris of the continual mistakes of so many others, ever puzzled you? I mean, doesn't your always being correct just seem statistically unlikely? Suspicious?) Ego defines "right" as what is good for the individual, and "evil" as any force that works against one's will.

A positive ego enhances potential for one to achieve his or her genetic desires, as one acting with confidence is more prone to succeed. Genetics' triumph can equate to cultural difficulty if by achieving, one violates any of the myriad social taboos.

As a personal example of the mischief ego running out of control, working against genetic and cultural demands, can precipitate, consider how one becomes addicted to alcohol and other drugs. The mind (ego) craves pleasure and convinces one the experience is positive. Did you think alcoholics were held down and force-fed to the point of addiction? Or perhaps he or she wasn't aware these chemicals could be harmful? Addiction, (be it to drugs, booze, sex, money, food, tobacco, gambling, etc.) results from one's brain demanding pleasure, regardless of the cost to the body.

The greatest fear of ego (self) is rejection. As we've discussed, in ancient times, banishment from society resulted in isolation and almost certain death. Most fear conflict and failure due to the possibility of social renunciation that may follow.

Rejection anxiety also explains why people consistently accept the advice of "experts"—to have a large office, or a "right-sized" office—to market, or not to market—blown like a balloon in the currents of prevailing thoughts, rather than freely following one's unique and carefully considered plans. It seems more admissible to fail within the constraints of accepted wisdom than to succeed based on one's own plans.

Humans need to belong! Yet, such an externally focused mind-set creates an existence akin to a horse wearing blinders. One is pulled this way and that, throughout life, by forces one doesn't fully comprehend. (Doesn't it seem a shame to dedicate eight years of college to prepare one for a lifetime pulling a cart?!)

The combined drive of the above three forces is so pervasive, while most remain unaware of their existence, genetics, culture and ego determine the great majority of behavioral decisions without one's conscious knowledge. **To live a joyful life mandates one be aware of these forces, be able to control their**

influence by one's volition, and thus be liberated to lead an existence chosen by careful thought . . . not reflex.

Yet awareness alone doesn't lead to joy. It merely allows one the **opportunity** to freely choose a path toward wisdom and happiness. But enough of the "old news." Let's consider a definite method to achieve joy within a dental office. Recall that the examples listed, while confined to our profession, can illustrate the pathway to joy in any endeavor.

The first ingredient for achieving joy in the work-place is to attempt to create an atmosphere of **FLOW** in one's every effort. (This is a concept to which I was first introduced by Dr. Mihaly Csikszentmihalyi's fine books *Flow* and *The Evolving Self*. I'd recommend reading these books—especially *The Evolving Self*—to everyone who desires joy.) A sign flow activities are occurring is when one is so involved in what he or she does that awareness of time is lost. Personally, these events most often take place while I'm engaged in sports, hunting or writing, but any activity may result in flow if properly structured—including practicing dentistry.

To obtain flow, some precise criteria must be met:

1. The activity must have CLEAR RULES: The tennis ball lands in bounds. One wishes to produce an average of $2,000 per day, see 20 new patients a month, collect 99%, seat 15 crowns a week.

2. PRECISE FEEDBACK must be available. "I want to feel good," fails this definition. In each example listed above, it's easy to ascertain if one has achieved his or her objective.

3. CHALLENGES AND SKILLS MUST BE IN BALANCE. There's little enjoyment in losing a tennis match 6-0 or winning by the same score. This balance of skill and challenge is so critical in dentistry it will become the entire second step of our three-legged joy formula.

4. A SENSE OF CONTROL is possible, but can only be maintained through concentrated effort. Think back to moments in sports, music or other activities when one experienced

flow. Every dentist has treated patients where he or she enjoyed a sense of mastery. Feels good . . . doesn't it? Yet if one's concentration falters, this dominance can quickly disappear. (This disruption of flow may partially explain the unpopularity of hygiene checks.)

Thus, to enhance joy within the office, one must create flow situations. This means establishing clear goals—not just surviving each day—that are meaningful and easily measured. As one labors to achieve mastery, he or she has created a game situation, within a pressure-filled office, that can lead to pleasant, flow experience.

These "games" can involve the entire staff, and are winnable contests. One not only enjoys the moments of triumph, but experiences growth and success as a result of one's labors. **Understand that joy comes to those who are actively seeking to obtain appropriate and realistic self-set goals**, with full awareness of one's genetic drive to never acquire enough. But joy rarely happens to horses pulling a cart directed by others.

The second portion of our joyful triad deals in greater depth with the third step of flow, the **balance between challenge and skill**. I believe this step is more essential, within the discipline of clinical dentistry, than in most endeavors.

If one's skills for a given task greatly exceed the challenge the activity presents, he or she is bored. Consider a day of nothing but recall examinations.

If one's skills are inadequate to the challenge, he or she suffers anxiety. The image of an endodontic procedure performed on the upper second molars of an obese, gagging-prone, apprehensive patient who is "hard to get numb" flashes through my brain—raising a fine sheen of perspiration on my entire epidermis. (Please feel free to select the clinical nightmare of your own choosing.)

While dentists can't totally avoid either boredom or anxiety, one can learn to control them. Certainly one can enhance dental skills with education and effort, but the wise refer treatment too challenging for one's current level of ability. (The anxiety these too-difficult procedures foster is not consistent with joy, or the maintenance of reasonable mal-practice insurance rates!)

Be aware of the negative effect to one's sense of wellness from both boredom and anxiety. Be certain each daily schedule contains a mixture of simple and complex procedures—not all elementary one day, all intricate the next. This balance is easily achieved by setting daily production goals. A day containing all simple procedures is low-production and boring, while all complex treatment results in a day of high production and possibly fatal hypertension. Seek the golden mean by attempting to schedule each day near one's carefully set production average; this targets an important portion of one's practice vision.

The third segment of one's quest for joy is the knowledge that **an appropriate increase in life complexity leads to personal growth which, in turn, leads to joy**, be it in relationships, skills, hobbies or dentistry.

Fearing the new and unknown is a natural protective reflex, similar to humans' fear of snakes. Knowledge that within feelings of anxiety are the seeds of growth can cause the enlightened to seek out challenges lying within the range of their abilities, thus maximizing success and bliss. (Climbing Mount Everest lies beyond the pale of most, and setting such an impossible goal is unlikely to enhance joy.) Many activities are pleasant, but only those resulting in growth lead to meaningful and lasting enjoyment and an enhanced sense of self (ego).

In modern America, self-esteem seems to have become something that is granted. Another of Americans' burgeoning list of rights and entitlements, of promised gain without strain or pain. As if the mere fact of existence carries with it an innate and perpetual self-worth. Nothing could be further from the truth.

If one wishes to feel good about himself or herself—to enjoy an authentic and sustainable positive self-image—do the right things . . . avoid the bad. If one leaves decay under a restoration, or seats a crown with an open margin, low self-esteem should result. One's behavior has earned the distress, despite his or her

382

brain's most ingenious efforts to create excuses, by the short-sighted behavioral selection made. Such discomfort serves as a guide to direct one back toward the pathway to right action and happiness. (Alcohol allowed me to ignore many such warnings of impending disaster, until my life pulled a *Titanic!*)

On the other hand, when one confronts a difficult situation and grows in the act of dealing with the obstacle, be it an honest sharing of feelings with another or a complex procedure performed well, authentic growth has occurred. Once the challenge has been faced (or, on occasion, endured), the positive feelings that result have substantiality. (Unlike the fleeting joys of addictive behaviors.)

Seneca told us long ago that, "The good things which belong to prosperity are to be wished, but good things that belong to adversity are to be admired."

Enjoy the pleasant things of life—the nice day, the quiet talk of sports and the mundane—the good things of prosperity. But understand that reliable and abiding joy comes from meeting challenges and thus earning, by one's extraordinary efforts, the seeds of growth contained within.

Failure doesn't exist—it is merely another of many illusions. There is only effort and outcome. Each adversity courageously faced offers a chance to grow—to become more complex within the fabric of one's being—and thus to earn true and lasting joy. Not the fleeting pleasure of a nice meal or kind word, but the internal glow of well-deserved self-contentment that is THE ingredient most essential to a joyful career and life.

Summary

The pathway to bliss begins with awareness. Study one's behavior with a new alertness to genetic, cultural and ego-driven bias. Are one's actions consistent with his or her carefully elucidated beliefs and values, or controlled by forces beneath one's conscious awareness? (It is culture, assuming the guise of peer pressure, that advises one to be just like everyone else in order to gain acceptance . . . even if this means being miserable!)

Apply this new clarity to one's profession (and life). Attempt to create flow activities within the office by focusing on carefully selected and defined goals and achievements. Be aware of the essential need to balance skills and challenges to obtain happiness. Boldly seek obstacles appropriate to one's current skill level, identifying them as opportunities to grow and thus earn enduring joy. Set aside the foolish fear of failing that restricts one's personal potential, and toil to become more.

The path I recommend requires bravery and prodigious effort. I hope the topics of this book will present a blueprint of meaningful challenges to many. By undertaking these suggested exertions, one will provide excellent service and be rewarded by an existence replete with happiness and excitement; a career and life blessed with success, wealth, internal peace and joy. Choose to make life a courageous adventure. Settle for nothing less.

Chapter Eight

Financial Freedom

I've written a lot about money (my utterances revealing where my mind and heart often lie). There are probably as many concepts concerning the purpose and use of money as there are people, but to me, **money is a form of stored energy**. Energy, in its many guises—food, shelter, drink, mutual funds—is the substance all modern citizens must labor to achieve to maintain life. Having the energy of money stored relieves one of the need (not necessarily the desire) to work. Thus money is the coin of the realm with which I purchase my most precious possession: **Freedom!**

I'd encourage every reader to make a conscious effort to consider the place and function of money in his or her life as one studies this chapter. Ask yourself, "Do I understand, am I comfortable in my relationship to currency?" "Does my existing financial situation fill me with joy?" and "If not, what exactly do I need to change?" Such an in-depth, personal awareness concerning money—an unavoidable source of so much pain and joy—is foundational to achieving success, wealth and joy.

Allow me to briefly describe my previous writings on money. The final 80 pages of *Focus* defines money market funds (henceforth MMF), bonds—government, corporate and municipal (tax-free), stocks, and how, why and where one can purchase each of these assets.

In Chapter 20 of *Focus*, I also discussed my utilization of retained corporate earnings. I successfully employed retained earnings for 15 years, but no longer use them, as the potential returns from the lengthy bull market in American stocks, with average annual returns during the last few years of 30%, made tax sheltering of a stock paying a 7% dividend within my professional corporation not the best possible use of resources.

In Chapter 23 of *Focus* I also reveal how I financed my four children's education, using the least expensive and most effective possible method, by investing for them, virtually on the day each was born, employing the Uniform Gift to Minors Act (UGMA).

I add a personally painful chapter on financial losses I have experienced (Chapter 24 of *Focus*), hoping others might learn from my errors. I'm delighted to inform one and all I have no financial failures to add to my ledger since that chapter was written, around 1993, mostly due to the seemingly unstoppable bull market. I know a bull market is not to be confused with genius, but its bountiful fruits may be enjoyed just as much as if one had earned the returns by his or her sagacity!

I also devoted 36% of *Freedom* to financial concerns—creating an "everydoctor investment guide"—an asset ladder used to identify the proper investment during all the various situations and segments of one's life. I contend there is no one perfect investment, for if there were, no other choice would exist. But there is an ideal investment for any individual, at a given point in time. This optimal asset can be identified by considering such variables as the person's investment acumen, time devoted to finance, personal interest in the subject, amount of money available, and appropriate risk at any given life juncture.

The topic of mutual funds was also addressed in *Freedom*, and I included 25 pages of dialogue concerning a variety of hypothetical investment situations whose examples are meant to guide investors of every ilk.

These two resources, and virtually countless other books, are available to explain the bedrock of investing. I won't repeat a word of the basics here. Instead, I will present a series of essays on finance, each related, yet each with a unique message.

Please forgive some deliberate redundancy. (Feel free to take umbrage over accidental repetitions!) Certain points are so critical to developing a useful relationship with money and achieving fiscal success, I have chosen to repeat them, in variations of the same powerful, basic theme. (Raising kids tends to enhance one's tendency to reiterate important messages.)

I don't comprehend everything (closer to nothing) the first time I'm exposed to information. I assume most are like me in this regard—and pray none are worse—and these reverberating vital messages are central considerations that **I have observed, from dentists' behavior, the great majority need to have strongly, repeatedly reinforced.**

We'll begin by examining several versions of a personal relationship with wealth, dealing with the development of a general philosophy concerning money. We'll proceed to the vital need and techniques that assist one in getting out of debt. These behaviors naturally flow into saving and building toward financial independence.

Allow me to clearly state that I react to debt as most people react to poisonous snakes, and I've saved money steadily since my first job at age 8.

However, as a portion of my evolving philosophy of money, I made a deliberate choice, shortly after undergoing treatment for my alcoholism and enduring the terror of Megan's head injury, to no longer make a conscious effort to save. At that time, my annual investment returns already exceeded yearly savings, and it seemed appropriate (and still does) to **enjoy the wealth I'd worked so hard to obtain.** I hope each reader will someday be allowed similar financial freedom, but my nature urges each to be certain one's status makes such a decision realistic.

I define "financial freedom" as having sufficient wealth that one no longer is forced to work for a living. As having attained sufficient net worth to live the lifestyle of one's choice until all material needs have ceased. (That's a sensitive, rather poetic way of saying DEAD.) I can promise all the joy of never having to worry about funds again is an experience worthy of the profound efforts we are about to contemplate. It frees one's mind for an entirely NEW, refreshing, challenging and exciting set of problems!

Please understand, and here the redundancy begins, that **developing a PERSONAL VISION OF WEALTH is the key to obtaining the amount of riches one desires, as well as finding peace and happiness with money.** (History is replete with cautionary tales of the wealthy and miserable—not a goal any sensate being desires.) **Creating an image in one's mind is the first vital step to all meaningful achievement.** (All creation begins with thought, proceeds to words, then is achieved through action.) It is this carefully defined understanding as regards personal finance that allows one to be resolute in his or her chosen course, and persist in a discipline, in times fat and lean, that will lead to the level of wealth appropriate to one's wishes and values.

Lacking such an empowering central vision, one might make decisions based upon whim and emotion. Capricious choices frequently prove to be mistakes in any circumstances, but in no venue is an unblinking focus more critical than in the unforgiving realm of finance.

(I trust the parallel between forming an essential vision of the office one desires, and the same integral discipline being necessary regarding money, is not lost. **Any meaningful accomplishment begins with the formation of a detailed and powerful vision of a precise goal that is consistent with one's carefully and clearly defined values.**)

We'll end this chapter with two short, but interesting financial topics:

How one can GUARANTEE each of his or her children will become millionaires—if such an achievement is deemed desirable—even if their parents never obtain that lofty goal, and

The ideal way to fund one's charitable giving to focus efforts in a more meaningful manner, maximize tax deductions, be absolutely certain each charity is legitimate, and have all tax chores and record-keeping performed for you at no charge.

Let's commence our study with a story about my 25th-year dental-class reunion that I hope will challenge and stimulate your thoughts concerning a personal philosophy of money, as this event did mine.

The Reunion

It was great fun visiting with my dental-school classmates at our 25th reunion in the fall of 1997. I had drifted out of touch with most, and hadn't seen some since graduation. (Insecure as I am, I was keenly disappointed to discover **none** were bald or fat!)

Late Friday night, as a group of six or so hoary dental veterans sat around a table, I was asked, based on my writings, how the heck I was financially able to work so few days and be almost ready to retire? (I was hardly selected as even remotely likely to succeed—especially by my classmates who slept at night, while I walked an eight-hour beat as a campus policeman—so the note of incredulity in the query was understandable to me.)

You've read enough of my history to know the answer, but I was embarrassed to be suddenly put on the spot. Working hard, avoiding debt, saving and investing are answers lacking the charm to which I felt members of the country-club set are entitled. So I explained I had married into the Coca-Cola family fortune. (I don't know why Coke. I was probably drinking a diet one.)

Allow me to complete the history of my delusion episodes. (At least the ones to which I'll admit in writing!) I was Christmas shopping with Jo a few years ago, in an out-of-town mall, when a comely young clerk, who had just sold us a sweater, looked at my credit card and asked, "What kind of doctor are you?"

When I replied, "A neurosurgeon," Jo, who was standing right next to me, about spit up! A delightful conversation ensued about the pro and con of cutting into brains for a living, but when we exited the store, Jo was understandably puzzled. "Why did you say such a thing?"

"I don't know. I'll never see that girl again, and for that moment, I just didn't feel like being a dentist."

389

The Coke thing was meant as an obvious joke. (Like I'd work had I married millions! Maybe my classmates thought we lived in $60-per-month, rat-hole student housing because we were eccentric?) Until Jo was asked about her "fortune" by a classmate's wife the next day, I didn't realize others took it seriously. (Even I am forced to admit my on-the-spot fabrication seems more likely than the true story!)

I will admit Jo is heiress to a successful farm family, her personal fortune differing from the level of a Coke inheritance, only by the number of zeros at the end. (Perhaps I'd better confess this too is intended as a joke. Seems I learned little from what Jo refers to as the "reunion incident.")

Anyway, my weak attempt at humor allowed me to escape the embarrassment of trying to give a serious explanation to my former classmates, although two did ask to be sent copies of my books, so they now understand my path. After we returned home, I fell to reflecting about how I did—seemingly against all odds—achieve wealth, at least by my definition.

(I have a net worth, in liquid assets, in excess of $2.5 million—not considering the value of my home, dental practice, the office space in which I practice, cars, gold fillings, hunting dogs, etc.—and no debt—in case one wonders exactly what an Iowa boy might consider wealth. Perhaps owning two hogs?)

I hope by now—because there ain't much book left—readers accept my candor as disclosure, not hubris. I grow perpetually more frustrated by wasting my time reading the thoughts of dental "experts" who reveal their supposed qualifications only in glowing but incomplete generalities. Such a dearth of hard data makes it impossible to quantify the value of their assertions, and I'm getting too old to squander precious moments trying to determine if these experts have actually achieved that of which they speak and write. (While I'm venting, having to urinate around 4 a.m. is also growing tiresome!)

I'm unsure why American culture has determined sex and money are two topics not to be discussed in polite company, as I don't think either are "dirty," and this societal censorship diminishes understanding of these two vital subjects. I am honestly relating who I am, and this should be understood in a similar manner to a dog's rolling on its back, exposing its soft under-belly . . . as a gesture of trust.

Readers know my humble history; my fears and insecurity. **It was never my goal—not even my dream—to become wealthy. I did have a POWERFUL DESIRE never to be poor.** It is said that great athletes, in championship games, often hope only to not embarrass themselves. That's pretty close to my thinking concerning finances. It would be wonderful to excel, but I didn't want to make any horrendous blunders that would provide a source of amusement for others.

What follows are my thoughts concerning how I did achieve wealth. I trust my reflections will advance each reader's consideration of his or her personal philosophy about money. (Recall that developing clarified financial values is your ASSIGNMENT FOR THIS CHAPTER.)

All 20 or so of my classmates who attended the reunion, with the exception of myself and two other bottom-feeding general dentists, were specialists. Many of them probably had more successful practices than I. (All had nicer clothes!) I don't know the details of any of my classmates' financial situations, other than what I gathered from scraps of conversation, but none seemed near retirement. But, after speaking to numerous dentists for several years now, I understand many spend to purchase things—luxury homes, expensive cars, even trophy spouses—in a doomed attempt to assuage a sense of emptiness and dread with objects.

At some point, even the ultra-successful, big-dollar producer practitioners discover, often to their horror, that they haven't achieved joy, yet have incurred mountainous debt resulting from failed attempts to purchase happiness. They sense their strength beginning to ebb, yet must continue to produce at the same level to service debt. (The expression, "service debt" should, by itself, cause one to pause, for two reasons. Who would choose to be debt's servant? Also, in farm country, we say the male animal services the female.)

The possessions—once a hoped-for source of joy—and the accompanying financial obligations now feel like millstones tied around their necks. Aware they aren't physically and emotionally able to produce at this level much longer, and knowing debt service makes it impossible for them not to, they grow fearful, finally aware of the self-set snare into which they have fallen.

Is there a single individual in recorded history who has achieved happiness through possessions? I know of none, and yet so many try, seduced by the *Maya*—the illusion—of the material world. The failure of wealth to create happiness is the message of the ancient myth of King Midas and the curse of the golden touch, as well as among the main teachings of every spiritual master throughout history of whom I'm aware.

I hope the REFOCUS segments prove meaningful, as the rest of the book is little more than a complex excuse—a carrier—to allow these thoughts to appear in print. (It's easier to worm a cat than to get dentists to read philosophy!) As a millionaire who once longed for death, let me assure you, if one is unable to achieve a working philosophy of life, nothing else matters, least of all material possessions.

I return, somewhat reluctantly, from the comfortable arms of philosophy to the mundane explanation of how I was able to become wealthy. I believe the single most important factor in achieving my financial freedom was the **unconscious decision** I made to **OBJECTIFY MONEY**.

(In complete candor, the following ideas didn't occur to me until after the reunion, so I realize this mind-set did not consciously lead to my financial freedom. However, had I been blessed with a carefully reasoned, values-based, balanced awareness of the purpose of money earlier in my life, I feel I could have avoided great pain, and still attained wealth. Remember, our clear goal is to achieve success, wealth and joy **simultaneously**. I attained each separately, and as a result, suffered greatly during the process.)

For reasons we'll explore, but which may never be completely clear, **I made money my "TOY," my object—the primary source of my sense of self.** In the early days of my savings, purchasing a $5,000 municipal bond replaced clothes, new cars, bigger homes, country club memberships, trips to Hawaii, extramarital relationships—whatever attainments and/or objects those who seek to purchase happiness choose as a medium of exchange.

Certainly the pain and suffering I endured (most convincingly demonstrated by my addiction) showed I too had lost my way, but when my pain diminished, I had over $1 million in the bank, not merely a collection of aging and depreciating status symbols. (I guess I'm suggesting money as a superior delusion to those who remain unenlightened?!?)

Money is too integral to the functioning of contemporary society to be ignored. In the modern world, having no clear concept of personal finance is akin to driving on the Interstate with one's eyes closed. The only question is where and when disaster will strike. (Wager on soon and near.)

There exist two basic ways in which one interacts with currency. Which method one chooses defines the most critical philosophical decision one ever makes concerning money . . . and eventually everyone's behavior falls predominantly into one of these groups.

1. **One can work FOR money**, as do all who owe debt and pay interest. (The serviced!)

2. **One can have money work FOR THEM**, as do all who save and invest. (The servicers!)

Take a moment right now—an interlude of honest and courageous insight—to define into which group you belong. Ask yourself, is this where you wish to remain? Consider the words of the brilliant P.T. Barnum (yes, the circus guy), who advised money is a wonderful servant (member, Group 2) but a terrible master (member, Group 1). **(Do you understand this critical point!?!)**

It seems to me THIS is the clear fork in the road. (Who said, if one comes to a fork in the road . . . pick it up?) The watershed decision each must make concerning his or her relationship with money. Either one **chooses** to employ money on his or her behalf, and delay gratification (much more on the trait/ decision to delay gratification will follow) or one attempts to achieve joy by purchasing stuff, and risks being forced to exist as money's servant. (As most dentists are BLESSED with relatively prodigious incomes, achieving wealth is usually a choice one can realistically make. This is a precious truth many grasp too lightly!) This single decision determines if one will spend a lifetime swimming with or against financial currents.

This may also be seen as a fundamental psychological decision to choose substance and lasting internal gratification over appearance and the need to impress (fool?) others. The general choice of working hard to achieve, or attempting short cuts to joy, overlaps into many other life venues in addition to finance.

It might provide clarity, at this early juncture, to ask oneself how buying things one can't afford to achieve happiness is working to date, if such is the choice one has made in his or her quest for success, wealth and joy? (It is certainly the majority decision in American culture!) I've stated I know of no one who has ever purchased his or her way to happiness. I believe it is IMPOSSIBLE to use debt to achieve these critical ends, although, should it be done, I'm confident it will be an American who achieves such a breakthrough, as we are working so diligently toward the unlikely end of **owing one's way to success**!

Allow me to summarize my retrospective realization of the subconscious choice that led me to wealth. By some legerdemain I found the genetic, cultural and ego gratification I (ALL) need to be (at least marginally) happy by focusing on the process of storing energy in the form of money. I presume the vigor of my drive is partially explainable by my soul-deep need for freedom . . . to choose, to express (the carrot), and my terror of failure—of which poverty may be my most haunting example (the stick).

Let's consider the forces of genetics, culture and ego as regards wealth. Simultaneous forces urge one to attain, (genetic), to share (culture), and to do nothing that will lead to rejection, while still being admired as an individual (ego). (I never claimed attaining balance was easy . . . merely essential!)

394

It's obvious how my **genetic** needs were fulfilled by wealth accumulation. Working hard and obtaining money—a potent form of contemporary power—maximizes my personal, and my genetic legacy's (children's), opportunity to continue to survive and reproduce. (Studies have illustrated that wealth enhances reproductive opportunities. That hasn't been the case for me, and, as essential as such information may be, for once I'm going to heed society's—and my wife's—wishes . . . and just not go there!)

Culturally, I've always had to walk a tightrope. Civilization's forces suggest that reaping the rewards for working one's brightest and hardest makes one guilty of the sin of greed. Today it is politically correct in many circles to believe that all people should be equally rewarded, regardless of effort or achievement. You know how I feel about such road apples! (That's Iowa talk for the odoriferous debris that periodically cascades from the aperture beneath the tail of a horse.)

Yet, obtaining success will result in one's being judged and criticized for hard-won achievement (in spite of the fact that the Christian faith considers jealousy—the act of coveting—to be a sin). I'm aware of this fact, but prefer paying the price of others' resentment of success, rather than settling for achieving less than the utmost of which I'm capable. Let's consider possible ways to reduce this "social cost of success."

Visible signs of wealth act as a lightning rod for such censure. While many go into debt to procure such trophies (borrowing money to purchase the resentment of peers?), I'm not a showy guy by nature; thus—though insecurity gives me a tendency to brag—I've never suffered greatly the need to acquire objects to impress others. (We still live in the home we purchased in 1975. I've always maintained there is no reason to ever wear clothes in which one would hesitate to skin a squirrel, although—thanks mainly to Jo—my formal wardrobe has evolved beyond this earthy description, if only marginally).

On the other hand, this lack of interest in others—or preoccupation with introspection and personal achievement—has resulted in my facing societal rejection due to lack of sensitivity to others' emotions.

I suspect wealth would be more socially acceptable in one who has learned to be aware, or who, due to his or her nature, is naturally more keenly aware of others' thoughts and emotions. I'd don't anticipate living long enough to become such a person, and thus ever being in a position to prove or disprove my hypothesis.

However, the Bible instructs that from whom much is given, much is expected. I accept this wisdom, and feel richly blessed, in many ways. I have tried to return some small portion of my bounty to the community from which it came.

A powerful spiritual nature has led me—admittedly sometimes reluctantly—toward charity. (The final segment of this chapter deals with forming Charitable Gift Trusts, illustrating it is not contradictory to be both charitable and SMART!) This seemingly innate metaphysical drive to help others, for which I claim no credit, may be the only trait that has allowed me to co-exist within community!

Be aware of the substantial cultural forces that seek to punish success. (Dr. Paddi Lund and his associate and editor, Mr. Fletcher Potanin, have shared with me what is referred to as the "tall poppy syndrome" in Australia. This is the tendency for people who achieve above the norm to be destroyed by their peers, as a poppy that grows above its mates is surely demolished by the winds. This is a powerful metaphor!)

Understand these attacks are not personal, and if you crave the company and esteem of others, avoid an ostentatious lifestyle. Personally, my nature saved me from being overly flamboyant, and having no desire to purchase "trophies," allowed accelerated enhancement of my wealth. But I've never made any conscious effort to hide my prosperity, and it's a decision for which I—and my family—have paid a price in social rejection.

While the relationship of culture and my personal success has always been ambivalent, **ego** may be the key to my successful personal philosophy of wealth. I've been able to create a satisfactory sense of self—a positive identity—through money accumulation. This deep sense of security and well-being has freed me from much of the need or desire to impress others (except for the aforementioned tendency to boast, that sickens me afterwards as much as alcohol ever did).

For instance, I've always purchased new, quality cars, but usually drive them for a decade. (I love my five-year-old Lexus, and have no plans to trade it. This is the only vehicle I own, so it serves as my "hunting truck." I especially appreciate the ability to fit two dog kennels into the back seat!)

As I mentioned, I don't care for clothes—other than to cover a body increasingly less seemly—and have no desire to join a country club. I'm most happy hunting, gardening, writing, reading—usually alone, except for my family and hunting buddies. (I KNOW I would have been much happier born 200 years ago, except the guns of that era weren't very accurate. Anybody else feel misplaced in time?)

Why money satisfies my ego needs so completely, I don't pretend to fully understand. Could be genetics (I share with my father a downright fierce hunter/gatherer nature), my impoverished upbringing (strident need bequeathed to me what Dr. Earl Estep—one of my heroes—refers to as a "death grip on reality," at least as pertains to money), or a mean streak so virulent that it keeps me away from others and thus any risk of adopting behavior based on their conceptions of right or wrong. Whatever the reason, I'm delighted that it works for me, as being generally free of concern and fear of the thoughts and opinions of others is as wonderful a gift as is financial independence.

I'm not even vaguely suggesting my path to be ideal—for me, let alone anyone else—merely attempting to assist the reader (and myself) to develop an understanding of what might have resulted in a personal philosophy that has dictated wealth, or how one's values concerning money could lead to a lack of same. I hope these thoughts will be helpful for those who desire the freedom of wealth—money is only an obligation to those who choose to make it so; as for most, I believe financial freedom to be an essential ingredient of joy.

While my motivations to wealth are admittedly less than lucent, I make no pretense of understanding debt from a genetic, cultural, ego or any other standpoint. It seems the entire status of one who purchases with debt, or with funds one can't afford, is DELUSION, CHIMERA, SELF-DECEIT. Perhaps I'm missing something?

Genetically, debt is counter-productive to survival, almost a form of negative energy. Perhaps reproductive opportunities are enhanced by the appearance of wealth? (And never underestimate the power of this innate reproductive drive, despite culture's dictates that it not be discussed.) True wealth would be a more effective genetic force, but takes time, effort and talent to achieve. Debt may be perceived as a short cut to enhanced sexual opportunities, but it seems to me a gain consummated (the word used advisedly) at the cost of one's future. Debt bequeaths no positive impact to the fate of one's progeny.

Culturally, the leased luxury car and heavily mortgaged home lend the appearance of success, but it is this very demeanor of affluence that can lead to rejection. I'm uncertain as to the motive of those who wish to be envied, thus disliked, especially when the success for which they are ostracized is counterfeit. I believe the concepts we are exploring have not been carefully considered, and the net result is one living a lie, and being rejected and isolated for the wealth he or she doesn't possess.

(Does anyone believe one is liked because of his or her riches? Others may choose to hang around, or seek employment with the affluent, but not due to affection. They are merely attempting to fulfill their genetic mandates by trying to capture some of the wealth for themselves. Think of the relationship as akin to that of a shark and blood, the wealthy person being the blood, those in need the sharks.)

Ego may prove the essential argument to illustrate that achieving happiness by using debt is impossible. How can one hope to evolve a powerful, enduring, positive sense of self, when continually aware he or she is deceiving others? Life can't be fulfilling and wonderful when one exists with the perpetual awareness he or she is living a lie.

398

I believe only achievements that are honestly earned can result in the consistently untroubled sleep of the just all desire—all need—to possess hope of achieving peace and joy. It is possible to fool others, but I'm amazed at the lengths to which people go toward the impossible task of deluding themselves. Devote that deceptive energy into a quest to become the kind of person one pretends to be, thus earning the abiding peace of mind so craved.

These thoughts are humbly presented in an effort to stimulate one to create a conscious, value-based, proactive mind-set as regards money. As we proceed to consider economic strategy and reality, one should continue to reflect and refine one's vision as to the ideal role money will play in one's life.

The topic of this chapter is money, so by necessity, we'll focus on that single subject. Again I plead, please don't lose sight—as I did years ago—of the essential need for balance in one's life. Money is a necessity in modern culture and can't safely be ignored, but one must not be seduced into over-valuing currency either.

One must grow socially, in one's work, spiritually, as well as in the realm of finance and material objects, to achieve bliss. Only when all these facets of one's life have been optimally developed has one maximized personal growth—the task I consider to be the **purpose of existence.**

Let's continue on this path by considering some of the more commonplace steps essential to the achievement of wealth.

Money Just Shouldn't be a Problem

That's right, money should be no problem, at least for dentists. Compare our income to the average of the world's population, the mean of Americans' remuneration, one's capital resources as a student or—for many—the income with which one's parents purchased a home and raised a family. Granted, achieving success takes time and effort, but we're wealthy by virtually any standard of comparison. Contemporary dentists are indubitably documented as among the highest revenue generators in the history of humankind.

But cold reality belies the above bold assertions. Few dentists consider themselves wealthy. Most struggle with personal and professional financial matters, often being unable to comfortably afford even equipment that would enhance their ability to provide care. One repeatedly hears the stark statistic that only 5% of dentists can retire and maintain the lifestyle they enjoyed while practicing. How can this be? What is the problem?

Thousands of erudite pages, hundreds of hours of lectures, are annually devoted to the issue of dental financial well-being. Yet, over my years in the profession, whatever change has occurred in dentists' collective fiscal situation has been to the worse. (Dentists' net incomes continue a steady annual decline in terms of inflation-adjusted purchasing power—the only accurate measure of financial status.) Perhaps the answers offered have been too complex, diverse and difficult to implement.

One ideally begins any project with a solid foundation. I will demonstrate in four indelibly clear steps how each and every member of our profession can place himself or herself on a sound underpinning upon which enduring financial independence can be constructed. What follows is not a shortcut to wealth unearned and thus undeserved; no bag of magic beans is offered. It is a concise plan that anyone may grasp and implement which, when nurtured with effort and time, will achieve the objectives of professional success and personal financial freedom residing along the pathway to the ultimate goal of bliss.

Step One: Clearly comprehend that one is engaged in the business of dentistry!

Our profession has been exempt from many onerous fiscal realities for decades due to a shortage in supply of our brethren, the fiscal stimulus provided by the advent of dental insurance—at first as generous as it now is constricting—and the LEGAL MONOPOLY WE ENJOY. But, as we've examined, the halcyon days of guaranteed financial achievement in dentistry are ending. The competitive pressures of an over-supply of dentists, escalating government intrusion, insurance and third-party plans with effects that steadily reduce one's profit margin, plus the ubiquitous forces of taxes and inflation, are eroding our profession's profitability.

But what industry can survive and not pay attention to the business that is its livelihood? Dentists' days of indulgence in this regard have ended, as they have for the professional monopolies of medicine and pharmacy, and every other industry of which I'm aware. Today each dentist who hopes to survive must volitionally embrace the mantle of businessperson.

One must be aware of and control expenses by diligently and thoughtfully challenging every outlay of capital. One must precisely comprehend every nuance of monthly profit and loss statements, making needed adjustments as these documents dictate. One must perpetually seek methods to enhance his or her office's stream of revenue by becoming more efficient (refining systems with the aid of accurate monitors) and adding increased patient services to treatment options.

One must refuse to be deluded by such fool's gold as production or new-patient flow, focusing energies unerringly on the penultimate measure of practice success: NET PROFIT. In short, one must act like **every other successful business in the world.** Surely this mandate is not unreasonable?

Step Two: As a result of this business orientation, a steady stream of practice profits will eventually be forthcoming. One must then create a precise plan to get out and stay out of debt, from which NO circumstance will allow one to vary.

Debt is the act of mortgaging one's future to pay for the present. Look at the precarious position in which spending money not earned has placed our nation, or consider the fiscal collapse of the Soviet Union. Individuals go readily into debt, yet this very behavior decimated the great bear of Russia, threatens to destroy America, and YOU AND I DON'T ENJOY THE POWER TO LEVY TAXES.

(I know it can't happen here—because we are different— but do you ever consider the lifestyle changes occurring within the last decade to dentists residing in the (ex-?) superpower nations of Russia and Japan? In the event of a complete national collapse, I can shoot and grow all my family requires to survive. What's your plan?)

The method to recover from the shameful and painful debt that strangles many dentists is simple: **Begin spending less than one makes**. How did one ever assume a right to enjoy the use of money he or she had not yet earned?

The *discipline* of debt repayment leads naturally into the act of saving. With every pay period, the FIRST CHECK WRITTEN goes to debt reduction, then, when one's financial ledger is cleared, the next to savings. One deposits not what is left when he or she has eaten and drunk their fill, but the **first dollars earned**. No level of earning power exists that will allow one who spends more than he or she makes, to achieve financial freedom! IF ONE FAILS IN THIS STEP OF DISCIPLINE ONE HAS VIRTUALLY NO CHANCE TO ACHIEVE FINANCIAL FREEDOM AND THE PEACE IT OFFERS.

Forgo forever the dishonor of spending what one has yet to earn—a behavior I consider a form of moral dishonesty—even if legal. Dedicate a specific amount of money each pay period to the first check of savings. Realize that with this payment, one is purchasing a passage to financial freedom. What else could one possibly buy that contains greater value? When you run out of money before you run out of month, do without and learn from the experience. Accumulating wealth is just this simple and is essential if one has no wish to be a "rich doctor" who can't pay his or her bills.

Consistent saving is an integral facet of creating a life structured around discipline and moderation. In all aspects of one's life—diet, exercise, spending, relationships, managing one's office—one must strive for this equilibrium of work, play, friendship and spiritual presence. **Undisciplined behavior of every ilk—be it spending, drinking, eating—is an attempt to soothe the pain occasioned by a life out of balance.** These efforts always fail and often increase the very pain one is attempting to attenuate. (I diligently tried to drink myself happy. Sadly, the

402

effort didn't prove successful, despite high initial hopes, amazing creativity and unflagging effort devoted to the task.)

Step Three: Debt reduced, and a steady flow of savings now guaranteed (see how simple—if not easy—a successful life really is?), one must understand investing at a level that is ideal for his or her unique financial status.

A description of the "ideal investment" depends entirely on each individual's situation. How much **time, interest, ability and capital** does one bring to the table? Inappropriate investments can rob one of growing savings and peace of mind. (Again, an in-depth discussion of ideal investment vehicles and choices comprises the final third of *Freedom* and *Focus*, and won't be repeated here.)

Step Four: Time will make one wealthy.

This is the final factor in our equation. Create a successful dental business, get out of debt and save with discipline. Invest sagaciously in a manner consistent with the unique individual one is. The more one saves, and the greater the return on one's investments, the faster he or she will accumulate wealth. But once one is on this trail, only time separates them from the attainment of whatever financial goals they have established. (We'll observe an example of The Eighth Wonder of the World—compounding interest—most carefully later in this chapter.)

Completion of each and every one of these four steps is essential to achieve one's goal of fiscal independence.

The awareness that one is free of debt and growing in wealth and stature will give one a sense of pride and a deserved peace of mind more profound than even Prozac can provide. This will prove a welcome respite from the sleep-robbing dread of a life filled with potential, yet remaining unfulfilled. The laws of nature have not been repealed, even for dentists. It remains essential that one DO THE CORRECT THINGS to earn a life of joy. Within right action lies the pathway not just to wealth, but to peace and happiness.

With these four steps an immutable, concise, stable foundation upon which one may build financial freedom has been established. Let's proceed to employ this foundation as it is meant to be used—as a base upon which to further build one's understanding of success, wealth and joy.

Six Fundamental Habits of Wealthy Dentists

As you already know, I worked my way through eight years of education, paying virtually 100% of my expenses. In 1974, after a two-year military hitch, I began a practice from scratch. I borrowed $10,000 from my Grampa Kehr, had saved $10,000 during my two years in the army (on a salary of $16,000 per annum) and paid off the remaining $10,000 required to build the office from the first two months' cash flow. Eight months after first opening the office doors, my practice was completely debt-free. Thirteen years later, I no longer needed to work for income, as I had accumulated enough wealth to achieve lifetime financial security for my loved ones and myself.

I'm often asked—as I was at my reunion—how I achieved financial freedom so quickly and in a less than wealthy (an example of damning with faint praise) section of our nation. I continue to share my thoughts on the subject hoping I can guide others who desire work to be a choice they make, and freedom the defining characteristic of their life. What follows is a carefully garnered master list of principles or fundamentals—shared experiences and characteristics from the many doctors I know, or of whom I've read, who have attained money in abundance.

One may emulate this recipe to achieve financial freedom, if he or she chooses, but one must flavor it with unique personal ingredients. These include applied labor and diligent study, but ideally also encompass honesty and a sense of joy and wonder at the rich fabric of life itself.

Wealth alone is empty, meaningless. Of what benefit is a billion dollars in gold to someone stranded on a deserted island? Never lose track of the primary ingredient of existence—joy.

Money in abundance does provide a savory seasoning to virtually any life-time repast, but one must not become so disoriented that an all-consuming quest for money becomes one's master. Such a narrow focus will unfailingly lead to loneliness, if not despair.

(I know you've read this before. Guess what? You'll be reading it again! If this message, so essential to achieving one's bliss, isn't internalized into the very fiber of one's being, what else matters?)

Affluence now assigned its proper place within the universe, let's examine **six common characteristics of uncommonly wealthy dentists**:

1. *Started saving and investing early*

My first memory of saving was as an 8-year-old, putting the profits from my paper route and odd jobs—grass cutting and snow shoveling being the "big ticket" items—into a glass fruit jar, stored safely on a high kitchen shelf. That humble and frugal beginning proved essential in my efforts to work my way through eight years of college. Had my parents not instilled the habit of saving in me at this tender age, I would never have been able to accumulate the necessary financial resources to attend a university.

We'll deal with investments that offer returns superior to those of a fruit jar shortly, but ponder one vital question now: What financial example am I currently setting for my children? And always . . . is this displayed prototype consistent with my true values? (Again, one must devote the effort and time needed to define his or her beliefs before answering this central query becomes possible.)

Virtually every person of self-made worth I know has a history of very early—and often very difficult—labor. My father told me I would learn to play, but children need to be taught to work. Do you agree? And, if one's offspring aren't tutored in this vital topic by their parents, then by whom?

For those without a history of saving and investing, your "early start" must begin *NOW*. We'll deal with the specifics of the accumulation process in the course of the following discussion, but with savings—as with most good habits—tomorrow never comes. If one can't commit to vigorously saving and investing, quit reading! I can't help you achieve wealth . . . and I doubt anyone else can, either.

2. Run highly profitable businesses

The key word, to the financially successful dentist—or one who desires to be—is once again **business**. Dentists who succeed are acutely aware—and demonstrate their perspicacity with every decision—that they manage a dental business. I'm frequently contacted by dentists who haven't achieved the success to which they aspire. As we discuss the particulars of their situation and possible remedies to improve their finances, they often explain they don't "like" the business aspects of practice. "It's just not me. Not something I'm **comfortable** with."

I guess that's fine, if dentistry is your hobby. For me, it's the method I've chosen to provide for my family's well-being. Let me again relate this concept to our shared educational backgrounds. In my college years there were a plethora—some semesters it seemed a universe—of courses I didn't "like." Success in these subjects was integral to my plans of later achievement. Despite the lack of interest or enjoyment, I worked hard at mastering these unpleasant academic requirements. Were we supposed to enjoy dental school? To find it a place where we were "comfortable"? If so, I really missed something.

(Those of you who were academically gifted, lived in nice homes, drove late-model cars, wore nice clothes, honeymooned in the Caribbean—all paid for by Daddy and Mommy—and were liked by the instructors, please have the good manners to remain quiet. The rest of us broke our respective asses getting through school!)

Here is the bottom line, as unpleasant as it may prove: **staying within one's comfort zone almost always means forfeiting any chance of meaningful growth.**

It has been said that successful people are those sufficiently motivated to perform the tasks, essential to achievement, that unsuccessful people decline to do. Fear of failure paralyzes many, stopping them from even attempting their best. One's aspirations must be sufficient to overcome his or her fears.

Do you desire wealth enough to become a student of the science of obtaining it? To challenge your fears and discomforts, and ethically perform whatever tasks are required to succeed? To contribute the labor necessary to attain the personal stature to become deserving of receiving your wishes?

To obtain anything of value, one must first grow as an individual until one becomes worthy of possessing that for which he or she yearns. To obtain that which one hasn't yet earned—as when buying with credit, or by accepting the performance of sub-standard dental care, not returning fair value commensurate with one's compensation—is certainly not a point of passage on the journey to success, wealth or joy.

3. Spend less than one makes

Most of my readers live in America, so let's examine this point carefully! I didn't say spend less than one's credit card maximum, or spend until the bank refuses one's loan request— but less than one's income.

The average savings rate for a Singaporean is 47%. Japanese save 17%, Europeans 13% and Americans 4%. The above-listed facts are NOT typos. They ARE a disgrace to our country and its proud pioneer heritage. They also explain how this generation of Americans has become the largest debtor nation in Earth's history!

How much should one save? A **minimum** of 10% of his or her before-tax net income. I'd strongly suggest one save 20%. I paid off my office, school and home loans after less than three years in private practice, and then began to save 50% of my income, and still lived on 10 times the money I had available as a student.

A close veterinarian friend banked 100% of his practice's income for several years after he joined an existing clinic, and lived almost entirely on his wife's receptionist salary. They are a young and very wealthy family today, handsomely repaid (by my boon companion, compound interest) for their few years of sacrifice.

By what method should one save? There is but one effective way: Saving MUST be given the singular honor of being the first act of one's regular financial strategy—as it is undeniably the **most essential**. Don't save last, from the pittance that's left after one has spent his or her fill. How has that approach worked for you to date? Have you managed to attain the lofty 4% American average?

I told you there would be no magic answers to achieving wealth provided here. **I lied**. There is one true bit of sorcery I wish to share. It is the wizardry of tax-free compounding. (Works a lot better than a fruit jar.) Allow me to illustrate this essential point with a simplistic example.

Toilet paper is 1/1000 of an inch thick. (It is considerably less in some facilities I've endured, but after having employed magazine pages—tip of the chapter, avoid the shiny picture-pages—tree leaves, corncobs and half a handkerchief for this unsavory task of most personal hygiene, one becomes appreciative of toilet paper of any thickness.) If one doubles tissue paper (compounds it) 50 times, the resultant pile will be 17,769,895 MILES high. Enough to reach the moon and back over 17 times!

True, unless one's gastrointestinal system is in total uproar, one is unlikely to need this much tissue! But, the same growth outcome occurs with money. The key is having the time to allow one's finances to compound multiple times. This is what's meant by "having your money work for you."

The earlier one starts saving, the longer one's money labors on his or her behalf. The higher one's investment yield, the more quickly, thus frequently, one's money will double. Historically, the stock market has returned 10.7% per year over the last 70 years. At that rate of earnings, money doubles approximately every seven years. At a 12% return, money doubles roughly every six years. Let's examine what happens to $10,000 invested at the above-listed returns over time.

At a 10.7% return	at a 12% return
$10,000 at age 30	$10,000 at age 30
$20,000 at age 37	$20,000 at age 36
$40,000 at age 44	$40,000 at age 42
$80,000 at age 51	$80,000 at age 48
$160,000 at age 58	$160,000 at age 54
$320,000 at age 65	$320,000 at age 60
$640,000 at age 72	$640,000 at age 66
$1,280,000 at age 79	$1,280,000 at age 72
	$2,560,000 at age 78

These are the returns from a **single investment of $10,000**, made at age 30, compounding at a rate of 10.7% or 12%. Is there any dentist who feels investing $10,000 to be beyond his or her capabilities? That total represents approximately **one month of the average dentist's profits**.

Check the math yourself. Can you see that if the 10.7% investment was made at age 23 the total at age 79 would be $2,560,000? If one can achieve a 12% return, the same initial $10,000 deposit made at age 24 nets $5,120,000 at age 78. With $5.12 million here, $5.12 million there (because, once one grasps the power inherent in compounding, he or she will save more than once, right?), pretty soon we're talking real money!

4. Excellent advisors

Few attain great success, in any endeavor, without receiving help from others. Accurate information is vital to achievement, and skilled counselors can provide one with essential knowledge. The advisors may be dental consultants, financial experts, physical trainers or spiritual guides. Mentors also come in the form of books, magazines, lectures, newsletters, or meetings attended—any resource that provides one with knowledge that helps one attain his or her desires. As we've discussed, success-oriented people will go to whatever lengths are required to achieve their goals. (Even reading books!)

Having an advisor assist one does not mean checking one's brains at the door. The counsel of these experts enhances and accelerates personal growth; it does not replaces it. No matter what form of assistance one seeks, the RESPONSIBILITY for the successful outcome of whatever ventures are pursued remains his or hers alone. (All together now: One can delegate authority, but not _____.)

We'll deal with investing concepts in our discussion of the two remaining fundamentals. Certainly accountants, lawyers, brokers and other professionals can be invaluable sources of information in the specialized, ever fluctuant and challenging field of finance. But, never make the mistake of allowing others to make final decisions that affect one's future. Listen and learn, then perform the lucubration required to independently develop optimal solutions.

I'm aware of many doctors, sporting a variety of degrees, who have been conned, defrauded, extorted from. In each case, it was the doctor's failure to assume personal responsibility—whether occasioned by lack of education regarding finance, distraction, laziness or uncertainty—that led to the horrific result.

5. *Diversify*

Let me be crystal clear: We're discussing diversity in one's investments, not one's business. Many dentists begin second businesses that can't possibly prove as profitable as their existing office. As superior income can't be the motive, I assume he or she opens the second business out of boredom with the dental profession. If one decides to begin a second enterprise as a hobby, you must be aware that the time, thought and energy taken from your practice will make this second business a very expensive pastime.

We are privileged to be members of a professional monopoly, with income of the average dentist ranking in the top 1% of our wealthy nation's wage-earners. To take one's eyes off this golden goose of a dental practice, to open an ice-cream shop or child-care facility is to, I feel, have truly lost touch with financial reality.

Napoleon's tragic mistake was to open a second front—don't let it be yours.

(I fully realize and accept that if I dedicated the energy I invest in writing to my practice, my income would be many times greater. That I can choose to make such a sacrifice is a gift of financial freedom. My concern is for dentists who make similar concession of income without the awareness or the ability to afford such forfeitures.)

To recap, one has saved, established a profitable business and become familiar with advisors to help one achieve his or her goals. Our efforts have succeeded! Money is accumulating and our hero's enthusiasm and ability to invest is expanding. Again, the exact form one's investments take should vary depending on one's interests, amount of wealth, available time, and personality. Regardless of one's choices, be they MMF, stocks, bonds, mutual funds, real estate, collectibles—all desire to invest in a manner that gives the greatest return for the least risk. The final two principles assist one in achieving the goal of every knowledgeable investor, to attain an **enhanced return with reduced danger**.

Financial diversity results from investing in contrasting assets. Many scholarly tomes have been penned to describe how a **dissimilar group of investments** can **increase return**, while **decreasing risk**. The essential variable is the degree of difference among assets held by the same person or entity. (This concept of investment diversification is referred to as "cross-correlation" by financial professionals and is identified by a symbol that looks like the Nike logo.)

Owning stock in two different American companies gives but a small diversity, due to the inherent similarity of these investments. One can decrease resemblance by investing in differing industries, or in a mixture of large and small companies within the U.S. stock market, but correlation remains fairly strong. Owning stock and art or precious metal would greatly increase diversity, as events that impact one entity would have reduced impact on the other.

Let's study an example that illustrates the essential relationship of diversity to successful investing. Factors that affect American companies, such as U.S. rates of interest and inflation, will have smaller correlations with businesses of other nations. By investing internationally, one can achieve the necessary diversity to allow increased returns, while decreasing the volatility of one's investment, and thus reducing risk. But, is international investing wise? Let's review some basic facts.

In 1984 American industry accounted for 54.1% of the world equity market. In 1993 that percentage was reduced to 37.0%. The average American laborer makes $18 per hour. In China, Russia and India the average labor remuneration is $.25 per hour. These facts indicate other nations may possess a competitive advantage over American businesses.

It seems conceivable to improve returns by investing outside the borders of America, while at the same time increasing the safety of one's nest egg, as a steep decline in American fortunes might be balanced by an increase in growth outside our borders. Also, an international meltdown might be countered by a strong American market, as occurred in 1997.

(For whatever it's worth, based on this premise, I've gradually increased my international holdings over the last several years, using international mutual stock funds, finally holding my international investments steady at 10% of my total invested dollars. My average annual return over approximately three years of international investing has been 19%, a return higher than most international funds have attained, but lower than the Dow Jones industrial average over the same period. Key to this relatively strong return from international investments over this period has been avoiding any fund that invests in Japan, a black hole for investments for close to a decade.)

6. *Choose long-term investment winners*

Significant success, in any venue, comes from an accurate and consistent long-term focus. Outstanding achievers in any field don't wish to be a cowboy one day, a fireman the next. One must carefully and deeply reflect to discover his or her true

412

values; what it is one sincerely desires. One then creates **written plans** to help achieve these goals and monitors progress towards them, making adjustments as situations dictate.

The same strategy must be employed for successful, profitable investing. One studies various opportunities and carefully chooses the financial areas he or she feels best correspond to one's individual talents and needs. Be it stocks, commodities, real estate, one sets goals, then invests long term while monitoring and adjusting as befits the circumstance. ONE DOES NOT flit from investment to investment, tossed by the fickle tides of emotion, rather than the steady currents of reason and guiding values and beliefs. Explicitly defined values allow one to defy emotions of the moment and continue in his or her commitment to a steady financial course.

Intelligently applying the above six principles, in combination with time, will reward one with wealth. But allow me to mention the force most likely to defeat efforts to achieve one's financial objectives: that ancient, but lately subdued and ignored foe . . . INFLATION.

Despite several recent quiet years, U.S. inflation for the last 25 years has averaged 5.7% annually. The rate for the last 40 years has been 4.4%. Pay careful attention here. In the last 20 years, 62% of the dollar's purchasing power has been lost. $100,000 of 1976 money had the purchasing power of $37,700 in 1996. In the last 30 years, 77% of the dollar's power has been eroded so $100,000 has the purchasing power of $22,100. (Do any of you remember the nickel Cokes of 1950? What will the cost of that venerable beverage be in 2020? And will you be able to afford to have one?)

Now, let me attempt to arm one against the implacable foe of inflation. Roger Ibbotson and Rex Sinquefield's classic study revealed the following facts about investments since 1926:

Stocks have out-performed inflation over that time period by an average of 7.7% per year.

Long Bonds have out-performed inflation by an average of 1.7% per year.

413

Real Estate has out-performed inflation by an average of 3.5% per year.

Which weapon would you select in your lifetime struggle against inflation's pernicious effect on assets?

Happiness, not wealth, is the goal of life. Yet, nothing does the job of money as well as lucre itself. If one doubts my word, try getting a Coke from a machine using some instrument besides coin of the realm! (One might be successful employing a hammer, but such a choice could lead one to encounter a spot of trouble with the forces of culture.) Yet, always remember, when money has served you—and the icy beverage is in your hand—enjoy the drinking.

Let's now consider the thoughts of two experts who have devoted their lives to the investigation of wealth, in an effort to further comprehend the philosophy and behavior of affluence. I've always believed in studying the behavior of extraordinary achievers, as I contend **success leaves clues** from which the motivated may learn. (This book is intended as a series of less-than-subtle hints for those willing to work to achieve any of the author's attainments you may desire.)

Achieving Financial Independence

Allow me to repeat my contention that few deserve wealth more than dentists, after investing exhausting years and thousands of dollars in education, enduring the lonely struggle required to develop as successful, independent business-persons, and expending the effort continually demanded to provide excellent dental care. Yet, even after overcoming these daunting challenges, few within our profession ever achieve complete financial freedom. Why is this so?

Invaluable information has recently been published to instruct those who would like to become wealthy, or wish to provide services for the affluent. The best-selling, compelling book, *The Millionaire Next Door*, by Thomas J. Stanley, Ph.D. and William D. Danko, Ph.D.—available at any bookstore—is the source of much of the information within this article. The book is extremely readable and I recommend it highly. Let's

414

begin our efforts to understand how wealth is achieved, with a study of this species called millionaires.

The Typical Millionaire

Of the approximately 100 million existing American households, roughly 3.5 million have a net worth in excess of $1 million. The typical millionaire is 57 years old, male, married with three children. **Their average taxable income is $131,000.** (Approximately the average for American dentists! Are most of us then destined to become millionaires?) The average income of all U.S. families is $33,000.

The **average total income** of millionaires (including investments and other unearned income) is **$247,000.** Their median net worth is $1.6 million. These wealthy individuals typically work 45-55 hours per week and dedicate an average of eight hours per month to investment matters. **They invest 20% of their income on average and tend to make their investment decisions personally.**

Traits That Lead to Wealth

Having defined these individuals, let's examine the methods whereby they achieve wealth. The authors repeatedly emphasize this theme: study of these wealthy folks, the great majority self-made millionaires, reveals **lifestyles of hard work, perseverance, planning and self-discipline.** (See . . . I'm not the only drudge insisting one must labor diligently and wisely to achieve success, wealth and joy!) How are these values illustrated by their behaviors?

1. Millionaires **live well below their means.** They save a minimum of 15% of all income, and they save first—not what's left after spending. They typically occupy the same home for years, surrounded by neighbors in similar dwellings, who have lower net worths. They understand that "the opposite of frugal is wasteful."

2. **Millionaires allocate time, energy and money efficiently, in ways conducive to wealth-building.** They begin investing and

415

planning early in life, working on a set schedule within both their business and personal lives. They have clearly defined lifetime priorities and goals that are rigorously pursued, leading to the achievement of prosperity.

3. **Millionaires believe financial independence to be more important than displaying elevated social status.** The book explains a colorful Texas description of someone having a BIG HAT, BUT NO CATTLE. These are folks who enjoy luxury cars, homes, clothes, club memberships and vacations (BIG HATS) but, often despite excellent incomes, have accumulated little net worth (NO CATTLE). Millionaires typically care little for "hats," but are deeply concerned with the size and health of their "herds."

4. **Millionaires' partners are planners and budgeters**, often more frugal than their spouses. Husband and wife work as a team, sharing a mutual goal of wealth accumulation.

Jo's hard-scrabble upbringing on her parents' Iowa farm strongly instilled in her an appreciation—a reverence—similar to mine concerning money. Her efforts have been essential to our family's financial success, and sharing similar values concerning money has significantly reduced the topics over which we might fight. (Never fear, sufficient points of contention remain to keep our relationship "interesting.")

It is nearly impossible to achieve financial freedom without both partners in a relationship exhibiting the values and behaviors that lead to wealth. **Husband and wife need to engage in frank discussions until a basic agreement concerning family financial policy is achieved, or both peace and wealth will elude them!**

Are You as Wealthy as You Should Be?

Enough abstraction—let's get personal. **DOCTOR, ARE YOU AS WEALTHY AS YOU SHOULD BE?** Performing the following simple calculation will provide the answer:

Multiply one's age by one's pre-tax annual income and divide by 10. This number is what **one's net worth should be.**

For example, if you are a 40-year-old dentist whose pre-tax income last year was $140,000, your net worth should be:

$$40 \times \$140,000 / 10 = \$560,000.$$

Take a moment to complete this calculation. The proper figure to use can be found on line 32—Adjusted Gross Income— located at the bottom of the first page of income tax form 1040. Is your net worth consistent with your age and income?

(If you are curious, my 1997 pre-tax income—including earned income and investment income, but not tax-sheltered returns from my retirement account—was $304,811. Doing the math, my net worth should be: {$304,800 x 51 / 10 = $1,554,480.} I seem to have gotten lucky and found an additional million or so somewhere along the way!)

The Millionaire Next Door predicts many doctors will fall short of the level predicted by this net-worth calculation. Their studies found **the relationship between education and wealth accumulation to be NEGATIVE.** The higher one's level of formal education, the lower one's net worth tends to be! Why? Part of the answer is the lost years of income production forfeit to schooling and the accompanying education-related debt. But another significant factor is that higher education leads to an elevated lifestyle. (Big hat-ism!) Society seems to expect excessive spending from its "educated elite," and many well-schooled high-earners comply with these expectations.

Not only is money consumed no longer available for wealth accumulation, but spending increases the **largest single expense for most American families—income tax.** (Taxes consume more revenue than food, shelter and transportation expenses combined for many American families!) Consumption = taxation. Tax must be paid on all income spent.

An integral portion of realizing financial independence is achieving a reduction in taxation, as through tax-sheltered saving and investing. (Basically we are discussing IRA, 401-K, corporate and other forms of tax-deferred retirement plans, or investing in tax-free municipal bonds.) The United States taxes earned income, but does not extract a tariff from accumulated

417

and tax-sheltered wealth until death (in the form of estate taxes). Limiting the dilution of savings that results from taxes being paid, and establishing an environment where savings grow free of annual taxation, tremendously enhances the return of invested dollars.

Why do so many high annual income-earners forfeit a chance to achieve accumulated energy, in the form of wealth, by indulging in the deadly combination of spending and the resultant taxation? Often they choose to trade financial well-being for social status, **working, planning and sacrificing for the short-term goal of purchasing to IMPRESS OTHERS.**

In contrast, the greatest joy of the millionaires interviewed came not from possessions, but from the **SELF-SATISFACTION DERIVED FROM THEIR ACHIEVEMENTS** and **FREEDOM FROM FEAR.** (To which I might add a heartfelt AMEN!)

Attaining wealth—achieving greatness in any venue—is difficult and involves more than just inner (cattle) or outer (hat) focus. Evidence exists to indicate key traits required to accumulate money, or excel in many endeavors, exist by age four. (In fairness to Drs. Danko and Stanley, let me alert readers we are about to stray from the guidance of their excellent book, for a moment, to consider a few thoughts of yours truly.)

The Marshmallow Test

I believe a famous psychological study conducted years ago can shed light on key behavioral choices that accompany achievement. Preschool children were offered a marshmallow that they were allowed to eat, but told if they would wait to consume the sweet until the adult returned from "running some errands," they would receive a second marshmallow. Their conduct during the few minutes they were left alone with this treat was filmed.

Many ate the marshmallow, often within a few moments of the adult's leaving. The ones who waited, and "doubled their return," visibly suffered, often putting their hands over their eyes, singing, walking around—in courageous, Lilliputian efforts to delay gratification.

The children in this study were followed throughout their school careers. The ones who earned the second marshmallow outperformed those who ate theirs by significant margins in school grades, test results—virtually every factor measured. **The ability to delay gratification is a vital component of any success, including wealth accumulation.** It is also an act of strength and courage.

Take a moment to evaluate your personal history. How have you fared in your lifelong battle to deny short-term pleasure, secure long-term gain? You may measure yourself by such criteria as tendency toward debt or savings; choosing exercise over eating; affairs or working on relationships—any of the common life situations where the options are immediate, transient pleasure, or choosing to endure distress now to achieve significant rewards later.

If personal history shows one has been a sucker for immediate gratification, and one wishes to change, what can he or she do?

1. **Awareness.** The first essential ingredient is recognizing one's behavior pattern and realizing other options exist. Without achieving this understanding, there is slight chance for meaningful change.

2. **Determined effort.** Aware, and wanting to change, one can work to obtain his or her desires. Set clear goals, such as saving BEFORE purchasing that next car (I have never in my life purchased a car in any manner except by writing a check for payment in full on the day the sale was closed), or major piece of office equipment, rather than using debt. Or, going to the gym four nights a week instead of home to drinks, a heavy meal and a night spent in a semi-stupor in front of the television.

3. **Monitor progress.** Measure one's debts as they melt away, or savings as they grow. Observe how one's body responds to the gym as inches disappear and energy increases. Be ready to adjust your program if you realize change is needed to obtain your goal.

Achieving Financial Freedom

Returning to *The Millionaire Next Door*, the authors break financial matters into offense and defense. **Financial Offense** is earning power. On average, dentists enjoy excellent offense, with average annual earnings in the top percentage points of American wage earners. A correlation between earned income (offense) and wealth accumulation does exist, but the relationship is not nearly as direct as one might assume.

Financial Defense concerns personal spending habits—how well one can fortify himself or herself against the urge to consume (successfully delaying gratification). Those who have participated in any sport know defense creates champions. **It's not what one earns nearly as much as what one does with it that determines financial outcomes.** In part due to the confiscation of wages by the American tax system, **saving and effective investing are more critical to wealth accumulation than is earning ability**.

Cutting through the data and stories, this is the point: Will one choose vanity (HAT) or substance (CATTLE)? Few are able to afford both. Will one's life's focus be exterior—centered on the impression one makes on others and the fleeting pleasure this provides? Or will one concentrate inside—on the joy of lasting accomplishments that bequeath enhanced self-esteem, of achieving freedom from fiscal anxiety by assuring the financial well-being of his or her loved ones?

Reflect on your life's goals. If financial freedom is a major target—not a wish, but something you are willing to work to obtain—these thoughts, and *The Millionaire Next Door*, contain a clear prescription as to how one can achieve these desires.

The good news? Dentists have average incomes approximately four times those of the general population and thus most have the opportunity to achieve financial freedom.

The bad news? This accomplishment requires courage, strength, persistence and determination—a two-marshmallow existence!

420

But, take heart. Don't the above traits describe the very person you wish to be when you grow up?

(An astute reader might note the book's proposed path to millionairehood is very similar to my personal journey. Allow me to assure one and all, my values resulted not from this book—published in 1996—but from 51 years of severe trial and egregious error! However, it is extremely comforting to read the words of acknowledged experts who agree with my personal beliefs.)

Let's revisit the land of marshmallows. I believe one can glean much from the general lessons of delayed gratification that are foundational to significant achievement in any venue. Let's attempt to further enhance our understanding by considering examples of decisions of postponed satisfaction versus immediate enjoyment that are familiar to all dentists.

Within the Humble Marshmallow, a Key to One's Future?

This is a cute story, but why tell doctors of 4-year-olds and marshmallows? The preponderance of dentists are out of pre-school—at least physically, if not emotionally and psychologically—and most have matured to an age when sugar is generally consumed in its liquid form. I'd like to advance the theory that all our fates rise and fall within the same vessel carrying these children—our proficiency in delaying gratification. (Maybe one really does learn all they need to know in kindergarten?)

Is this ability to resist the siren song of temptation, so vital to happiness and achievement, inherited or learned? I'd guess both. Not much you can do to alter the genetic soup that formed you, at least until scientists improve that sheep cloning stuff, but let's examine the venue one can control—behavioral possibilities.

We've discussed how behavior can be altered through **en-lightened awareness, determined effort and monitored goals.** One must recognize the need to cultivate delayed-gratification capability by realizing how possessing the strength and courage required to prolong pleasure can enhance one's life, or how lacking this trait can rob one of achievement and happiness. Once this awareness is achieved—and I trust the examples we're about to consider will convince any doubters of the importance of delayed gratification—one can create deliberate plans to make the changes required to attain this essential personal strength and/or moral character, then monitor progress and adjust behavior as indicated to achieve one's desired results.

One may evaluate delayed-gratification proficiency by observing one's ability to tolerate distress for the sake of achievement. Disappointment and frustration are unpleasant but necessary portions of the human condition, as postponing enjoyment, or prolonging suffering to achieve a worthy goal, is essential to achieve meaningful growth and gain. (Dental school represented a prolonged exercise in delayed gratification for most.)

Inability to endure the discomfort incumbent to frustration can result in hasty, poorly throughout, short-term-focused behavioral decisions such as anger, lying, alcohol or other drug abuse—all choices that may result in pain to the individual and those around him or her, while working against ideal achievement and the development of personal strength.

Cultivating the ability to withstand distress allows one the precious time required to solve problems—not merely react to them. Being able to delay gratification means having the power to embrace thoughtful choice over emotional panic, exercise over addiction, understanding over conflict, relationship growth over divorce.

Let's examine some common contemporary situations where lacking the courage to delay gratification reduces the quality of one's life and threatens to rob one of success and joy.

An inability to tolerate stress can result in deficient clinical dentistry. A sub-par crown is seated, because the dentist, perhaps despite a strong personal desire to provide excellent care, lacks the courage to tell the patient a remake is required and suffer the feelings of embarrassment, guilt and self-doubt that accompany painful reality. (Both time and financial constraints might further weaken a dentist's resolve and increase the difficulty of revealing the truth to patients in such situations.)

Short-term, this dentist must live with a sense of un-ease, aware he or she provided less than the service promised and paid for. Long-term, the results of a failed crown might include an unpleasant confrontation with an unhappy patient, loss of the patient, the patients' family and all future referrals, or legal action; all possible sequelae resulting from a poor decision made in a moment of weakness.

Unable to tolerate short-term financial pressure, the dentist may accept a third-party plan, rather than pursuing a long-term, more difficult, but eventually more profitable strategy of practice development. A restorable tooth is removed because the doctor can't confront the patient's uneducated and pain-motivated demand for extraction and the possible personal rejection the insecure dentist fears may ensue.

When faced with a dissatisfied patient, a dentist unable to tolerate stress might blame staff, patient, lab, the weather—anything to relieve the pressure he or she feels incapable of tolerating. Under such circumstances, a deliberate lie can be told, and the respect of the dentist's staff—those he or she must interact with daily, and upon whose shoulders the fate of the practice rests—be diminished.

(Enjoying positive self-esteem is the end result of consistently behaving in a manner worthy of respect. This means accepting personal responsibility during times of distress. A positive sense of self cannot be derived from wearing an expensive, pure silk "power tie," leasing a luxury automobile, or hiding from one's obligations behind the title of doctor.)

In these and many similar scenarios, temporary relief of distress is purchased at the cost of forfeiting a lasting, significant gain. Dishonesty is a sure step on the pathway to failure and is often chosen—not to cheat or gain unfair advantage—but due to personal weakness resulting in the inability to tolerate excruciating reality.

Honesty is the best way to assure success—but often requires the wisdom and power to accept short-term distress in exchange for long-term gain (two marshmallows!) and the strength and courage to look someone in the eye and tell a difficult truth.

Financially, those unable to delay gratification, and work and wait to become worthy of the objects they covet, choose an outer focus—spending money in an attempt to convince others of the very self-worth they have yet to earn and which their immediate-gratification behavior demonstrates they doubt they possess. The money nightmares resulting from purchasing items one can't afford to impress others of one's worth do little to relieve an already acutely inflamed lack of self-respect. **Remember, DEBT is sacrificing the future to pay for the unearned joys of the present. CREDIT is debt dressed in a suit.**

As witnessed when considering the typical behavior of millionaires, those who possess the required personal power to delay gratification prolong purchases, preferring achievement and accumulated wealth (a form of stored energy) to conspicuous consumption of possessions to which they have not yet earned the right.

(Until recent years, one acquired the right to possess something when he or she had earned whatever was required to obtain their desire—and not before. This need to become worthy by one's efforts and achievements before possessing is an essential truth our debt-driven culture has buried deeper than a junkyard dog's only bone. It is a cancer eating at the heart of our culture.)

To be concise—a modern dentist's marshmallow is a luxury car, fine clothes, or a home located to the north of what he or she can currently afford. The choices: "eat" it now, or wait, save, then purchase this desire without the burden of debt.

Let's review our road map to achievement: To reap the benefits of delayed gratification, one must first understand its power and make a **conscious decision** to increase one's ability to prolong the amount of distress he or she can tolerate. Then, as did the kids in the marshmallow study, one must WORK AND SACRIFICE to achieve what he or she values. Clear goals established, one works to strengthen delayed gratification, monitors progress (debt is reduced, savings grow, pounds are lost, days of sobriety pile up), and adjusts course as indicated by events.

Valor consists of **DELIBERATELY FACING ONE'S FEARS**—not in having no fear. THUS COURAGE IS AN ACT OF WILL, AVAILABLE TO ALL! The ability to defer pleasure requires fortitude to develop and, like a muscle, must be frequently worked, thus strengthened, to have a significant impact on one's life.

One "exercises" this muscle by driving his or her car another year, even if a sibling and a neighbor both purchase new vehicles; by choosing a workout over a drink to reduce stress; by helping with homework instead of channel surfing or playing on the Internet; by dealing head-on with system and staff problems, not hoping they will go away; by facing dreaded rejection (there is no documented case of a dentist dropping dead after a patient refused suggested treatment!) and, after working to help a patient clarify his or her values, consistently recommending the care one feels to be in the patient's best interests.

Facing fear and delaying pleasure isn't easy, but the benefits of developing this trait are immeasurable, whether one deals with dental practice success, financial attainment, quality of life enhancement, or benefits to family and friends.

Self-esteem and confidence soar as one grows to realize he or she can handle the difficulties that all who live must endure. Business success and wealth will occur as a result of this basic behavioral choice, and are pleasant attainments, but they pale compared to the peace of mind, the freedom from fear which accompany the knowledge that one possesses the personal power necessary to consistently do the right thing in difficult situations.

(The battle to strengthen one's delayed-gratification ability is a major confrontation in which every alcoholic must prevail to survive, as within the bottle exists an easy, certain and predictable answer to dealing with stress; so please forgive any excess of zeal on my part concerning this topic. The realization that I must face the trials of life sober stands out among the more terrifying events of my life! Since I'm sharing, the second horrifying realization is that each activity, each friendship based on liquor consumption—which is every one for a drunk—must also be abandoned. An addict who quits abusing is suddenly faced with, not only a sober reality, but a great deal of open time!)

Accept this challenge and **become the kind of person you portray yourself to be to others** . . . strong and wise. The kind of person you wish to be in your heart—a man or woman with the power, especially when faced with adversity, to consistently act in a manner consistent with his or her personal values.

Let's change focus from the beliefs and behavior of millionaires and the development of delayed-gratification abilities to examine the more easily defined manner in which every dentist can assure each of his or her children will become millionaires.

How to Guarantee One's Children Become Millionaires

Parents love and cherish their children, wishing to protect them, even at the cost of Mom and Dad's safety and comfort, working to do everything possible to assure the brightest future for their unique genetic legacy to the ages. To assist in the fulfillment of this natural impulse I'd like to discuss a concept and course of action that can:

1. **assure all one's children will become MILLIONAIRES!**

2. **teach one's children the VALUE OF WORK.**

3. **educate one's children as to the importance and power of SAVING and INVESTING.**

(Please peruse the above-listed three attributes again. These are accomplishments I believe all parents would dearly wish their children to achieve.)

We'll get to the million dollars soon enough, but I contend learning the value of working, saving and investing to be of greater worth than mere fortune. A person with a modicum of talent, willing to work, save and invest a portion of the fruits of one's labor, will be more than just financially rewarded. He or she will

426

BECOME a person of confidence, achievement and poise . . . as well as wealth.

Take money from such an accomplished individual and he or she will soon earn it back. Give money to a person who hasn't developed these attributes and he or she will often squander the assets. (This is similar to the venerable homily, give a man a fish and feed him for a day; teach a man to fish and feed him for a lifetime . . . only without the fish!)

However, as critical as I believe values to be, a million dollars in the bank comes in handy for darn near anyone!

One's Millionaire Children

There is an easy, inexpensive, predictable method to assure one's children will become millionaires, even if their parents never achieve such lofty financial heights. The Taxpayer Relief Act of 1997 (don't you love the irony with which our Washington solons name these mystifying mountains of legislation?) has made the task easier with the introduction of the **Roth IRA.** What is the investment required of parents to assure a **seven-digit after-tax net worth** for their offspring? Naught but a few thousand dollars, an hour or two of time and a modicum of erudition.

Let's consider a hypothetical example. Dr. Sagacious has a 10-year-old son. Dr. S. employs Junior in his office: cleaning, folding statements and stuffing envelopes, helping with yard work—whatever tasks are necessary and appropriate to the child's skills and strength. (These wages are tax-deductible business expenses for Dr. S.) Junior's 1997 earnings for his labor are $2,000. Dr. S. puts this single year of earned income into an IRA where it will compound free of the pernicious influence of taxes. This **one-time, $2,000 contribution, compounding at 10.7%** (I've assumed this 10.7% rate, as that is the average return of the stock market over the past 70 years) **will be worth $1,091,899 at age 72.**

Let me be precise: one contribution of $2,000, made at age 10—thus experiencing 62 years of the blessing of compounding—returning 10.7% per annum, will grow to $1,091,899 by age 72.

Let me buttress Junior's hypothetical example with a true story near and dear to my heart. The youngest of my four children, now 14-year-old Rachel, has been employed by my office for three years. (My four children all began their working careers as preteens, and all have retirement accounts. I'm using Rachel's example because as my youngest, the magic of compounding within the new Roth IRA will bequeath greatest benefits to her.)

After three years of IRA contributions, Rachel has a 1997 balance of $5,820. This total is a composite of contributions and earnings. I pay Rachel a competitive wage, commensurate to the tasks she's asked to perform and hours worked, thus compensation for her first two years of work was less than $2,000. This deficiency—paying a salary below the maximum IRA contribution allowed—is foolish based on total effect of her compounding investment, but consistent with what I claim as the more profound lesson—the value of work.

Every parent who chooses to employ his or her children must make a personal decision whether to emphasize total return (and pay $2,000, regardless of the child's effort) or work ethic (pay a reasonable wage, allowing the child an opportunity to earn $2,000) by the manner in which he or she chooses to compensate their progeny. Rewarding a child—even an 11-year-old—for work he or she didn't do is not consistent with my personal values or the lessons I wish my children to internalize, no matter how powerful the effect of compounding.

(When I was 11 I gave up my three-year-old paper route career to begin a summer job at the marina located directly across the road from our home. The pay was only 35 cents per hour, but I got to work 70 hours a week. This is a bit more of a "value lesson" than I desire to inflict on my children.)

Let's assume Rachel continues to contribute $2,000 per year (because I can now insist she do so) until age 18—four more years—then never places another dime in her retirement fund for the remainder of her life. (An unsettling thought, but there is little I can do to force contributions—other than through the influence of the educational experience we are discussing—after Rachel attains age 18.)

Employing our assumed 10.7% rate of return (Megan and Rachel's mutual funds' actual 1997 IRA returns were in excess of 26%), her account will be worth **$4,629,188** should she have the good fortune to attain 72 years. As Rachel now has a Roth IRA, all $4.6 million-plus will be **tax-free.** Even at Rachel's tender years, awareness of this potential reward provides significant insight and motivation for what her daddy devoutly hopes will be the creation of a lifelong work, save and invest ethic.

Allow me to also employ Rachel to illustrate the educational process as regards the power of saving and investing. The day she first opened an IRA, then 11-year-old Rachel and I sat on a couch as I illustrated, with rough calculations scribbled on the back of an envelope, how one $2,000 contribution would grow to $512,000 (assuming a 10% return), by age 68. Rachel perused my figures for a heartbeat, then looked me in the eye and asked, "So if I put in another two thousand dollars, I'd have a million?"

The power of compounding or the true cost of spending that my daughter grasped so succinctly, despite her tender years, is a double-edged concept that **most dentists reveal by their actions they don't understand.**

To illustrate my contention, assume a 25-year-old dentist chooses to reward himself or herself for graduation from dental school by purchasing a $30,000 car. Ignore the total cost of the vehicle in interest, depreciation, maintenance and repairs, fuel and insurance—assume our new graduate somehow pays cash for the car and all subsequent expenses are paid for on his or her behalf (the most rosy possible scenario)—but our youthful protagonist chooses to put all possible assets into a quality vehicle, rather than funding a retirement account. (For those with daughters, a wedding of similar expense can serve as a viable—and for those of us blessed with three lovely daughters, a frightening—example.)

Again, using 10.7% to age 72, the loss from that one failed $30,000 retirement contribution is $3,564,999. That's a very expensive ride! Is it possible for one to accurately understand the $30,000 purchase has an ultimate cost in excess of $3.5 million, and still fail to save? Can one also begin to perceive the total expense of education to include the opportunity cost of investments not made?

Roth Versus Traditional IRAs

I hope the above examples irrefutably demonstrate the power of compounding investments, but questions remain as to what is the best way to harness this financial energy. The advantages of tax-deferred (traditional) IRAs or tax-free (Roth) IRAs as opposed to saving after-tax dollars are too well appreciated to require documentation. But let's contemplate and compare the Roth IRA (first available in 1998) versus the traditional IRA. Both can be used for children, so long as income is EARNED (not gifted) and each allows for contributions of 100% of earned income up to a maximum funding of $2,000 per year.

When one funds a traditional IRA, he or she may receive a federal tax deduction for the contribution, if one's income falls within limits listed shortly. In 1998, the first $4,250 of earned income for children (not investment income) is tax-free. Few children achieve earned income in excess of this figure; thus, having no taxable income, no tax deduction usually accompanies the traditional child IRA. However, when money is withdrawn from the traditional IRA—which must be delayed until after age 59½ to avoid a 10% penalty—taxes are paid on all distributions as ordinary income (not capital gains) at the current tax rate of the individual making the withdrawal. (Hence traditional IRAs are **tax-deferring** vehicles.).

Roth IRAs allow NO tax deduction when contributions are made, but money may be withdrawn **tax-free!** Withdrawals taken before five years in the Roth IRA or before age 59½ (non-qualified withdrawals) can be subject to a 10% penalty, but Roth IRAs allow tax- and penalty-free withdrawals in cases of death or disability, and a one-time withdrawal of up to $10,000 to use towards the purchase of a first home.

(Enabling one's child to be able to make the down payment necessary to purchase a home from the fruits of his or her early labors, combined with the parent's wise guidance, is a significant—and life-enhancing—benefit not available without paying tax plus a 10% penalty in the traditional IRA. For many of today's youth, such a financial arrangement may prove the difference between being able to afford a home of his or her own, or being forced to pay rent, possibly for a lifetime.)

If non-qualified Roth IRA withdrawals are made (those occurring before age 59½ or before five years in the plan, with the exception of death, disability and first home purchase), the assumption is automatically made that contributed dollars—not earnings—are withdrawn first. These contributions can be withdrawn free of penalty or tax, our government graciously allowing one to reclaim his or her own, already taxed, money.

Establishing an IRA

There are some eligibility limits that influence IRAs, but these shouldn't concern any but the most fortunate and precocious of children. For the traditional IRA, federal tax deductibility of contributions is phased out between:
Single Adjusted Gross Income $30,000 and $40,000.
Joint Adjusted Gross Income $50,000 and $60,000.

If one enjoys income beyond these levels, he or she may still contribute to a traditional IRA, but will receive no tax deduction (thus creating a non-deductible IRA). Considering employment of a Roth IRA to enjoy tax-free asset growth, in circumstances where no tax deduction for traditional IRAs is available, would certainly be appropriate.

Eligibility to make a Roth IRA contribution is phased out between:

Single Adjusted Gross Income $95,000 and $110,000.
Joint Adjusted Gross Income $150,000 and $160,000.

Individuals are eligible to participate in a Roth IRA even if they have a retirement plan at work, and for couples, EACH may contribute earned income up to $2,000 annually. Unlike traditional IRAs, Roth IRAs not only don't require mandatory distributions to begin at age 70½, but one can continue to contribute earned income after attaining 70½ years—a potentially powerful estate-building tool, for those blessed by such longevity.

Due to income limitations detailed above and the $2,000-per-year modest amount that can be contributed, the value of either a traditional or Roth IRA is reduced for most higher-income-earning dentists. (One can attain financial freedom from $2,000 per year savings, if he or she can discover a technique to earn an annual return of 1,000%, or live to be 200!) But as the projections we've examined show, thanks to the marvels of compounding, for dentists just beginning in practice and youngsters with earned income, the fiscal rewards of a relatively small investment are staggering!

One can **convert a traditional IRA into a Roth IRA** if his or her Adjusted Gross Income (AGI) is less than $100,000 in the year the conversion is made. In 1998 ONLY, taxes due from the conversion can be spread over four years. (The individual making the rollover can elect to pay 25% of taxes due in each of the next four years, as opposed to all taxes being paid the year of the conversion.) I'd strongly recommended one choose to pay these rollover taxes with non-IRA funds (as Jo and I have for Rachel and 17-year-old Megan) so the value and earning prowess of one's IRA isn't diminished by tax payments being withdrawn from retirement accounts.

IRAs of either type are simple and easy to open through almost any financial institution. Fees are customarily charged to open and/or maintain an IRA. These assessments vary, each bank, brokerage firm or mutual fund that offers an IRA setting its own tariff. As a basis of comparison, my investment-broker daughter Heather Wilde's firm, A.G. Edwards, charges nothing to open either a traditional or Roth IRA, but assesses a $30 annual maintenance fee. Even this modest fee is waived under some circumstances.

Many possible outcomes exist for IRA investments based on individual situations and assumptions made. Please consider the above examples for illustration purposes only. Anyone contemplating an IRA should consult his or her tax adviser and investment professional to evaluate the specific situation, but I believe every parent should be aware of, and consider implementing, this powerful strategy that can assure wealth for one's offspring.

There remains one last concern I feel duty-bound to mention. Parents must determine if it is wise for their children to have such assets available. Once funds are placed in an IRA, parents can't legally prevent their offspring from withdrawing funds, paying taxes and penalty, then spending the money as the child chooses, once they have attained an age of legal majority.

The key variable is the character of the child. I have no qualms concerning any of my four children. (And I hope I don't live to regret that statement!) Remember, kids must be employed to earn the money eligible for IRAs. I feel this work orientation to be at least as valuable as the funds. My suggestion would be to NOT OPEN an IRA for any child unwilling to work and earn the income. (All offices have a plethora of tasks perpetually in need of doing, providing employment opportunities for every dentist's child.) As previously discussed, giving money to a child who refuses to work is a powerful lesson about which I'd think long and hard before committing, no matter how great the potential financial rewards. Once again, it's a matter of acting within the guidelines of one's clear values.

(Ms. Heather Wilde supplied much of the information within this article. As I've mentioned, Heather is a registered investment broker with a master's degree in finance who has a special interest in retirement and education investments. Heather will be glad to answer questions and provide further assistance, and can be reached by calling 319-524-5946 during regular business hours.)

Now let's scrutinize a final topic that has greatly enhanced the quality and joy of Jo's and my lives over the last three years. Here I will fulfill my promise to illustrate how one can be both charitable and smart.

Support Charity . . . the Smart Way

Dentistry is a profession of givers in a nation with a heritage of caring and helping. To buttress this contention, consider that there are over 600,000 IRS-approved American charities. (And I seem to be on each one's mailing list!)

For decades I've tried to do my part, giving to carefully selected causes I felt to be of worth, trusting they were legitimate entities (being "taken" by two bogus charities of which I'm aware), dealing with increasingly more strict IRS demands concerning record-keeping and documentation, hoping my gifts resulted in some good, although never able to witness that they did.

Wouldn't it be ideal to assist worthwhile charities, while an independent third party assures they are legitimate, receiving a major tax incentive in return for one's contribution, while all the bookkeeping, tax documentation, even mailing of checks is done for you, free of charge? Too good to be true? I would have agreed, until I discovered charitable gift, or donor-advised, funds.

How Charitable Gift Funds Work

One may establish a charitable gift fund with various forms of assets—cash, bonds or stocks—but once gifts are contributed to the fund, they are irrevocable. While any asset may create a fund, it is ideal to use stocks that have appreciated in value, and upon which one will owe significant taxes when they are sold, to establish the charitable account. Such equities can be sent directly to the fund, as allowing the fund to sell the stock assures there will be no confusion regarding tax liability. One deducts the full value of the shares contributed on the day they are sold (not just their initial cost) from his or her taxes the year in which the gift is made.

The fund I've used assesses no loads or fees from one's donations. The only expenses are the normal fees charged to manage mutual funds that vary from 1% to .45%, based on one's choice of financial instruments in which to hold his or her contribution.

Once the fund is established, the donor selects the charity and the timing of his or her gifts. When you decide to donate to a charity, you mail a simple one-page form to the fund indicating the desired amount of your gift and the cause you wish to support. The fund verifies you have selected an IRS-approved charity and sends them a check along with a letter explaining your gift (unless the donor chooses to remain anonymous). You receive statements that verify your giving according to the new, more stringent IRS standards.

For Example

Assume you purchased shares of stock some time ago for $2,500. While grateful that the equities have appreciated to be worth $10,000 today, you are unhappy to owe a capital gains tax on the $7,500 profit of $1,500 (20% capital gains tax rate x $7,500 profit = $1,500 of taxes due) if the securities are sold.

Rather than sell the stock and contribute after-tax dollars, (money remaining after federal, state, local, FICA and medical taxes are paid), you decide to gift these stocks directly to charity. By so doing, you avoid the $1,500 capital gains tax and IN ADDITION, receive a deduction for the entire $10,000 face value of the stocks in the year you make the gift. The dollar value of the deduction depends on your tax bracket, which could be as high as 39.6%, providing a $3,960 deduction to accompany the $1,500 capital gains tax savings. Not bad for an initial $2,500 investment!

Personal Value

Saving significant tax dollars and hassles on personal giving is wonderful, but the reason one contributes to charity is to help others. The money in the fund can be used to concentrate one's giving and best aid charities and organizations of his or her choosing. Before establishing the fund, our family used a "shotgun" approach, firing little pellets of after-tax charitable dollars toward most who asked. Since opening our fund, we've chosen to focus our giving, like a high-powered rifle, to maximize its effect.

Joann and I decided to keep the money near home and support our financially challenged school district that has been jettisoning programs as a floundering ship does cargo. Our funds allowed the establishment of a fine arts department that has produced plays the past three years—the first theater our high school has enjoyed for over a decade.

We also instituted a writing program that involves students from elementary through high school. Annual writing contests are held, the winning works published in an area newspaper and every entry compiled in booklet form by a local printer for the students and parents to keep. Prizes—gift certificates and government savings bonds—are given to first, second and third place entries.

We also support a weight training program that is new to our school system and struggling to begin. My lawyer-son, John Jr., assists some of the high school athletes in weight training. As I mentioned, John finished second in the nation in power lifting in 1997—not a gift he inherited from his weak, pudgy father!—and is a serious student of the sport.

Dentistry and the community in which we live have blessed our family financially. Reading the winning essays, watching students (many of them patients) perform in plays—none of which would have existed if not for our support—are rewarding sources of personal satisfaction I never received from dropping a check in the mail. (I have no plans to watch the kids work out with weights, and absolutely no desire to lift a single one myself! I hope the facility will help the participants in football and basketball achieve their full potential.)

I present the above examples of our experience only to illustrate possible uses of donor-advised funds. There are many worthy causes desperately seeking money on a local, national and international level. I believe you'll find the process of determining which causes you'll support to be a pleasant and interesting exercise.

While we make no effort to advertise our giving, we live in a small town, and word trickles out. Supporting local activities reflects well on our office. I believe such endeavors enhance our bond with existing patients and may result in new patients seeking our care . . . a not unpleasant side-effect.

One could easily employ such efforts as part of a marketing plan, by having the office award a scholarship under its name, or requesting public notice be given with each event one sponsors. Certainly this would generate wonderful publicity for one's office and our profession, while one helps his or her community in a tax-wise manner. Jo and I simply made a personal decision that we did not wish to have our names mentioned.

How to Begin

Fidelity was the first financial services company to sponsor a donor-advised fund, having begun operations in September of 1992. Similar funds are beginning to be offered by other firms (I imagine motivated by this fund's success) but Fidelity Investments Charitable Gift Fund is the company with which I've dealt and the only one, to my knowledge, with any existing track record.

Opening a charitable gift fund takes only a few minutes—about like opening a checking account. There is a minimum $10,000 initial contribution, but while one deducts the entire amount from his or her taxes the year the gift is made (subject to deduction limits set by the IRS), one can use these contributed dollars and the income they earn to fund giving for as many years as one likes—even after his or her death.

Fidelity offers a choice of four pools of funds in which one can place money. The growth pool, which we selected, has returned an average of 15.3% annually since its 1992 inception. While one receives no further deductions from these additional earnings, the income the fund generates means more assets are in your account, available to give to causes one selects.

Please consult your tax adviser to see how this strategy can best work for you. You may reach Fidelity's Charitable Gift Fund by calling 1-800-682-4438 or faxing 1-617-476-7824. Ask for information on the charitable gift fund and begin supporting charity, the smart way.

(I have no interest in nor do I receive any form of compensation from Fidelity Investments . . . which seems a darn shame after the heartfelt recommendation I just gave them!)

REFOCUS EIGHT: FAILURE!!

You stare at lunch with unfocused eyes, unable to eat due to a queasy stomach and throbbing knot constricting your throat. Your eyes flicker tentatively toward "the letter," replaced in its envelope, tossed to the far corner of your desk, to afford some sense of distance and protection, as your mind races through the whole sorry affair yet again.

The patient was extremely apprehensive and initially did request number 14 be removed. Maybe you pushed too hard in your belief this tooth could and should be retained for a lifetime? You found and treated a fourth canal, even though it meant another visit, with no additional fee. Perhaps, to the patient, your selfless dedication was just an additional miserable experience? Should you have explained the anatomy of the root more carefully, or stressed your commitment to excellence?

You did advise the tooth needed a crown, but knew in your heart there was little chance this patient would accept the additional care. Was placing a post and bonded restoration at no additional charge a mistake? So often, over the years, work you've done for a reduced or no fee has come back to haunt you. Maybe there's a curse on dental care not paid for?

You glance at your lunch, then at your watch. My God—15 more minutes and it all starts again! Despite desperate efforts to repress them, phrases of the letter lash your mind: "still suffering," "you wasted all my insurance dollars," "I asked to have the tooth pulled," "I'm telling everyone—all my family and friends—how unfairly and unprofessionally I was treated!"

You sip now-cold coffee and chew a bite of tasteless sand-wich—the lettuce as wilted as your self-esteem; must have some strength for the afternoon. The patient has refused your offer for a no-charge office visit. Could the filling be high? The tooth cracked? Other than an unusually modest insurance payment, you haven't received a penny for performing the procedure and probably never will. Is everything fine and the patient just trying to avoid fair financial obligations? You hope and pray the next letter isn't from an attorney! It's not right—not fair—to work as hard and well as you can, only to receive a slap in the face as reward for your efforts!

Dealing with Pain and Failure

During the course of the several calls a week I receive from dentists who have read my books or articles, I'm occasionally asked, "How do you deal with failure?" "Failure" might take the form of a patient leaving the practice, the discovery a bridge you placed three years ago has marginal caries, or the above fecal quandary of post-endodontic sensitivity I dragged you through. Usually the doctor prefaces his or her query by stating, "I bet you've never been asked this before." Does everyone be-lieve all others know how to handle disappointment, or that everybody else is perhaps too embarrassed to confess to less than perfection and inquire as to how best to address this universal situation?

Let's begin large, with another brief effort to grasp this broad concept: **There exists no such thing as failure, only effort and outcome**. Think of your past, how often seeming blessings be-came disasters (possibly weddings! or when a promising new staff member joined the team?), and seeming disasters contained the seed that launched one's life in a positive new direction. (Perhaps divorce or an "indispensable" staff member leaving?) Humans label events in a feeble and failing attempt to regulate that which can't be controlled . . . life.

One's penchant for "mislabeling" of good and bad is due to humankind's limited ability to fully comprehend the long-term consequences of even critical situations. In these instances, one

440

reacts mainly to the emotion of the moment. Consider the concept that **every event is supposed to happen exactly as it does, and occurs for a reason**. There is great peace inherent within such humble acceptance of reality, and we understand the presence of tranquility to be an indication one has acted with wisdom.

But cold philosophic insight does little to quench the burn of emotional pain. Consider the above hint of a world existing with a definite purpose, but how to develop faith in the workings of the universe is beyond the scope of our discussion. Let's attempt a more immediate, if less pervasive anodyne.

I offer no panacea, no salve to allow instant healing, as in some science fiction saga. **I've reached a point in my life where I distrust simple remedies for complex problems**. But allow me to share some thoughts garnered during my stay in this vale of tears. I believe I can help those who care so much they often awaken at 4 a.m. to ponder and ruminate.

When faced with adversity, how should one optimally proceed? The first critical step seems counter-intuitive: **DON'T BLOCK ONE'S FEELINGS—NO MATTER HOW PAINFUL.** But, one wants the pain to stop! Isn't it best to distract oneself with other thoughts or activities?

First, accept the fact that emotions exist. One can choose to deal with them honestly or attempt to ignore them, but no one can alter the immutable truth of feelings being present.

Let's examine a disingenuous approach to emotions, where one attempts to block them from his or her consciousness. Feelings don't disappear when one denies them, but instead seep ever deeper into one's brain, one's gut. At some point they will resurface. (Often this happens at 4 a.m., to end a badly needed night's rest, or when you "take someone's head off," as repressed feeling explode and some innocent staff or family member, who has the misfortune to be in the vicinity, suffers a seemingly unprovoked outburst concerning an unrelated matter.) Denying feelings allows their influence to expand. **Emotions must be acknowledged to be exorcised**.

During office hours, dentists seldom enjoy the luxury of dealing with unpleasant emotions the instant they occur, due to

441

the demands of other patients' treatment. Swallow your distress, fix a smile and keep going, doctor! Such is the reality of our profession.

But, as soon as the pressure is off, find a quiet place, relax and **concentrate on the physical presence of emotional pain**. Do you feel it as pressure in your chest, or a sharp pain in your stomach? Be brave! Urge this discomfort to give you all it's got, because after its best shot, it's going to be thrown out of here! Instead of cowering from pain, and continuing to endure its presence, one can choose to employ suffering as a catalyst to propel one toward understanding and growth and, by this courageous choice, banish distress.

Emotions must be openly, honestly dealt with for optimal learning to occur. If one allows defensiveness to cloud one's judgement, reason will be tainted by self-protection and an opportunity to learn and grow forfeited. One will be too deafened by the roar of internal rationalization and self-defense to hear the whispers of truth. In the calm eddy of reflection that follows the torrent created by deliberate exposure to one's feelings, meaningful discernment can allow one to make mental and behavioral changes that will expand one's understanding and **decrease the likelihood of a similar event again causing misery**.

Emotions dealt with, one can now think—and think one must. Consider the painful event with perspicacity, but detachment. **WHAT CAN ONE LEARN?** In the above drama, should you have helped the patient clarify his or her values more thoroughly before treatment? Were all insurance and payment concerns openly addressed, with proper financial arrangements agreed upon, and placed in writing? Was adequate time scheduled for the procedure, and was treatment provided during a portion of the day when one's strength allows ideal performance of this demanding care? Was a legal release for endodontics signed?

In the post-emotion calm, glean all possible information and insights. Authentic learning will occur first within the heart and head of the dentist. The next staff meeting offers an opportunity to explain this understanding and implement changes one believes will improve the business systems and people that comprise a dental office.

Personally, I'd rather be swindled than ever cheat a patient. "The customer is always right" is good business and keeps my blood pressure W.N.L. The chief enemy of this enlightened philosophy is the insecurity that makes one need to "win." It's the most hollow of victories when one pounds a patient into submission and collects $100, while losing the patient, their family and a career of referrals to one's practice. Many such "victories" and third-party plans start looking damn attractive!

When a patient is unhappy, I do everything within my power to make it right—refund, re-treat at no charge, apologize. Some feel displaying such empathy opens the door to successful malpractice suits, as one's concern can be interpreted as an admission of guilt. Once again, I'm no legal authority, but contend such behavior is perceived as fair, even generous, by patient and staff, and more likely to help one avoid legal ramifications. It is my little secret that this choice also best serves my self-interests. If one agrees with my philosophy, adjust office systems as needed, but be sure every staff member understands one's wishes.

But often, after painstaking reflection, I find I have done everything to the best of my abilities. In such a case, I still do whatever is within my power to satisfy our unhappy patient, but our procedures and systems require no adjustments. My most focused consideration has shown no factual basis exists for feeling badly about myself or my office. Even one's best endeavor doesn't promise perfection, and an optimal effort is all anyone can give. One must accept the fact that times exist when nothing he or she can do will satisfy another.

When this is the case, it is time to make every deliberate effort to **LET GO** of the predicament and the **accompanying feelings**. Calm, reasoned consideration has allowed one to drain every drop of possible learning from the situation. To continue to torture yourself because you can't control the outcome of every situation is nonsensical and dangerous.

Control

There are two portions to our blessed universe: those things one can control, and those one cannot. In part, wisdom consists of understanding the difference between these two great spheres. Powers and principalities exist that one's most determined efforts are unable to influence—some of these dwell at the root's apex, or the base of periodontal pockets—more within my wife's, children's and other humans' minds. To attempt to control everything is irrational and leads to madness (or alcoholism).

Perfectionism—the attempt to bend the outcome of all things to one's will—bequeaths many positive benefits. Always striving to do one's best moves one along the path toward peak potential. It's a great trait to exist in one's doctor or dentist. If I'm ever critically ill, I want a perfectionist physician worrying about my well-being at 4 a.m.! But perfectionism isn't much fun within one's skin, or for others to be around.

These folks are frequently burrs under life's saddle, as perfectionism is delusional—impossible to obtain—a form of mental illness that must be recognized as such. This unremitting quest leads to achievement, then **misery and often total breakdown and failure!** Reap the desired benefits of working to be one's best, then, when one has done all one can, LET GO! Realize the difference between using the pain of "failure" as a guide, and the foolish futility of beating yourself up because you've failed to control every facet of the universe.

Seek the wisdom within this famous poem:

THE SERENITY PRAYER

God grant me the serenity
To accept the things I cannot change,
The courage to change the things I can,
And the wisdom to know the difference.

A very few who read these words recognize pain as a friend sent to guide them. He or she feels equally blessed by sorrow or joy. Souls who rejoice alike in anguish and pleasure are called

enlightened—a destination worthy of the long, difficult life's journey required to achieve such complete peace of mind. Though few realize it, the ability to remain calm, under any circumstances, is the life the spiritual masters of all cultures have modeled, and the manner of existence all seek.

Conclusion

The world is changing, and dentistry must become more facile in adjusting to the altered influences with which it is confronted. I've done my utmost to describe the form I earnestly, ardently believe dentistry should adopt to remain viable in the face of existing third-party, government and business challenges.

Yet, continued existence is not my reader's goal. The book's central assumption is that every dentist desires professional success, financial freedom and JOY . . . whether he or she is aware of these aspirations or not. Furthermore, I contend these three objectives are interconnected and symbiotic—none can be meaningfully complete in the absence of the other two.

A portion of reaching this tripartite objective includes establishing a dominant practice, that creates a bountiful cash flow, which is optimally employed. It also requires mastering self-awareness and value clarification techniques with which one may develop a precise personal philosophy that serves to guide one toward decreased stress and enhanced joy within home and office. Deliberately choosing a value-based life leads, one thoughtful decision at a time, to the development of **wisdom**. (Correct data and knowledge are important, but one knows he or she has acted with wisdom when they are HAPPY.)

One must become aware of the influence genetics, culture and ego exert on life decisions. These forces can't be banished, but once their consequences are understood, one's ability to reach decisions consistent with one's beliefs and values is optimized by this conscious awareness of normally subconscious forces.

This book was begun with the idea of creating a short, concise tome. In that regard I've obviously failed! The text I first envisioned is contained within, if one removes all portions dealing with the author and his philosophy. (Those so inclined better get scissors and glue at the ready. This book is meant as a guide to one's future, and as such, to be read and re-read over the years, so feel free to condense until one achieves the form he or she currently desires.)

I've revealed my personal history and philosophy extensively—unwavering in pro and con—as my **intention is to change lives**. Aiming for any lesser mark is not worth my time or trouble; not capable of engaging my interest. To have such a profound effect, my story must be believed and internalized on a deeply personal level.

To achieve the degree of faith necessary to facilitate authentic growth, each reader must know, understand and **TRUST ME**. It is to realize this goal that I've shared with such candor, willing to open myself to the "rejection that is as a sentence of death," about which I've blabbered on throughout the text. One may choose to risk a form of death to obtain an objective about which he or she cares intensely, passionately. (Perhaps my "hardest truth" was revealing 1997 monitors with personal production of $4,000 per month! I looked a lot more like a dentist—at least on paper—in 1996!)

To the best of my comprehension I've not lied—not even exaggerated—a single fact. (Dizzy Dean—Hall of Fame pitcher, ex-broadcaster, singer of "The Wabash Cannonball," and legendary raconteur, said, "It ain't bragging if you done it." According to the gospel of Diz, I ain't bragged either.)

I am guilty of being proud of my achievements. Certainly, many have done more, but few started with less, or paid as dear a price as I. But, beyond any physical attainments, I'm most grateful for finally being blessed with the wisdom that has granted me peace. This took a long, agonizing time to achieve, and I still vividly recall the living nightmare that was "peacelessness." It is not a state of being I'd wish visited upon anyone, yet might well represent the common ground of contemporary humankind.

448

This chronic loss of equilibrium, with the resultant pain and fear, was a price I once felt one must pay to obtain success. I was wrong—one can achieve both success and joy together—and I suffered greatly for my error in judgement.

Let me hasten to add, I'm well short of being a spiritual or enlightened person. My life lacks complete peace, although I grow steadily closer to this most central of goals. I still devote an inordinate amount of time to the pursuit of wealth, although money has never brought me security or happiness. I hope to grow to the point where material possessions are of no great concern to me, but I'm not there yet, and believe the overwhelming majority of my audience is still concerned with the mundane events of life—like making a living. (I will once again offer a small gift to the enlightened minority at the end of this chapter.)

My overall purpose restated, let's briefly review the eight building blocks that, when employed in synergistic combination, allow for the fulfillment of a dentist's dreams.

Clinical excellence—achieved by an act of will, a decision to do nothing less than one's best, that is available to all—is the foundation upon which any successful dental practice must reside.

Yet the most expert clinical skills offer no advantage unless patients accept offered care. Becoming behaviorally adept is essential to practice success and personal happiness, as the basis of all people skills resides in a profound understanding of human nature without which those living in society are lost.

Yet clinical and behavioral excellence are of no benefit unless one has patients on which to employ these talents. Every successful business markets, and I've illustrated inexpensive, fun, ethical and professional ways in which one may concisely identify his or her practice's purpose to the public, to facilitate its rapid growth.

Every business is comprised of a series of systems. Dentistry has some catching up to do, as compared to other industries, in our awareness and refinement of systems. Personal turmoil will decrease, happiness and efficiency increase, when dentists develop the wisdom necessary to allow them to stop blaming people and begin to refine systems.

Profitable expanded hygiene is the fiscal base upon which modern dental practice success rests. An office with no hygiene, or with a hygiene department resulting in a net loss to the practice, will be eliminated from competition in *Dentistry's Future*. Let me be unmistakably concise in stating my belief: Without efficient, profitable expanded hygiene, no dental office can remain competitive.

The above five segments successfully implemented, one has created a solid footing upon which to construct a group practice. The increased production, coupled with decreased overhead percentage available in a well-run group, is the mantra of *Dentistry's Future*.

Practical advice concerning locating, hiring and successfully employing associates has been included. I capped our discussion with an effort to help readers in the development of a personal philosophy concerning money. One must harvest, then employ fiscal assets—safely yet effectively—to achieve the portion of freedom in our modern world that consists of having sufficient wealth to allow choices.

SUCCESS is the answer to third-party pressure and a bountiful future for independent dental practice. Dentists must come to see themselves as business-people, entrepreneurs profiting from their minds, not just technicians employing their fingers. A busy office with a 50% overhead can continue to thrive in the increasingly more competitive dental environment. **At 65% overhead, the battle is lost!**

None of the above listed fragments of information—valuable as they are—possesses sufficient power to safeguard our profession from the miasmas that threaten it. Integration of each of these eight facets, and the geometric compounding of energy thus created, results in a whole possessing many times the power of its parts.

But, as you strive to achieve the level of success you desire, please don't forget that my existence has demonstrated no achievement has value if not accompanied by peace of mind.

450

Success, wealth and bliss must all be achieved simultaneously. Delaying the attainment of joy to gain success and wealth is a fool's bargain . . . more likely to lead to a mausoleum than a mansion.

Let me conclude with the "graduate level" information concerning a philosophy of life about which I earlier hinted. I fear few can comprehend this knowledge on a precise and personally meaningful level—I'm not sure I'm able. I hope this brief discussion will serve as food for thought, and perhaps help create an inspiring vision of the glory of a world free of worry and strife, attainable for all, that will empower those so influenced to continue their quest to more fully understand these concepts.

A master of life remains centered under any circumstance: pulp exposure, root-tip fracture, IRS audit, OSHA investigation, lawsuit, bankruptcy, divorce . . . even death. Such equanimity requires faith that there exists a plan, a definite purpose to existence. That everything which happens occurs **exactly as it should**. That no accidents, no coincidences, no luck—good or bad—no tragedies exist.

Such erroneous definitions and labels applied to events are the result of illusions caused by the frailty of the human senses and perceptions. Only experience—the essential happening that must occur to enable one to define himself or herself and thus grow—abides within the universe.

With this awareness one understands that he or she can't fail, as life will continue to provide occasions to master essential lessons, until the needed task is complete. (Life gave me repeated, painful opportunities to learn from my drinking for 15 years.)

Fear of problems disappears when one realizes that where he or she stumbles, there lies his or her treasure. When I was finally able to summon the courage to face my foe—alcoholism and the fears that repeatedly drove me to the mindless oblivion of drink—I was blessed beyond my ability to comprehend.

Upon what do you currently falter in life? Be it marriage, addiction, practice struggles . . . can you visualize the form into which you will have grown when this hurdle is overcome? If

451

one can comprehend such a revelation, he or she will feel blessed by pain, and excited by the opportunity crisis represents!

Masters understand there exist only two forces in the universe:

1. **A divine power**—called by whatever name to which one can best relate—that is the force of oneness and love. (I choose to call this force God. Alcoholics Anonymous discusses "a Power greater than ourselves." Other sages, in other cultures, have referred to Buddha, Krishna, Allah and numerous additional terms. I believe the power to be identical, but wise men and women over the ages have called this entity by many names.)

2. **The other**—basically varied responses to fear—be it anger, lust, jealousy, terror, etc . . . all similar in that they are states of non-love, in which one has lost contact with the purpose and oneness of the universe and, shrouded in this ultimate and most intimate blindness, trembles.

With every situation in which one is involved, reflect. Has one's reaction been guided by love, or by a form of fear? This identification can be reached by making the effort required to become accurately aware of one's feelings! Emotions serve as beacons to assist one in choosing a path away from pain, toward a more abundant existence. The presence of happiness demonstrates love and wisdom exist. Any emotions other than peace and joy are based on "the other"—on a construct of fear.

If joy isn't present in ANY SITUATION, contemplate . . . then **select another choice** of thought and behavior consistent with love. This process of awareness, followed by carefully chosen action, is called learning, and is only frightening and painful when one fails to understand these essential truths. It is through such deliberate consideration and disciplined behavior that one grows.

This thumbnail sketch is overly simple, but I believe the thoughtful can sense, within it, a guide to peace. Please understand, these are merely my personal beliefs—not presented as divine revelation. I pass them on, not to challenge other doctrines, but because they have enriched my life and I truly desire to share my joy.

The effort to grasp and implement this awareness has changed the fabric of my life, pushing other concerns into the background. The comprehension that one may control—not events or emotions—but his or her actions by seeking always to discover the **highest response of which one is capable**, can lead one to heaven on earth.

When troubled by any aspect of your life, please put this proposed doctrine to the test. Consider, in this difficult matter, are my habitual actions based on love, or a form of fear? To achieve peace and joy, one must **ABANDON BEING RIGHT, or winning, choosing instead to be happy.** If one's behavior doesn't result in peace, it is not based on love. In such cases, one can consider and implement other, higher choices. This growth, so contrary to our contentious human nature, requires great awareness and effort to attain, but such is the certain path to bliss.

Thanks for your attention and patience. I'm certain I've tried both many times. I believe in each of you, as God makes no mistakes. Each of you is a spiritual being, capable of accomplishing whatever you desire. **PLEASE CHOOSE YOUR GOALS WITH THOUGHT AND CARE.** God will bless your sacred journey.

Give the Gift of Dentistry's Future to Your Friends and Colleagues